SOCIAL AND ACADEMIC ABILITIES IN CHILDREN WITH HIGH-FUNCTIONING AUTISM SPECTRUM DISORDERS

Social and Academic Abilities in Children with High-Functioning Autism Spectrum Disorders

NIRIT BAUMINGER-ZVIELY

THE GUILFORD PRESS
New York   London

KH

© 2013 The Guilford Press
A Division of Guilford Publications, Inc.
72 Spring Street, New York, NY 10012
www.guilford.com

Printed in the United States of America

This book is printed on acid-free paper.

Last digit is print number: 9 8 7 6 5 4 3 2 1

The author has checked with sources believed to be reliable in her efforts to provide
information that is complete and generally in accord with the standards of practice
that are accepted at the time of publication. However, in view of the possibility of
human error or changes in behavioral, mental health, or medical sciences, neither the
author, nor the editors and publisher, nor any other party who has been involved in
the preparation or publication of this work warrants that the information contained
herein is in every respect accurate or complete, and they are not responsible for any
errors or omissions or the results obtained from the use of such information. Readers
are encouraged to confirm the information contained in this book with other sources.

Library of Congress Cataloging-in-Publication Data

Bauminger-Zviely, Nirit.
  Social and academic abilities in children with high-functioning autism spectrum
disorders / Nirit Bauminger-Zviely.
      pages cm
  Includes bibliographical references and index.
  ISBN 978-1-4625-0942-3 (hardcover : alk. paper)
  1. Autistic children—Education.   2. Social skills in children.   I. Title.
  LC4717.B38 2013
  371.94—dc23
                                                                    2012051199

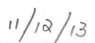

11/12/13

About the Author

Nirit Bauminger-Zviely, PhD, is Associate Professor in the School of Education at Bar-Ilan University, Ramat-Gan, Israel. She serves as Head of the Graduate Program in Special Education, specializing in autism spectrum disorders (ASD). Dr. Bauminger-Zviely's research focuses on social-emotional development of higher-functioning children with ASD and on the design of relevant interventions that promote social-cognitive processes, social relationships, and peer interactions. She has been at the forefront of basic and applied research on affective and cognitive correlates of social relationships and interactions in these children and has pioneered new and effective methods of cognitive-behavioral treatments, including multimodal individual and group social-cognitive behavioral interventions. Dr. Bauminger-Zviely is the author of numerous book chapters and journal articles in such publications as the *Journal of Autism and Developmental Disorders*, *Autism Research*, and *Child Development*.

Preface

For well over a decade, I have been trying to put together the pieces of an intriguing puzzle exploring a unique subgroup of individuals within the autism spectrum, namely, those with relatively normative or even high cognitive capabilities. These individuals with high-functioning autism spectrum disorders (HFASD) may resemble their lower-functioning counterparts with autism in their shared diagnostic profile, but the higher-functioning individuals differ not only in their normative cognitive functioning but also in their more active social participation and understanding of the social milieu. Much has been written and said about autism, but as I worked day in and day out over many years with these high-functioning children, adolescents, and adults, their families, and my colleagues in the field, I identified a deep need for a comprehensive summary of theory and research focusing expressly on their social and academic lives—the distinctive ways in which they see the interpersonal world and maneuver within it, and the unique ways in which they learn. Many individuals with HFASD operate in inclusive educational settings where they interact with peers and adults who do not have disabilities, as well as with other individuals with HFASD, and where they must tackle a diverse range of academic and social demands.

Uncovering this subgroup's mixture of high capabilities alongside their major deficiencies in basic skills, both in the social and the academic realm, poses an interesting and challenging puzzle for empiricists, educators, and interventionists. This book's aim, therefore, is to provide an extensive description of the state of the art in the field of social-emotional and cognitive-academic abilities among individuals with HFASD, mostly school-age children and adolescents. My underlying goal is to help the stakeholders in these youngsters' lives to understand the complexities of high-functioning individuals' unique social-emotional and cognitive-academic patterns and thereby to facilitate the development of optimal treatments to improve their quality of life.

The book opens with an introductory chapter in which diagnostic characteristics of HFASD are described, along with major theories that guide understanding of the social, as well as the cognitive-academic, profile of children with HFASD. Then the two main sections of the book comprehensively review the unique abilities of individuals with HFASD and pinpoint their implications for intervention.

Part I includes three chapters outlining the social-emotional profile of the targeted subgroup and two further chapters describing the cognitive-academic profile and comorbid aspects of HFASD. Chapter 2 focuses on the social-cognitive and social-affective profile of youngsters with HFASD, which establishes the foundation for their capacity to develop peer relations. The latter, comprising peer social interactions and culminating in friendships, is discussed in Chapter 3. The developmental trajectories of the social deficit from infancy up to adulthood are described in Chapter 4. Although the book focuses mainly on children and adolescents with HFASD, the developmental perspective provides a rich contextual framework for understanding how social deficits are manifested over the lifespan and also offers fruitful information in terms of intervention goals. Chapter 5 presents the major cognitive and academic characteristics of these high-functioning children. Due to the high comorbidity of HFASD and other psychiatric conditions, such as attention-deficit disorder, anxiety, and depression, Chapter 6 addresses the major psychiatric conditions found to co-occur with HFASD. These comorbidities have implications for understanding both the social and the academic characteristics of youngsters with HFASD.

Part II furnishes a wide-ranging discussion of intervention models in both the social (Chapter 7) and the cognitive-academic (Chapter 8) realms. The description of social interventions in Chapter 7 comprises a review of the state of the art in treatment models for HFASD, with special emphasis on cognitive-behavioral interventions (see especially Appendix A). Moreover, Chapter 7 strives to help readers move from theory to practice by offering demonstrations and practical examples derived from many years of continual implementation of my own ecologically based social intervention model, as detailed in Appendix B. Chapter 8 reviews existing cognitive-academic strategies that have been implemented in the field and have undergone empirical examination.

Those seeking additional information on assessment measures while reading the book should find Appendix C particularly helpful. This appendix presents a comprehensive but not all-inclusive list of the most frequent standardized and nonstandardized assessment tools that have been employed in the field to evaluate social characteristics and social intervention outcome results for HFASD. These measures tap a range of social-cognitive and social-affective skills, as well as peer-relations capabilities. This appendix does not directly relate to any specific book chapter but, rather, spans all of the chapters pertaining to the social deficit for HFASD, offering a wide perspective of measurement options in the social realm.

I conclude with Chapter 9, highlighting major issues that were raised in the book. This chapter also emphasizes some future domains for exploration.

As I work with and investigate children with HFASD and their families through the years, they never stop surprising me with their capabilities, sensitivities, and enormous potential for learning. I have learned to see their affective bonding with friends and parents, as well as their jealous expressions, social isolation, and feelings of despair in school with their peers. It is a challenge to learn about the world through their eyes. In this book, I have attempted to provide an extensive overview of the literature with regard to their whole gamut of capabilities and disabilities and to suggest diverse ways for helping them cope with such a multifaceted profile. I conclude this preface with the hope that the readers of this book will gain theoretical, as well as practical, knowledge about this unique subgroup of children within the autism spectrum.

ACKNOWLEDGMENTS

I would like to express my deep gratitude and appreciation to the people who helped turn the dream of writing this book into a reality.

To my close and beloved family:

> Chico, my husband, for being the rock of my life since forever.
> Hagar, my daughter, for teaching me things that cannot be found in any book.
> Ben, my gift, for his kindheartedness and for his endless willingness to help.
> My parents, for teaching me to cherish caring.

To my dear friends who made this possible:

> Dee B. Ankonina, my dedicated, brilliant editor, who put my thoughts into better words.
> Yael Kimhi, my colleague and friend, who generously helped me to enrich this book with her expertise in cognitive and academic profiles for high-functioning autism spectrum disorders.
> My dear colleagues/friends who enriched me with their wisdom, especially Connie Kasari, who kindly opened the window to the

autism field for me and sustained me in hard times; Peter Mundy, for encouraging me to write this book; and Sally Rogers and Marjorie Solomon, for their friendship and support.

Last, but definitely not least, to the children with high-functioning autism spectrum disorders and their dear families with whom I met and worked throughout the years: For opening their hearts to show me where I should look, I dedicate this book to them.

Contents

INTRODUCTION

1. High-Functioning Autism Spectrum Disorders: 3
Definitions and Theoretical Explanations
Diagnostic Criteria: Moving from DSM-IV-TR to DSM-5   4
Theories for Understanding Social-Emotional
and Cognitive-Academic Characteristics in HFASD   8
Summary and Conclusions   28

I. SOCIAL-EMOTIONAL AND COGNITIVE-ACADEMIC PROFILES

2. Social-Cognitive and Emotional Competence   31
Social Cognition   32
Emotional Competencies   40
Summary and Conclusions   57

3. Peer Relations   59
Social Interaction in HFASD   60
Social Relationships: Attachment and Friendship
in HFASD   72
Peer Relations in HFASD: Integrative Thoughts   84
Summary and Conclusions   86

4. Developmental Changes in Social Functioning   88
Overview of the Social Challenges
Experienced during TYP   88
Social Functioning across Development in HFASD   89

The Beginning of the Social-Emotional Deficit:
Early Markers in Infancy through
the Preschool Years   90
Early Peer Relations: Social Play and Friendship
in the Toddler and Preschool Years   93
School Transitions: Trajectories and Predictors   100
The Transition from School to the "Real" World:
From Adolescence to Adulthood   103
Summary and Conclusions   108

5. Cognitive Strengths and Weaknesses   110
   with Yael Kimhi

   Cognitive Characteristics of HFASD   111
   Academic Abilities   121
   Summary and Conclusions   130

6. Associated Comorbid Conditions   131

   Major Comorbid Diagnoses   132
   Measures to Assess Comorbidity in HFASD   144
   Summary and Conclusions   150

II. INTERVENTION MODELS

7. Interventions to Facilitate Social Functioning   155

   Major Challenges and Components
   of Social Intervention   155
   Conceptual Basis of Social Intervention   156
   CBT-Based Studies in HFASD: Literature Review   159
   CBE Intervention: Taking CBT from Theory
   to Practice   163
   Social Implications for CBT-Based Treatment
   of Comorbid Anxiety Disorders   178
   Interventions to Improve Social Relationships
   in HFASD   182
   Summary and Future Directions   183

8. Interventions to Facilitate Cognitive   187
   and Academic Functioning
   with Yael Kimhi

   Frequently Used Strategies to Facilitate General
   Academic Skills in ASD   188
   Structured Teaching   188
   Strategies Targeting Memory Skills   191
   Strategies Targeting Question Asking and Answering   194

Strategies Targeting Reading   197
Strategies Targeting Writing   206
Strategies Targeting Mathematics   209
Selecting Appropriate Strategies   210
Summary and Conclusions   210

CONCLUSION

9. Where Are We Now and Where Do We Want to Go?   217

The Social Realm   217
The Cognitive-Academic Realm   225
General Future Directions and
   Concluding Remarks   229

APPENDICES

Appendix A. Cognitive-Behavioral Therapy Techniques   233
   and Settings

TABLE A1. *Definitions of Major CBT-Based Cognitive*
   and Behavioral Techniques for HFASD,
   with Examples   234
TABLE A2. *Role Description of Main Change Agents*
   in Interventions   240
FIGURE A1. *CBT-Based Social Intervention Techniques*
   and Settings   241

Appendix B. Multimodal Cognitive-Behavioral-Ecological   243
   Interventions

TABLE B1. *Main Curriculum Topics for CBE*
   Dyadic Intervention   244
TABLE B2. *Main Curriculum Topics for CBE*
   Small-Group Intervention   245
TABLE B3. *Criteria for Selection of Peer Aide*
   with TYP in CBE Treatments   246
FIGURE B1. *CBE Intervention Model   247*
FIGURE B2. *Excerpts from a Sample CBE Curriculum*
   Unit for Combining Both Learning and Experiencing
   of Social Conversation   248

Appendix C. Assessment Measures to Evaluate Social   251
   Characteristics and Intervention Outcomes for
   School-Age Children and/or Adolescents with
   High-Functioning Autism Spectrum Disorders

TABLE C1. *Measures of Attachment   252*
TABLE C2. *Measures of Emotional Expressiveness*
   and Responsiveness   253

Contents

TABLE C3. *Measures of Emotional Understanding
and Recognition* 255

TABLE C4. *Measures of Executive Function* 258

TABLE C5. *Measures of Friendship* 260

TABLE C6. *Measures of Social Cognition:
Problem Solving* 263

TABLE C7. *Measures of Social Cognition: ToM* 265

TABLE C8. *Measures of Social Competence
and Social Adjustment* 267

TABLE C9. *Measures of Social Interaction* 272

References   275

Index   313

INTRODUCTION

Chapter 1

High-Functioning Autism Spectrum Disorders

Definitions and Theoretical Explanations

"I'm so lucky that I have Asperger ... because children with Asperger syndrome are really smart. . . . " This insightful statement was made by a 15-year-old with Asperger syndrome during his social skills group, which I facilitated. Indeed, children and adolescents along the autism spectrum who have high-functioning cognitive capabilities do form a unique subgroup that has been attracting growing attention from researchers and mental health professionals in recent years. According to the latest report from the Centers for Disease Control and Prevention (2012), the estimates for co-occurrence of intellectual disability with autism spectrum disorder (ASD) among all ages have declined from 75% to only 38% over recent decades.

The substantial subgroup of individuals who are cognitively high functioning with an autism spectrum disorder (HFASD) appears to reveal a unique social-emotional and cognitive-academic profile. In line with the core deficits of autism, children with HFASD generally demonstrate a poorer quality of peer relations and distorted or deficient levels of social cognition and emotional understanding, compared with their typical counterparts (see Chapters 2 and 3). However, compared with children with ASD who are less cognitively able, this subgroup of children with HFASD shows more engagement in social interactions, better ability to form friendships, and greater understanding of the social and emotional environment. The "compensation hypothesis" assumes that these children use their relatively high cognitive capabilities to compensate for their low social-emotional functioning (Hermelin & O'Connor, 1985; Kasari, Chamberlain, & Bauminger, 2001). Furthermore, children with HFASD are at risk of developing affective disorders, such as anxiety and depression, because they can recognize

3

their own social difficulties and identify the gap between their own social functioning and that of their typical peers (see Chapter 6). In addition, this subgroup of children is also unique in their cognitive-academic profile, exhibiting strengths alongside areas of major deficit, with a high percentage of comorbid learning disorders (see Chapter 5).

In this chapter, I first describe diagnostic characteristics of the three major diagnoses that constitute the HFASD subgroup: high-functioning autism (HFA), Asperger syndrome, and pervasive developmental disorders not otherwise specified (PDD-NOS). By examining these diagnostic criteria, I define the target HFASD population at the focus of this book (namely. HFA, Asperger syndrome, and PDD-NOS). Next, I present the major theories that have been expounded by scholars and researchers in this field to explain the functioning and deficits of individuals with HFASD. These theories include social communicative, social-cognitive, and cognitive conceptualizations, all of which hold significant implications for the social-emotional, as well as cognitive-academic, functioning of persons with HFASD.

DIAGNOSTIC CRITERIA:
MOVING FROM DSM-IV-TR TO DSM-5

The autism field now faces a period of change in the perception of autism diagnostic characteristics and in the terminology referring to this group of neurobiological disorders, which until recently was characterized by deficits in social relations and in verbal and nonverbal communication and by repetitive behaviors. This group of disorders, previously named PDD (pervasive developmental disorders), is now being termed autism "spectrum" disorders (ASD) to reflect a continuum of functioning along a spectrum (e.g., Lord, 2010). This shift in perception and terminology is clearly reflected in the transition from the DSM-IV-TR diagnostic criteria for autistic disorder (American Psychiatric Association [APA], 2000) to the definition of autistic disorder (APA, 2013) in the DSM-5. To clarify the diagnostic characteristics of the group of disorders that are the subject of the target population of this book—HFASD—as I compare the DSM-IV-TR and the DSM-5 definitions and criteria I focus on individuals with the diagnoses of Asperger syndrome, HFA, and PDD-NOS. In all these milder forms of autism, the individuals function above the intellectual deficit level (Gotham, Bishop, & Lord, 2011).

Historically, the definition of autism and related disorders began with the first clinical reports by Leo Kanner (1943) in the United States and by Hans Asperger (1944/1991) in Germany, each defining a group of children showing a unique profile of difficulties in social, communication, and behavioral characteristics. These two reports set the stage for extensive research aiming to achieve a valid definition for the disorders, one that would be specific enough to include only individuals with the relevant disorders but would also be sensitive enough to include all eligible individuals, despite individual differences and developmental changes in the disorders' manifestations. A historical review of definitions of autism is beyond the scope of this book; therefore, only the most updated definitions are described here.

Diagnostic Characteristics

DSM-IV-TR (APA, 2000)

According to DSM-IV-TR (APA, 2000), which served the mental health community for over a decade (since DSM-IV; APA, 1994), autistic disorder is defined by onset prior to age 3 years and by the presence of deficits or unusual behaviors within three areas: reciprocal social interaction; verbal and nonverbal communication; and restricted, repetitive interests and behaviors. The *social deficit* is manifested by at least two of the following: marked difficulties in nonverbal behaviors for regulating social interactions (e.g., eye contact, facial expression, gesture, body posture); problems in developing peer relations at the appropriate developmental level; failure to spontaneously seek shared enjoyment, interests, or achievements with others (e.g., infrequent use of pointing, bringing, or showing behaviors); and lack of reciprocity. The *communication impairment* is manifested by at least one of the following: failure or delay in spoken language without compensation through alternative communication methods; substantial difficulties in initiating or sustaining conversations; use of stereotyped speech, delayed echolalia, or idiosyncratic language; and limitations in the development of spontaneous make-believe play or social imitative play that is appropriate to developmental level. The *restricted and repetitive behaviors* include at least one of the following: unusual preoccupation with a circumscribed interest; inflexible observance of nonfunctional routines; motor mannerisms that are repetitive (e.g., hand flapping); and interest in parts of objects. To qualify for a diagnosis of HFA, the child must meet the criteria for autistic disorder but have an IQ level above the intellectual disability level (> 75), in comparison with classic or low-functioning autism (LFA), in which the child meets the criterion for autistic disorder but functions below the intellectual disability level (IQ < 75).

The DSM-IV-TR diagnostic criteria for Asperger syndrome resemble those of autistic disorder with regard to the social and the restricted/repetitive behavior criteria; however, the communication criterion differs. Individuals diagnosed with Asperger syndrome do not show clinical delay in spoken language (e.g., single words used by age 2 and communicative phrases used by 3 years), but they do show pedantic speech, as well as difficulties in developing a conversation. They also function above intellectual disability level in cognitive development and demonstrate adequate self-help skills and adaptive behaviors (excluding social interactions), and in childhood they show curiosity about the environment.

The DSM-IV-TR diagnostic characteristics for PDD-NOS include severe, pervasive deficiency in reciprocal social interactions or in verbal or nonverbal communication, or symptoms in the area of stereotyped behaviors, interests, and activities, but without a clinical profile that meets the criteria for a full diagnosis of autistic disorder or Asperger Syndrome. The PDD-NOS diagnosis is usually given to children who do not evidence sufficient symptoms to qualify for a full autism diagnosis, who were older at the time of onset, or who reveal milder forms of autistic disorder. These individuals are characterized by an average or above-average level of cognitive functioning.

As seen from these three DSM-IV-TR diagnoses for cognitively high-functioning children on the spectrum, the borders among HFA, Asperger syndrome, and PDD-NOS are very problematic. Thus, to date, difficulties are often encountered in forming differential diagnosis between them.

DSM-5 (APA, 2013)

In an attempt to address these problematic differentiations and inconsistencies between disorders within the autism spectrum, the first major change in the DSM-5 (APA, 2013) definition of autism is its lack of specific terminologies to denote differential diagnoses within the autism spectrum. Instead, DSM-5 uses a single category—ASD—that includes autistic disorder (spanning both high and low cognitive abilities, i.e., HFA and LFA, respectively), as well as Asperger syndrome and PDD-NOS. The rationale behind this single category is that a single spectrum disorder with expanded specifiers and ratings of severity better reflects the current state of knowledge about pathology and clinical presentation, thus eliminating subtypes of ASD (e.g., Lord & Jones, 2012).

The second major change appearing in the DSM-5 definition is its inclusion of only two symptom domains instead of three: the social-communication domain and the fixated, repetitive-interests domain. The rationale behind the integration of the social and the communication domains is that most symptoms are relevant to both. For example, difficulties in reciprocal social conversation, which appear in DSM-IV-TR's communication domain, certainly relate to social interaction too. Indeed, the communication and social domains constitute a single factor in prominent diagnostic tools such as the Autism Diagnostic Observation Schedule—Generic (ADOS-G; Lord et al., 2000) and the Autism Diagnostic Interview—Revised (ADI-R; Rutter, Le Couteur, & Lord, 2003).

Importantly, in DSM-5, individuals need to meet all three criteria for the sociocommunicative domain: noticeable deficit in nonverbal communication, lack of social reciprocity, and problems in developing peer relations appropriate to developmental level. They must also meet two of the following criteria for the repetitive behaviors and interests domain: stereotyped motor or verbal behavior, disproportionate adherence to routines or difficulties with change, restricted and fixated interests, and hyper- or hypo-reactivity to sensory input or atypical sensory interest in aspects of the environment.

The inclusion of sensory behaviors in the diagnosis for ASD is new. Sensory modulation impairments are frequently observed in conjunction with an ASD (e.g., Ben Sasson et al., 2009). Atypical responses to multisensory, haptic, and oral sensory/olfactory stimuli were identified as possible predictors of social deficit severity. For example, a positive relationship has been observed between the severity of the sensory modulation and social impairments experienced by children with HFASD (e.g., Hilton, Graver, & LaVesser, 2007; Hilton et al., 2010).

In both symptom domains (social communication and repetitive behaviors/interests), developmental referents for defining symptoms are a key feature of the DSM-5 definition. Individual differences in symptom severity according to chronological age (CA) and developmental level (mental age [MA]) are described for consideration. Relative to this, age of onset is also treated more flexibly in DSM-5 versus DSM-IV-TR. DSM-5 acknowledges the fact that symptoms indeed must be present in infancy or early childhood (as in DSM-IV-TR) but suggests that symptoms may be detected only later in development when social demands surpass the individual's restricted capabilities. This provides an avenue for diagnosing older high-functioning individuals. The ASD diagnosis can also be associated with other conditions, such as Rett syndrome, Fragile X syndrome, and various psychiatric conditions (e.g., attention-deficit/hyperactivity disorder [ADHD], obsessive–compulsive disorder [OCD]).

The major implication of the DSM-5 definition is the absence of Asperger syndrome and PDD-NOS as unique subetiologies within the autism spectrum. The definition of PDD-NOS is problematic, as mentioned earlier, with no clear floor boundaries (e.g., Volkmar, State, & Klin, 2009). A new category was added to the DSM-5, social communication disorder. This category encompasses children who exhibit deficits in social-communicative skills, but not in restrictive/repetitive behaviors necessary for ASD. Children, who in the past received the DSM-III category of PDD-NOS, may now form a substantial part of this new DSM-5 category. Moreover, the suggested exclusion of Asperger syndrome from the new DSM-5 definition has been debated due to its implications for parents and professionals (see, for example, Ghaziuddin, 2010; Kaland, 2011; Volkmar et al., 2009; Wing, Gould, & Gillberg, 2011), but empirical examinations have consistently failed to provide strong support for the differentiation between HFA and Asperger syndrome. These two subetiologies were assumed to differ in several ways, such as in Verbal IQ profile or levels of social interest and motivation; however, accumulative data, including a number of recent reviews and some of the former reviews, showed little evidence for this and other distinctions between the two (see, e.g., Frith, 2004; Klin, 2011; Lord et al., 2012; Macintosh & Dissanayake,

2004). It is difficult to predict the consequences of the final DSM-5 criteria in the field. Nevertheless, in this book I follow the perception of a spectrum of disorders, and I also adopt the term "HFASD" while reviewing studies on individuals who function above the intellectual disability level, integrating findings related to PDD-NOS, Asperger syndrome, and HFA. Also, individual differences in functioning in each area of symptomatology are described throughout the various chapters. When a review of findings in this book is not limited to HFASD but, rather, relates to the whole spectrum (also including individuals with IQ < 75), I use the term "ASD." In a like manner, when discussion relates only to individuals who function below the intellectual disability level (IQ > 75), I use the term "LFA."

The understanding of the diagnostic profile of HFASD is not complete before reviewing the major theories that have been suggested to explain the cognitive-psychological mechanisms underlying the social-emotional and cognitive-academic functioning and deficits of individuals with HFASD. These theories provide another channel for enhancing a general understanding of HFASD. In the next section I review these theories.

THEORIES FOR UNDERSTANDING SOCIAL-EMOTIONAL AND COGNITIVE-ACADEMIC CHARACTERISTICS IN HFASD

In this section, social-communicative, social-cognitive, and cognitive theories are described as possible explanations for the unique social-emotional and cognitive-academic profile of HFASD.

Social-Communicative Theories: Affective Theory, Intersubjectivity, Joint Attention, and Identification

In an attempt to understand HFASD, social-communicative theories strive to untangle children's ability to form interpersonal engagement with others based on emotions and shared attention. Four major theories uphold social-communicative underpinnings for HFASD: affective theory, intersubjectivity, identification, and joint attention.

Affective Theory

Historically, Leo Kanner (1943) was the first to define ASD as a disturbance in affective contact, as follows:

> We must, then, assume that these children have come into the world with innate inability to form the usual, biological provided affective contact with people, just as other children come into the world with innate physical or intellectual handicaps. If this assumption is correct, a further study of our children may help to furnish concrete criteria regarding the still diffuse notions about

the constitutional components of emotional reactivity. For here we seem to have pure-culture examples of *inborn autistic disturbances of affective contact.* (p. 250, emphasis in original)

According to Kanner's view, something is lacking in the emotional and interpersonal dialogue of the child with ASD. Kanner's perception of ASD as a disorder of affective contact and as a constitutional deficit in emotional reactivity laid the groundwork for extensive study exploring the nature and breadth of the social-emotional deficit in ASD (Hobson, 2005). Furthermore, it provided a social-affective explanation for these children's difficulties in forming friendship and attachment security, in understanding interpersonal relationships, and also in understanding and experiencing social emotions such as loneliness and jealousy. Such emotions obtain their meaning through interpersonal relationships and interactions or through social and emotional understanding processes.

Intersubjectivity

The difficulty in developing meaningful relationships among children with ASD has also been explained via intersubjective theory (Trevarthen & Aitken, 2001). Trevarthen and Aitken described typically developing infants as congenitally having social-communicative "interpersonal awareness," that is, as possessing primary "intersubjectivity" or "person awareness." This person awareness, through which the infant is specifically receptive to others' subjective states in person–person immediacy, enables the infant to share attention and to link his or her own subjective experience to the subjective experience of another person. Primary intersubjectivity assumes that the infant possesses conscious appreciation of adults' communicative intentions very early in life (Trevarthen, 1979). Secondary intersubjectivity, which typically develops around 9 months of age, comprises a cooperative intersubjectivity (person–person–object awareness) in which infants' interactions with another person begin to make reference to surrounding objects (Hobson, 2002).

Hobson (2002) emphasized the emotional nature of this person–person intersubjectivity: By coordinating patterns of behaviors with those of other people, infants become emotionally connected with others. Trevarthen and Aitken (2001) underscored the way that emotions between people (such as jealousy) have their foundation in the dynamic reactions of even young infants, who have limited neurological and cognitive development yet do experience "being present" with another—meaning that they experience someone else as a "person." A lack of intersubjective sharing, which seriously disrupts children's ability to experience, be sensitive to, or react emotionally within social contexts, is considered a core deficit in autism (Hobson, 2005; Rogers & Bennetto, 2001; Rogers & Pennington, 1991). Whereas infants with typical development (TYP) can recognize and share affective experiences with others very early in life (Dissanayake & Sigman, 2001), young children with autism have been described as having difficulties in turning to others to express their feelings or in responding to others when feelings are expressed (Hobson, 2005).

Identification

Expanding on the intersubjective view and providing a psychoanalytical perspective on the difficulty in developing social communication, Hobson and Meyer (2005) suggested that individuals with ASD reveal a specific deficit in identification—which is a mechanism that is responsible for human interpersonal connectedness (Hobson & Hobson, 2007; Hobson & Meyer, 2005). In TYP, through identification, one person is drawn to assume another's psychological self–other orientation; that is, the observer tends to copy the bodily expressed style of that person in feeling, acting, or relating to others. By assimilating or imitating the other's stance through the identification process, the individual shares that person's mode of relating to the self and others in such a way that it becomes possible for roles to be reversed between the two people, in behaviors and in attitudes (Hobson & Hobson, 2007). In ASD, this ability for identification appears to be problematic at both the nonverbal and verbal levels of interaction, thereby impeding their development of interpersonal engagement.

Joint Attention

Joint attention is a pivotal social-communicative skill that is developed based on primary and secondary intersubjectivity. The coordination of attention and the sharing of a common point of view between social partners are the core defining characteristics of joint attention (Mundy, 1995; Mundy & Newell, 2007). During their first months of life, infants with TYP spend much of their time in face-to-face dyadic interaction with people, engaging in mutual gaze, vocal interchange, and turn-taking games (primary intersubjectivity; Trevarthen, 1979). Gradually entering into this dyadic caregiver–child interaction is the infant's sharing of an interest in an outside object to form a triadic interaction, which develops between 6 and 12 months (secondary intersubjectivity; Trevarthen, 1979). Triadic joint-attention behaviors such as pointing and showing are considered an early preverbal form of children's representational capabilities, which form the basis for the evolvement of other, more complex representational capabilities such as theory of mind, which is described later (Mundy & Stella, 2001; Tager-Flusberg, 2001a). Coordination of attention is required for both social and academic learning (e.g., Mundy, Sullivan, & Mastergeorge, 2009). Thus poor ability in joint attention may affect children's capacity to succeed in pedagogical settings, as well as in social interactions, across development (Mundy & Sigman, 2006; Mundy et al., 2009).

Deficits in joint attention are considered an early, fundamental marker in the etiology of ASD (Mundy, 1995). Although the impairments are more severe in declarative joint attention (pointing for social purposes—to show and share an interest), deficits in imperative joint attention (pointing to express a request) are reported as well (Clifford & Dissayanake, 2008). However, impairment in joint attention is not total; these deficits vary with developmental level, as well as with symptom severity. Children with less severe autistic symptoms and higher IQs demonstrate earlier and more intact joint-attention behaviors (e.g., Anderson et al., 2007; Mundy, Sigman, & Kasari, 1994; Naber, Swinkels, Buitelaar, Dietz, van Daalen, & Bakermans-Kranenburg, 2007; Schietecatte, Roeyers, & Warreyn, 2012). Furthermore, joint-attention behaviors in ASD at younger ages, during toddlerhood and preschool, were found to predict later language gains (at age 5 years: Charman et al., 2005; at 8 years: Sigman & Ruskin, 1999; at 9 years: Anderson et al., 2007; in adolescence: McGovern & Sigman, 2005), as well as to predict later social interaction capabilities (at 9 years: Lord, Floody, Anderson, & Pickles, 2003). In contrast to the language and social development domains in ASD, which were both linked to joint attention, the domain of repetitive stereotypic behaviors was not (e.g., Delinicolas & Young, 2007; Uono, Sato, & Toichi, 2009).

JOINT-ATTENTION TYPES: RESPONDING AND INITIATING

It is important to differentiate between two basic forms of joint attention: responding joint attention (RJA) and initiating joint attention (IJA). RJA refers to the infant's ability to follow the direction of others' gazes, gestures, or verbalizations in order to share a common point of reference. IJA refers to the infant's spontaneous seeking of shared interests or pleasurable experiences with others, which involves infants' own use of gestures, eye contact, and vocalizations to direct others' attention to objects, events, or themselves (Mundy & Newell, 2007).

These two basic forms seem to have different developmental functions and trajectories in ASD (Mundy & Newell, 2007). Both are useful in early identification of ASD, but RJA becomes less evident as an ASD marker among children with a MA of 30–36 months or higher (Mundy et al., 1994) or among children with HFA at school age or older (Nation & Penny, 2008). Thus the RJA deficit seems to diminish with age. In contrast, the IJA deficit was observed in children from preschool to adolescence (e.g., Mundy & Jarrold, 2010; Sigman & Ruskin, 1999). However, IJA has been much less explored among children with HFASD at school age or older than among younger children with ASD. Only some indications of IJA in HFASD are available; for example, preadolescents with HFASD were found to perform showing and sharing behaviors to attract their main caregivers' attention to their own drawings or games during a jealousy-provoking experiment (Bauminger, 2004).

The correlates of RJA and IJA seem to differ as well. Both IJA and RJA are associated with executive inhibition and language development in

ASD, but RJA is a more robust correlate of language (e.g., Schietecatte et al., 2012; McGovern & Sigman, 2005). Moreover, only IJA is associated with differences in social and affective symptom presentation in ASD and with a preference for social versus nonsocial stimuli (e.g., Charman, 2003; Lord et al., 2003; Mundy et al., 1994; Schietecatte et al., 2012; Sigman & Ruskin, 1999). Thus IJA and RJA may display unique paths of associations with childhood social-communicative outcomes (Mundy et al., 2009).

ACADEMIC IMPLICATIONS OF JOINT ATTENTION

Joint attention and coordination of attention are cardinal for learning, inasmuch as learning situations require shared and coordinated attention (e.g., with the parent, teacher, classmate) focusing on an object or event to be studied and understood. Joint attention may also function as a self-organizer that facilitates information processing and enables spontaneous social learning from the environment, using both RJA and IJA. For example, Baldwin (1995) suggested that both forms of joint attention are used as a means to reduce referential mapping errors in spontaneous early language learning. Moreover, through RJA, infants guide themselves to the correct area of the environment. Through IJA, the child indicates to the parents that something is of immediate interest, which helps the parents follow the target of their child's attention in order to provide new information regarding that context. Indeed, the learning function of joint attention continues to operate throughout development (e.g., Nathan, Eilam, & Kim, 2007). However, to the best of my knowledge, the correlates of joint attention regarding specific academic capabilities in HFASD (e.g., reading, writing, mathematics) have not yet been explored.

SUMMARY OF JOINT-ATTENTION THEORY

Taken altogether, joint attention is a fundamental, early, preverbal capability for social, communicational, and academic growth. Deficits in joint attention characterize young children with ASD and have prognostic influences on later social and academic learning. These children are more likely to show a greater deficit in IJA than in RJA, including a deficit in the act of coordinating attention with another person. Yet less is known about the developmental trajectories of RJA and IJA in older individuals with HFASD. The understanding of the social deficit in HFASD requires the understanding of these older children's cardinal deficit in coordinating attention and in sharing behaviors, which are all based on joint-attention capabilities. Yet, again, joint attention alone does not provide a full explanation for the complexity of difficulties that older children confront during social interactions, such as the need to use executive-function capabilities to simultaneously process dynamic information in social situations. Neither does joint attention sufficiently explain the restricted and stereotypical behaviors observed in these children, which hamper their social and academic adjustment.

Summary of Social-Communicative Theories

The affective, intersubjective, identification, and joint-attention views provide explanations for the difficulties in social-communicative skills as well as in interpersonal engagement among children with HFASD. Indeed, many researchers agree that emotional engagement develops atypically in autism, but a gap exists in the literature regarding the unique characteristics and range of these children's emotional expressions in interpersonal contexts (Hobson, 2005; see also Chapter 2, this volume). More specifically, interpersonal capabilities in children on the spectrum are not an all-or-nothing phenomenon (see Chapter 3). Furthermore, the social-communicative theories reviewed here are not sufficiently useful in explaining individual differences in interpersonal engagement or in explaining the special cognitive-academic difficulties that characterize HFASD. A more complete understanding of the nature and breadth of the social-emotional deficit in autism requires taking into consideration the role of individual differences and the effect of mental capabilities on social-emotional functioning, as described in the different chapters focusing on social-emotional and cognitive-academic characteristics (Chapters 2–5).

Social-Cognitive Theories: Theory of Mind and Development of Self

One of the key components in determining how children conceive of relationships is ascertaining what children understand about themselves and other people—an understanding of "other minds" (Lombardo & Baron-Cohen, 2011). Social-cognitive theories, such as theory of mind and theories of self, have striven to illuminate the underlying psychological mechanism that explains the primary social-communicational symptoms characterizing ASD, as follows.

Theory of Mind

The theory-of-mind (ToM) hypothesis focuses on children's ability to differentiate the self from others and to attribute mental states to others— such as beliefs, desires, intentions, and emotions—and thereby to predict their behaviors accordingly (Frith & Happé, 1999; Liebal, Colombi, Rogers, Warneken, & Tomasello, 2008; Wellman, 1993). The ability to mentally depict the psychological status of others is called "metarepresentation," because it involves the individual's capacity to mentally represent another individual's mental representations (Mundy & Stella, 2001). Interactions between people involve representations about the other's mental states at several levels. First-order beliefs describe what people think about real events. However, social interactions can be properly understood only by taking into account high-order beliefs—what people think about other people's thoughts and even what people think that others think about their thoughts (Perner & Wimmer, 1985). According to the ToM approach, a disturbance in metarepresentational capabilities forms the basic psychological mechanism underlying social-pragmatic and academic deficits in ASD.

FALSE-BELIEF RESEARCH

Understanding of false beliefs (typically developed at around 4 years) has been perceived as a litmus test for ToM because false-belief attributions—understanding that an individual's belief or representation of the world may contrast with reality—can unambiguously reveal a distinction between self and others. The false-belief paradigm evaluates the child's (true) belief and the child's awareness of someone else's different (false) belief (Dennett, 1978). First-order false-belief understanding ("X believes that P") and second-order false-belief understanding ("X believes that Y believes that P") was extensively examined in ASD. Initially, using a classic first-order false-belief paradigm, Baron-Cohen, Leslie, and Frith (1985) showed that the majority of individuals with ASD (80%) failed the "Sally and Anne" puppet-play task (Wimmer & Perner, 1983), whereas the majority of individuals (85%) with Down syndrome and with TYP passed the task. According to this paradigm, after Sally left the room, Anne transferred the ball from its original location in a basket to a new location in a box; the question is where Sally will look for her ball upon returning, assuming she is unaware of the transformation. Most participants with ASD erroneously pointed at the ball's new location, whereas most individuals with Down syndrome or TYP pointed at the original location. This pioneering study established the basis for vast research on ToM (not restricted to false-belief paradigms) in ASD, in line with the notion that ToM may provide a unified explanation for the primary symptoms that define ASD (see discussion in Tager-Flusberg, 2001a). Employing a range of different verbal and nonverbal tasks and paradigms, ToM was used to explain children's major difficulties in reciprocity, in peer relations, in social conversation and pragmatics, in emotion recognition and understanding (specifically of complex emotions), and in pretend and symbolic play (see reviews in Baron-Cohen, 2000; Lombardo & Baron-Cohen, 2011).

TOM AND COGNITIVE-ACADEMIC CAPABILITIES

Scholars have also utilized ToM to explain these children's cognitive-academic difficulties because it was perceived as critical for children's academic achievement. In the classroom, children are expected to understand not only the teacher's intentions throughout the lesson but also the author's intention in any basic or complex narrative text. Moreover, in

TYP, ToM enables readers to interpret the protagonist's intentions, goals, thoughts, feelings, and actions, thereby enhancing understanding of the subtext's implied meanings in narrative texts (Mason, Williams, Kana, Minshew, & Just, 2008). In contrast, many children with autism have difficulty understanding that communication enhances interpretation of intended meanings (Hale & Tager-Flusberg, 2005; Happé, 1993). Tager-Flusberg and Sullivan (1995) found that children with autism showed difficulty in supplying appropriate mental-state explanations for story events, in comparison with children with TYP. Likewise, Losh and Capps (2003) reported that children with HFASD provided fewer explanations for characters' internal states, in comparison with children with TYP. Researchers also found that adults with HFASD demonstrated difficulty both in ToM and in comprehending narrative texts—specifically, in the ability to monitor protagonists' states of mind (Mason et al., 2008)—and therefore generated fewer explanations for characters' mental states in comparison with control participants (Beaumont & Newcombe, 2006).

LIMITATIONS OF THE TOM EXPLANATION

Although ToM is considered critical for social and communicational functioning, and although children with ASD are considered to have difficulties in attributing mental states to others, the ToM hypothesis has not yet been proved to apply specifically only to ASD (ToM difficulties have also been found in other populations, such as children with learning disabilities or attention deficits) and universally across the spectrum (e.g., Yirimiya, Solomonica-Levi, Shulman, & Pilowsky, 1996). For example, individuals with Asperger syndrome and HFA can pass false-belief tests yet remain subtly impaired in providing explanations for their answers, which necessitates a higher level of social understanding (e.g., Bowler, 1992). In a like manner, they can effortlessly and spontaneously infer others' traits from descriptions of behavior, but they exhibit tremendous difficulties during spontaneous everyday interactions that comprise ecologically valid applications of mentalizing. For example, they have great difficulty in inviting someone to play during recess (which requires consideration of the other child's preferences, moods, or fatigue) or in applying empathic behaviors when exposed to others' distress (e.g., Belmonte, 2009; Dahlgren & Trillingsgaard, 1996; Frith & Happé, 1999; Ramachandran, Mitchell, & Ropar, 2009; Tager-Flusberg, 2001a).

Both conceptual and methodological criticisms have been voiced about the ToM hypothesis for ASD. Various ToM measures were criticized for their narrowness, overreliance on verbal capabilities, or ecological invalidity. Authentic communication requires much more on the child's part than merely inspecting a story character's false belief, desire, or intention (see, e.g., Astington, 2003; Peterson, Garnett, Kelly, & Attwood, 2009). In real ongoing daily spontaneous interactions, children are exposed to multidimensional social and emotional cues that are constantly changing.

Therefore, the processing of real social information goes beyond mere understanding of individuals' mental states; it encompasses reading of the whole situation, shifting attention from one cue to another, and deciding which of the most salient cues is peripheral and should be excluded from one's processing while attempting to understand the situation. Thus, issues of executive function (e.g., planning, cognitive shifting, monitoring, goal-directed action) and central coherence (e.g., perceptual and cognitive abilities to grasp the "big picture" and to differentiate between relevant and peripheral cues) also play an important part in social information processing (see later in this chapter). Thus far, ToM measures have not captured the full complexity of understanding real, live social situations and interactions.

In line with the notion that the ToM social-cognitive theory does not encompass all aspects of understanding social situations, the ToM hypothesis does not provide a sufficient explanation for other features that characterize children on the spectrum, such as their repetitive behaviors, obsessive interest in narrowly defined topics, insistence on sameness, and unique cognitive profile (e.g., strong visual-spatial skills alongside impaired language). Furthermore, as seen next, understanding others' mental states involves understanding the self. Indeed, Lombardo and Baron-Cohen (2011) suggested that individuals with ASD are characterized by "mind blindness," meaning that the mechanism for representing or attributing mental states to both self and others is profoundly impaired in ASD (see also Frith & Happé, 1999).

Development of Self

In comparison with the substantial body of ToM research investigating attributions of mental states to others, the attribution of mental states to oneself (the nature of the self, self-reflection, self-awareness) has been less explored in HFASD. Some evidence has indicated that introspection is hampered in HFASD and that these children demonstrate difficulties recalling events pertaining to the self (e.g., Frith & Happé, 1999; Hurlburt, Happé, & Frith, 1994; Millward, Powell, Messer, & Jordan, 2000).

Indeed, it seems that some aspects of knowledge about self are more impaired than others in HFASD. Knowledge of the self as distinct from others, as socially effective, and as an object of others' regard (the "interpersonal self" according to Neisser, 1988) appears to be more damaged than the knowledge of the self that relates to the physical world (the "ecological self" per Neisser, 1988). Yet even this distinction does not fully capture the difficulties in development of the self in HFASD, because not all aspects of the self in relation to others are damaged. Specifically atypical are those aspects of understanding the self that are linked with emotional experience, which require projection about the self vis-à-vis the representation of social relations. For example, in a jealousy-provoking experiment in my Behavioral Research Laboratory (Bauminger, 2004), preadolescent children with HFASD could be clearly observed experiencing jealousy in a triadic interaction when the main caregiver deliberately focused exclusive attention on a peer rival—friend or sibling. However, these children were unable to tell about this experience, and we could obtain only indirect knowledge of their jealous feelings. For example, one preadolescent with HFASD said he was "happy" when his mother constructed a model with his brother (while ignoring him), but by inquiring a bit further and asking what he was happy about, we learned that the boy indeed "was happy when the big model crashed!" Other findings also indicate that individuals with HFASD show difficulties in reflecting about self-conscious emotions such as pride, embarrassment, and guilt (which require the projection of the self in relation to others), as well as in showing empathic concern for someone else (e.g., Capps, Yirmiya, & Sigman, 1992; Kasari et al., 2001).

It seems important to distinguish between experiencing and understanding interpersonal situations. That is, even if children exhibit some difficulties in explaining social emotions such as jealousy or pride, they nonetheless can feel and experience at least some of them. For example, Hobson, Chidambi, Lee, and Meyer (2006) found that even among children with LFA, most parents reported that their children did experience jealousy, pride, or shyness, whereas they could barely report on instances in which their children displayed such emotions as guilt, pity, shame, or embarrassment. The implication of this gap between experiencing and understanding social emotions for understanding the interpersonal self in HFASD requires further exploration. Furthermore, explanations of why certain social emotions are reported to be experienced in ASD whereas others are not are still very speculative, and their implications for the development of the self in HFASD are not quite clear (see Chapter 2 for elaboration on the emotional deficit in HFASD). However, atypicalities in the development of the interpersonal self may offer an avenue to understanding the difficulties that children with HFASD experience in social emotions and social relationships.

Summary of Social-Cognitive Theories

Social-cognitive theories suggest that the social-interpersonal and academic deficits in HFASD stem from atypicalities in the development of the self in relation to others (e.g., the interpersonal self) and from difficulties in mentally representing others' mental states, such as intentions and emotions (ToM). As reviewed, these theories do encompass some important aspects of social and academic functioning in HFASD; nevertheless, they do not sufficiently explain other difficulties, such as these children's cognitive rigidity and their perceptual preferences for piecemeal processing at the expense of global configurations. The latter deficits are better explained by a different theoretical direction, that of the cognitive theories.

Cognitive Theories: Executive Functions and Weak Central Coherence

Another perspective for elucidating the core deficits in HFASD originates in two more cognitive-oriented theories, namely, the executive-function construct and the weak central coherence theory. Both focus on the ways in which children with HFASD cognitively construct and process social and cognitive information.

Executive Functioning

Executive function is a cognitive construct that refers to a set of mental processes, thought to be mediated by the brain's frontal lobes (Duncan, 1986), that enable higher-order planning and underlie goal-directed behaviors in children's constantly changing social and academic environment (e.g., Ozonoff, South, & Provencal, 2005). Executive function processes that enable goal-directed behaviors include: planning of actions to achieve a goal and to approach a task in an organized, strategic, and efficient manner; mental flexibility to shift attention, disengage from the current situation, and guide new behaviors in order to relate to ongoing situational changes; self-monitoring of interfering thoughts and actions; focusing and sustaining attention to retrieve relevant information and generate responses; inhibition of prepotent responses; generating novel ideas and concepts, including the formation of abstract concepts; and use of working memory to maintain and manipulate information over brief periods of time (e.g., Best, Miller, & Jones, 2009). In TYP, executive function components seem to follow different developmental trajectories (see review in Best et al., 2009). Inhibition appears to improve significantly during the preschool years and to change less later on, whereas working memory and shifting ability seem to emerge during preschool but to mature only later. In contrast, planning seems to make major developmental gains only during later childhood or adolescence.

The different executive function components are important both for social functioning and for school academic skills (e.g., Best et al., 2009; Blakemore & Choudhury, 2006). In children with TYP, various executive function components were found to correlate with academic competencies such as reading comprehension (Cutting, Materek, Cole, Levine, & Mahone, 2009; Swanson, 1999); mathematical skills (e.g., Bull & Scerif, 2001; Cirino, Morris, & Morris, 2002; Espy et al., 2004; Sikora, Haley, Edwards, & Butler, 2002); writing and note-taking capabilities (e.g., Altemeier, Jones, Abbott, & Berninger, 2006; Hooper, Swartz, Wakely, de Kruif, & Montgomery, 2002); and school achievements in science and English (e.g., St. Clair-Thompson & Gathercole, 2006). Difficulties in executive functioning may hinder students as they progress to higher grades, which entail complex writing and reading assignments and require the use of novel skills and strategies (Estes, Rivera, Bryan, Cali, & Dawson, 2011). Executive functions have also been linked to different aspects of social functioning in TYP, such as self-regulation, ToM, and social cognition (e.g., see reviews in Best et al., 2009, and Blakemore & Choudhury, 2006).

EXECUTIVE FUNCTIONING AND HFASD

Executive function deficits characterize individuals with ASD at different ages and levels of functioning (e.g., Ozonoff et al., 2005). Despite disagreement as to whether executive functioning is a primary or secondary symptom of ASD, vast consensus exists about its centrality to the understanding of the disorder. Some executive function subcomponents have been consistently identified as more deficient (e.g., planning and cognitive flexibility) than others (e.g., response inhibition), whereas research on some subcomponents (e.g., working memory, generativity of novel ideas, verbal fluency) has yielded mixed results (e.g., Bennetto, Pennington, & Rogers, 1996; Lopez, Lincoln, Ozonoff, & Lai, 2005; Ozonoff & Strayer, 2001; Robinson, Goddard, Dritschel, Wisley, & Howlin, 2009; Semrud-Clikeman, Walkowiak, Wilkinson, & Butcher, 2010; Verté, Geurts, Roeyers, Oosterlaan, & Sergeant, 2006). Interestingly, one recent study demonstrated sex differences in children's response inhibition; females ages 6–16 years with HFASD showed poor response inhibition, whereas males did not (Lemon, Gargaro, Enticott, & Rinehart, 2011). The authors suggested that the two sexes may have different neurobehavioral profiles in HFASD and therefore varying clinical needs regarding executive function, but this finding should be replicated in other studies to achieve a more conclusive picture.

Common characteristics of ASD, such as the need for sameness, the strong preference for repetitive behaviors, and difficulties in initiating new nonroutine actions, as well as switching between tasks, were all proposed as attributable to executive function deficits. Indeed, cognitive flexibility of various types seems to be especially affected, such as shifting from one response pattern to another; shifting from one set of concepts or cognitive set to another (extradimensional shift); inhibiting prepotent responses, which requires restraint of previously reinforced, well-learned responses, a particularly marked area of deficit; and shifting attention between different sensory modalities (e.g., visual to auditory), which requires disengagement from one modality and movement to a new channel in order to detect new targets (e.g., see review in Ozonoff et al., 2005). Planning is also impaired in individuals with HFASD; for example, in tests of planning and problem solving, participants used a larger number of moves to complete a problem and showed a higher frequency of rule violations compared with agemates with TYP (e.g., Lopez et al., 2005; Robinson et al., 2009).

Executive function capabilities are necessary for academic as well as for social functioning (e.g., Best et al., 2009); thus the executive function deficit may underlie some of the social as well as academic deficits characterizing

HFASD. Cognitive flexibility, particularly set shifting, was found to be a good predictor of social understanding and social competence in adolescents and adults with HFASD (e.g., Berger, Aerts, van Spaendonck, Cools, & Teunisse, 2003).

CORRELATES OF EXECUTIVE FUNCTION

Despite the theoretical rationale upholding the relevance of executive-function capabilities, especially cognitive flexibility, for social functioning, and particularly for areas that require information processing, such as social cognition, executive functioning has not yet been examined extensively in HFASD. The task of drawing integral conclusions from the research conducted thus far in ASD is also challenging because these studies varied in several ways: (1) in their targeted social functioning capabilities (e.g., joint attention, social understanding, ToM, adaptive skills, repetitive behaviors); (2) in their targeted executive function components (e.g., set shifting, attention shifting, working memory, planning, complex capabilities of working memory, inhibitory control); and (3) in their targeted participants' levels of functioning along the autism spectrum. In general at this time it may be concluded that some studies on ASD have identified links between executive function components and the following social-communicative components: social understanding, ToM, social competence, social interaction, adaptive skills (including communication and socialization), and pragmatic skills (e.g., Berger et al., 2003; Gilotty, Kenworthy, Sirian, Black, & Wagner, 2002; Joseph & Tager-Flusberg, 2004; McEvoy, Rogers, & Pennington, 1993; Ozonoff, Pennington, & Rogers, 1991; Pellicano, 2007).

Correlations of executive function capabilities with intelligence scores in ASD, more specifically with Verbal IQ, are interesting. IQ was found to play a role in executive function performance (e.g., Ozonoff & Strayer, 2001; Zandt, Prior, & Kyrios, 2009), where higher scores on Full Scale IQ were linked with better executive function performance. However, research on this correlation of executive function with Verbal IQ has yielded mixed findings. In Liss et al. (2001), differences in cognitive flexibility between children with HFASD and children with developmental language delay were diminished after controlling for Verbal IQ. The same pattern appeared in Lopez et al. (2005) with regard to group differences in the executive functions of cognitive flexibility and planning. Likewise, executive function's significant correlations both with adaptive capabilities and with autism symptomatology were no longer significant after accounting for Verbal IQ. However, the opposite emerged in Verté et al. (2006): Most of the correlations between executive functioning and autism symptomatology remained significant even after Verbal IQ scores were partialed out. Thus the role played by linguistic abilities in executive functioning merits further exploration.

Moreover, the developmental trajectory of the different executive function capabilities is also an issue for future study, because atypical age-related patterns have emerged on tasks tapping response inhibition and self-monitoring in children with HFASD versus controls with TYP (Robinson et al., 2009). That is, children with TYP showed the expected increase in these capabilities with age, whereas children with HFASD did not.

Very few studies have examined the correlations between cognitive-academic skills and executive function components. Bebko and Ricciuti (2000) compared the spontaneous use of a rehearsal strategy for a memory recall task among three groups: children with HFASD (mean CA = 9.7 years, mean verbal MA = 9.6 years), preadolescents with LFA (mean CA = 11.7 years, mean verbal MA = 6.7 years), and younger children with TYP (mean CA = 6). Their findings (see Chapter 5 for a full review of this study) showed that the rehearsal strategy was delayed in the HFASD group but almost absent in the LFA group. Bebko and Ricciuti (2000) asserted that these findings support the hypothesis of a delay in the development of executive function skills in HFASD and a potential executive function deficit in LFA. Importantly, when the task conditions were changed to supportive ones, more participants in both groups employed rehearsal strategies, leading the authors to conclude that external support enhances executive function skills.

Another cognitive-academic skill area that appears to be influenced by executive function is source monitoring, which refers to the set of cognitive processes involved in recalling the origin of memories, knowledge, and beliefs. Hala, Rasmussen, and Henderson (2005) reported that children with ASD (mean CA = 8.5 years, mean verbal MA = 6.7 years) revealed significantly poorer performance when required to identify the source of a given word, compared with children with TYP.

Regarding school success, it is important to stress that executive function is relevant not only to strictly academic learning but also to students' ability to participate fully in school activities. Participation in everyday life is crucial for children's development, rendering an impact on their future outcomes (World Health Organization, 2001). Zingerevich and LaVesser (2009) examined the contribution of executive function to participation in school activities among children with HFASD (mean CA = 7.6 years). They found that children with higher executive function abilities participated more in school activities. The authors asserted that children's ability to curtail certain behaviors, tone down impulsive responses, and regulate emotional reactions contributed to their more successful participation in the school setting. Altogether, executive functioning does seem to play a role in certain cognitive and academic skills, but empirical work in these areas remains at a very preliminary stage.

Finally, executive function was proposed as an explanation for the repetitive behaviors characterizing ASD (e.g., Turner, 1999). Indeed, several studies have examined the link between repetitive behaviors and executive function capabilities in HFASD at different ages (e.g., Boyd, McBee, Holtzclaw, Baranek, & Bodfish, 2009; Joseph & Tager-Flusberg, 2004; Lopez et al., 2005; South, Ozonoff, & McMahon, 2007; Zandt et al., 2009). In adults with HFASD, Lopez et al. (2005) found that some executive functions predicted restricted, repetitive behaviors, whereas others did not. Specifically, cognitive flexibility, working memory, and response inhibition were highly correlated with repetitive behaviors, whereas planning and fluency were not. In school-age children with HFASD, Boyd et al. (2009) reported that an executive function scale for behavior regulation (a composite score of inhibition, attention shifting, and emotional control) correlated with stereotyped repetitive behaviors such as self-injury, compulsion, and rituals/sameness and with the total repetitive score. In contrast, the executive function metacognition scale (e.g., working memory, planning, monitoring) did not correlate with these repetitive behaviors. In Boyd et al.'s (2009) regression analyses predicting repetitive behaviors, again the behavior regulation scale was one of the predictors, together with an ASD diagnosis, earlier onset, and higher scores on a sensory index.

Similarly, Zandt et al. (2009) demonstrated that higher difficulty rates in behavioral regulation and general executive function were related to higher rates of repetitive behaviors and compulsions in children with HFASD, whereas a test of sustaining and shifting attention was linked with lower levels of obsessions. In youth with HFASD (ages 10–19 years), South et al. (2007) found a correlation between executive function (preservation—difficulty adapting to a new sorting strategy) and repetitive general stereotyped behaviors as measured on the ADI-R (Rutter al., 2003) and the ADOS (Lord et al., 2000). Moreover, no significant correlations emerged between executive function and other repetitive aspects, such as circumscribed interests, object obsessions, motor movements, or rigid routines. Likewise, in verbal school-age children, Joseph and Tager-Flusberg (2004) failed to find significant correlations between executive function and stereotyped behaviors measured using the ADOS. Taken altogether, various aspects of executive function (as yet undetermined) may perhaps contribute to repetitive behaviors in HFASD; however, executive function deficits cannot fully account for these repetitive symptoms (e.g., Lopez et al., 2005).

SUMMARY OF EXECUTIVE FUNCTIONING

Overall, executive function does not appear to be a unique and specific marker for ASD because it has also been linked to ADHD, conduct disorder (CD), and OCD, among others (see review in Ozonoff et al., 2005). Hence an executive function deficit is probably not primary to ASD. Furthermore, executive functioning cannot provide an adequate explanation for the range of difficulties that children with HFASD encounter, especially for the less social, more instrumental quality of their social interactions and for their difficulties in coregulation and emotional expression. Nonetheless, research up to now has clearly indicated that comprehensive understanding of social and academic functioning in HFASD does require consideration of the influences of executive function impairments. Further empirical exploration of executive function's links with social cognition, social interaction, and diverse academic skills is very much needed, with important implications for future intervention.

Weak Central Coherence

A second cognitive explanation for ASD has been proposed, concerning the central coherence theory—a theory of global processing that refers to human beings' ability to see the whole, big picture rather than its parts when attempting to understand environmental stimuli (e.g., Happé, 2005). Historically, Frith (1989) proposed that individuals with ASD are characterized by "weak central coherence" (WCC), a cognitive style focusing on detailed, piecemeal processing or preoccupation with parts of objects and situations, which occurs to the detriment of global configurations and the extraction of higher-level meanings and thereby results in a failure to understand and use contexts efficiently. In a more recent review of 50 empirical studies concerning WCC in ASD, Happé and Frith (2006) underscored two major implications that should be considered when referring to the WCC theory. First, based on research indicating that individuals with HFASD can process global information when instructed to do so, this theory has shifted from an emphasis on global processing deficits to an emphasis on superiority in local processing. The implication of this shift is that we will need to administer open-ended tasks in intervention and evaluation, along with specific cueing to attend to the task globally. Second, according to the notion that WCC is not a deficit but rather a bias toward localized processing, a continuum approach should be advocated describing some individuals as more biased than others. Inconsistent findings regarding WCC suggest that it may characterize only a subset of the ASD population (as also found for ToM and for executive function). Indeed, a recent study by White and Saldan (2011) failed to show any significant differences between youths with HFASD (CA = 6–16 years) and youth with TYP on any of the measures (accuracy and reaction time) of the Embedded Figure Test, a frequently used visual-spatial WCC test (Witkin, Ottman, Raskin, & Karp, 1971) in which participants are required to detect simple objects embedded in larger, more elaborate figures. Due to the fact that this test requires special attention to localized processing, it was expected that youth with HFASD would outperform youth with TYP, but, as reported, this was not found.

In an attempt to understand whether a central cognitive mechanism is responsible for integrating information at both conceptual and perceptual levels, Lopez, Leekam, and Arts (2008) examined the relations between performance on a visual semantic memory task (conceptual level) and performance on a face recognition task (perceptual level) among adolescents with HFASD and adolescents with TYP. Contrary to expectations, only 2 of the 16 adolescents in the HFASD group showed difficulties on both tasks, which would support the WCC explanation. Another 2 adolescents revealed no difficulties on either task, but the majority of participants revealed difficulties on only one or the other task. Therefore, Lopez et al. (2008) failed to confirm the assumption that a central mechanism is responsible for integrating information at both the conceptual and perceptual levels, although they did substantiate the notion of subgroups within autism: those with weak conceptual coherence, those with weak perceptual coherence, and a few with WCC across domains.

WCC AND SOCIAL-EMOTIONAL ASPECTS

A bias toward detailed, localized processing according to the WCC hypothesis may interfere with the poor social functioning that characterizes people on the spectrum (Happé & Frith, 2006). For example, overly focusing on details may reduce the efficiency of schematization processes, thus affecting the organization of social-event knowledge. Event schemas (i.e., generalized knowledge of what happens at common real-life events, such as eating at a restaurant, going to a movie, or celebrating a holiday) enable the individual to structure social experiences and also to accommodate the variability of diverse social events. Loth, Gomez, and Happé (2008) tested the hypothesis that WCC (putting heightened emphasis on localized rather than global information about an event) and ToM deficits (having difficulties in predicting others' perspectives of an event) may conjointly contribute to difficulties in event schemas in individuals with ASD (of mixed cognitive functioning levels) compared with individuals with learning disabilities or TYP (CA = 8–28 years). Between-group differences were examined by dividing the ASD group into ToM-task failers and passers and comparing each of these two ASD subgroups with the learning disabilities and TYP groups. ToM/ASD failers showed profound impairment in event schemas, as compared with the TYP and learning disabilities groups. Specifically, these ToM failers showed difficulties in providing generalized descriptions of common events and in sequencing activities according to their naturally occurring causal–temporal order. This subgroup of ToM failers was more likely than the other two groups (learning disabilities and TYP) to describe common real-life actions at the subordinate level of specific exemplars ("slotfillers") rather than describing higher-order generalizations regarding the hierarchical structure of events ("global slots"), and they were less able to understand the global ideas behind why people go to restaurants or celebrate Christmas.

In contrast, the ToM passers in the ASD group resembled the learning disabilities and the TYP groups in their intact generality—an adequate ability to generate core elements of events in appropriate temporal–causal order and good understanding of why people go to restaurants or celebrate Christmas. Yet abnormalities did appear in the hierarchical structure of events furnished by the ASD group's ToM passers: Compared with the two other groups, their narratives mentioned significantly more specific examples ("slotfillers"), revealed more mistakes in judging how often optional loosely connected acts might occur in the context of an event, and also contained significantly more inappropriate acts. Thus both ASD subgroups—ToM passers and ToM failers—revealed more difficulties in understanding event schemas compared with the control groups, which may be partially related to their WCC (e.g., describing more subordinate, specific examples of real-life actions), but individual differences between the two ASD subgroups in processing event schemas were related to ToM capabilities. Thus WCC provided only a partial explanation for their difficulties in event schemas organization.

Another study supported Loth et al.'s (2008) research on the role WCC plays in processing event schemas in HFASD. Nuske and Bavin (2011) examined the extent to which children's WCC style affects comprehension and inferential processing of spoken narratives, in HFASD (mean CA = 6.7 years) versus TYP. In line with the WCC continuum approach positing a bias toward localized processing rather than global processing (e.g., Happé & Frith, 2006), children with HFASD were expected to perform comparatively poorer on inferences relating to event scripts in narratives and comparatively better on inferences requiring deductive reasoning. According to the authors, children can understand narratives as a coherent unit via inferential processing skills, which enable construction of a mental representation of the narrative. Indeed, this study's findings yielded no group differences regarding local processing. However, coinciding with Loth et al. (2008), in Nuske and Bavin's (2011) study the children with TYP significantly outperformed the children with HFASD on the following global narrative processing measures: The HFASD group had difficulty extracting the narrative's core elements, tended to refer to each event as a separate incident, and did not make spontaneous inferences concerning the event scripts. Interestingly, no group differences emerged in global processing regarding understanding of the main idea, probably because children were primed by the title.

The link between WCC and affect was also tested. In research on male adults with TYP, Basso, Scheftt, Ris, and Dember (1996) found that positive mood and optimism were associated with a bias toward global processing, whereas individuals with depression and anxiety displayed a tendency toward a localizing bias. Inasmuch as adolescents with HFASD are at risk for anxiety and mood disorders, Burnette et al. (2005) examined the hypothesis that preadolescents with HFASD would show increased levels of anxiety and mood disturbance in comparison with matched preadolescents with TYP and that those higher anxiety levels would correlate with a bias

toward a detailed rather than a global processing style. Their study findings did not affirm their hypothesis: Although the HFASD group displayed
evidence of anxiety, the anxiety measure did not correlate with any of the
individual differences found on the WCC measures.

Taking the existing research altogether, due to the fact that the links
between WCC and various aspects of social and emotional functioning
were not extensively examined and the fact that studies examining such
links mainly yielded only partial support, at the current stage it is difficult
to draw a conclusive picture. But it seems that an important area for future
empirical examination will be learning more about the extent to which WCC
may be helpful in explaining the difficulties in social-cognitive functioning
in HFASD, such as social understanding (event schemas) and social information processing, relative to other social-cognitive or cognitive theories.

WCC AND COGNITIVE-ACADEMIC ASPECTS

The unique contribution of the WCC explanation is its seeming relevance
in addressing aspects of ASD that are somehow overlooked by other theories, such as areas of special talent (savant autism—a superior specific skill),
pedantic and acute obsessions with details, or a lack of generalization ability. Indeed, as such, WCC provides a more comprehensive explanation for
the cognitive-perceptual deficits in ASD than it does for the social deficits.

Frith (1989) pointed out that "the meaning of any utterance in word
or gesture can only be properly understood by . . . placing it in context"
(p. 180). Indeed, WCC was found to be associated with poor performance
on various measures of reading comprehension in ASD (Frith & Snowling,
1983). Children with ASD who are classified as demonstrating WCC tend
to focus on single words while reading, rather than on the global meaning of the text (Happé & Frith, 2006; Randi, Newman, & Grigorenko,
2010). Therefore, they may encounter difficulties when trying to understand a text's meaning concerning events that are merely implied at the
level of a single sentence or multiple sentences. Furthermore, when reading
words with ambiguous meanings, these readers tend to turn to the word's
most salient meaning or pronunciation, and they less frequently use search
strategies regarding the sentence's general context, which could help identify words' appropriate meaning. For example, readers with ASD may pro-
nounce the homographic word "tear" in the same way regardless of its sentence context of either crying or ripping (Frith & Snowling, 1983; Happé,
1997). However, when cued specifically to look for context in the sentence,
children with ASD do manage to disambiguate the homograph's meaning
(Snowling & Frith, 1986).

A study (Norbury, 2005) concerning language impairment and context-
processing difficulties (requiring WCC) found that children with HFASD
performed at the same level as language-matched peers and that context
processing was related to the children's language ability (i.e., receptive

capabilities such as vocabulary and understanding of increasingly complex sentences; expressive capabilities based on a test of sentence recall). Thus children who had lower language scores had more difficulty selecting the correct interpretation of an ambiguous word in context, regardless of their HFASD or TYP diagnostic classification. Only those children with language impairment had difficulty using context to resolve lexical ambiguities in the text. Contrary to the WCC theory, deficits in contextual processing were not found throughout the HFASD group, but only within the subgroup of children with lower verbal abilities (Norbury, 2005). These experiments highlight individual differences in WCC among children with ASD based on children's language impairments, inasmuch as only those with ASD who had structural language impairment showed evidence of WCC in the verbal domain. Similar findings emerged in a novel eye-tracking study, which examined the eye movements of adolescents with HFASD and TYP, as they monitored spoken information for words displayed on a computer screen. Once again, only the subgroups of adolescents with poor language skills, whether HFASD or TYP, showed context-processing difficulties (Brock, Norbury, Einav, & Nation, 2008).

Another cognitive ability with a suggested connection to WCC is analogical reasoning. The question of analogical abilities in ASD was raised by Morsanyi and Holyoak (2010), because analogies involve relational integration, which is a form of coherence. Thus, according to WCC theory, a general impairment of analogical reasoning may be predicted in ASD. However, the authors found no support for this theory; their adolescents with HFASD solved the Raven Advanced Progressive Matrices test (Raven, Court, & Raven, 1983), a picture analogy task, and a scene analogy task on par with adolescents with TYP. Furthermore, when comparing strategy use, the HFASD group used the same strategies as the control group. Thus findings from analogical reasoning research do not provide support for WCC.

Studies have tried to tease out the relationship between WCC and impairments in other cognitive areas such as ToM, executive function, verbal abilities, and so forth. In their empirical review, Happé and Frith (2006) reported that the localizing bias characteristic of many individuals with ASD is not a side effect of executive dysfunction or of ToM deficits. Pellicano, Maybery, Durkin, and Maley (2006) also found that once age, verbal ability, and nonverbal ability were partialed out, the domains of ToM, executive function, and WCC seemed unrelated to each other.

In sum, many questions remain unanswered concerning the mechanism for weak coherence in both the cognitive-academic and the social-emotional domains (Happé & Frith, 2006). As such, the WCC explanation is helpful mainly in understanding children's cognitive style of information processing, but other deficit areas are not covered by the WCC explanation, such as quality of peer relations or difficulties in emotional functioning (expressing and understanding feelings).

SUMMARY AND CONCLUSIONS

As seen throughout this chapter, the social-emotional and cognitive-academic characteristics of individuals with HFASD are complex and heterogeneous and most likely cannot be accounted for by a single underlying cognitive, social-communicative, or social-cognitive theory. Indeed, Happé and Frith (2006) have stated that such a multilevel and multidimensional disorder as ASD cannot possibly be explained by one global theory. Instead, interplay between cognitive and social-communicative-affective theories is needed. Furthermore, as seen, the understanding of HFASD is also challenging vis-à-vis clinical diagnostic criteria. The implications of the DSM-5 in terms of ASD prevalence, the lack of subetiologies within ASD, and the links between the social-communicative and repetitive-restricted domains will still have to be learned throughout the next century (Lord et al., 2012).

Altogether, social-communicative theories seem to better explicate the affective quality of children's interactions and their difficulties in achieving interpersonal engagement and relatedness—and to explicate their deficits in collaboration and co-regulation during social interaction. On the other hand, social-cognitive theories appear to provide a more solid conceptual basis for these children's metarepresentation difficulties—making sense of the social world and of the people within it. Lastly, cognitive theories seem to furnish a good conceptual basis for these children's deficits within information processing, although they focus mainly on learning and cognitive functioning. That said, it should be noted that each of the theory groups strives to offer a comprehensive explanation for the social-cognitive deficit in HFASD. Thus social-communicative theories stress that interpersonal engagement is the "cradle of thoughts" and is related to language and cognitive development (Hobson, 2002). In addition, efforts have been made to explain how social-cognitive theories such as ToM and the development of self are relevant to children's development of both social and cognitive capabilities in HFASD. Likewise, cognitive theories (executive function, WCC) attempt to explain some of these children's social difficulties, too.

In all, the current review of the theoretical background of the core deficits in HFASD highlights the need for a multidimensional conceptualization of the social-emotional and cognitive-academic difficulties characterizing HFASD. That is, these individuals' difficulties in forming relationships, in understanding themselves, in understanding others, and in understanding themselves in relation to others must all be considered in conjunction with their unique way of processing information and learning, in order to obtain a full depiction of their social-emotional and cognitive-academic weaknesses and strengths.

PART I

SOCIAL-EMOTIONAL AND COGNITIVE-ACADEMIC PROFILES

Chapter 2

Social-Cognitive and Emotional Competence

In one of our studies examining peer interactions in HFASD, we wanted to investigate how preadolescents with HFASD would perceive and relay to us what they saw in a richly detailed color illustration depicting multiple dynamic social exchanges between various children in an outdoor setting. In the picture, several children were playing with a ball, others were walking while talking to each other, one child was swinging on a tree swing, and so forth. When presented with this rich social stimulus, one preadolescent boy with HFASD examined the picture closely, for a great length of time, but did not offer any response to my request that he give the picture a title or tell me "what was happening" in the picture. Finally, he asked me, "Nirit, do you see this boy swinging on the tree? Look at the tree and look at the ground. There's a white stripe between them [pointing to a white uncolored space in the illustration]. That boy is going to fall off the tree!" Of all the abundant social stimuli portraying companionship, shared enjoyment, and closeness between peers, this visual detail of empty uncolored space in the illustration is what caught this preadolescent's attention. This example from my Behavioral Research Laboratory illustrates the unique way in which children with HFASD may perceive complex social situations.

Complex, efficient interactions with peers are built upon the basic building blocks of social-cognitive and emotional capabilities (e.g., Lemerise & Arsenio, 2000; Saarni, 1999). Cognitive processes such as attention, information processing, and problem solving provide the essential structure for perceiving and understanding social behaviors, whereas emotional processes such as recognizing, expressing, and responding to feelings cast the communicative meaning of such social behaviors. For example, a single sentence such as "Tomorrow I'm going on a trip with my class" can be said with different affective intonations—whether enthusiasm, weariness, or anxiety—and each time it can carry different communicational-interactive intent. Both the speaker and the listener undergo complex processes while trying to communicate their own social and emotional needs and while attempting to comprehend the other's intents during the interaction.

How people make sense of the social world, including their understanding of self, others, and the interplay between self and others, is what we call "social cognition" (Beer & Ochsner, 2006). Many varying definitions have been proposed for this term, as well as different suggested components; however, vast agreement exists that the very thing that makes our cognition social is the core of what characterizes us as human beings. That is, the processing of social and emotional cues such as feelings, intentions, interpersonal relationships, and interactions is what sets people apart from objects (Beer & Ochsner, 2006).

This chapter focuses on social-cognitive and emotional competencies in HFASD. Children on the spectrum demonstrate genuine deficits in their intuitive reading of and learning about the social and emotional world. The first section of this chapter describes the social-cognition difficulties exhibited by children with HFASD in arenas such as social attention, social information processing, and problem solving. The second section below covers the major difficulties in emotional competencies exhibited in HFASD, namely in abilities such as recognizing, understanding, expressing, and responding to emotional input.

SOCIAL COGNITION

Social Attention in HFASD

In order to be able to take part in social interactions, people must first and foremost be attuned to them. Attunement means looking at other people's facial expressions and nonverbal gestures, listening to their verbalizations, and considering the social context in which the interaction is occurring. A critical aspect of social attention is the ability to select and concentrate on the relevant social and emotional stimuli that are helpful in making sense of the social interaction while excluding those stimuli that may be distracting. For example, when listening to a speaker, one should attend to the speaker's eye region to read expression rather than to focus on eye color (e.g., Ames & Fletcher-Watson, 2010). Although not a diagnostic feature, faulty social attention processes have been pinpointed as a characteristic of children with ASD that impairs their grasp of social situations and of others' mental states during such situations (Klin, Jones, Schultz, & Volkmar, 2003). Also, research (e.g., Elison, Sasson, Turner-Brown, Dichter, & Bodfish, 2012) has demonstrated that individuals with HFASD, from early childhood through late adolescence (CA = 2.6–17.25 years), tend to invest disproportional visual attention in nonsocial objects (e.g., trains, vehicles, road signs) relative to social stimuli (males and female of various ages displaying happy expressions). This atypical attention toward nonsocial information may potentially restrict developmental acquisition of typical attention patterns. However, a thorough understanding of social attention in ASD requires careful examination of the particular social-emotional stimuli, the child's level of functioning, and the specific methodology utilized to assess social attention.

Attention to Social versus Nonsocial Stimuli

A body of studies (e.g., Adamson, Deckner, & Bakeman, 2010; Dawson, Meltzoff, Osterling, Rinaldi, & Brown, 1998; Dawson et al., 2004; Riby & Hancock, 2008, 2009; Swettenham et al., 1998) has shown that across development, in toddlerhood, preschool, and middle childhood, children with LFA (with overall IQ level between 50 and 60) demonstrated a more robust social attention deficit than children with developmental delays and children with TYP. Children with LFA revealed a more severe deficit in orienting to social stimuli such as humming or name calling compared with nonsocial stimuli such as a phone ring or car horn (Dawson et al., 1998, 2004); they looked less at people and more at objects (Dawson et al., 2004); they shifted attention more often between object–object than between object–person or person–person (Swettenham et al., 1998); they showed little interest in the friendly examiner (Adamson et al., 2010); they lacked spontaneous gaze fixation toward the eye region (Riby & Hancock, 2008); and they paid less attention to facial stimuli (faces artificially embedded into a scene or scrambled scenes containing facial stimuli) compared with children with TYP (Riby & Hancock, 2009). Based on this series of studies, social stimuli and person–person interaction do not seem to be the focus of attention among children with ASD who function at lower cognitive levels (LFA).

Data regarding social attention in HFASD appear somewhat different and inconsistent. Several studies have compared visual attention in middle-childhood groups with HFASD versus TYP toward both animate stimuli (people, faces) and inanimate stimuli (objects; e.g., Kikuchi, Senju, Tojo, Osanai, & Hasegawa, 2009; McPartland, Webb, Keehn, & Dawson, 2011; New et al., 2010; Wilson, Brock, & Palermo, 2010). Wilson et al. (2010) implemented two main tasks: (1) eye tracking to explore visual fixation (i.e., the focus of the child's gaze) on 20 photographs depicting natural scenes, including people (ranging from one up to a crowd) and objects (e.g., pelican, ice cream van); and (2) matching tasks for identical or differing pair photographs of faces and of objects (shoe pairs), in which the differing photographs were taken with different cameras under different lighting conditions and transformed to gray scale. Interesting group differences emerged: Face and object matching were deficient in HFASD (mean CA = 10.13 years), but the eye-tracking results demonstrated that both groups showed a strong bias to orient toward people before objects, even though the children with TYP were quicker to fixate on the people. In addition, viewing preferences differed between the groups. In the TYP group, fixa-tions throughout the trial focused primarily on people and secondarily on objects, whereas in the HFASD group, fixations throughout the trial were divided equally between people and objects, and overall they looked less at faces than did the TYP group. Also, only in HFASD, a preference to look first at people was associated with facial recognition on the face-matching task.

In Kikuchi et al. (2009), children with HFASD (CA = 9.4–15.2 years; mean = 12.7 years) were equally good at detecting changes in stimuli for the human head region and for objects, whereas children with TYP were faster to detect changes in heads than in objects. Rather differently, chil-dren and young adults with HFASD (mean CA = 10.8 years) and a group of children and adults with TYP in New et al. (2010) revealed the same prioritized social attention to animate static stimuli (people, animals) over inanimate static stimuli (plants, artifacts). Also, both groups' response times and accuracy levels in detecting change to animate static stimuli exceeded those of inanimate static stimuli. Similar results regarding static stimuli emerged in McPartland et al.'s (2011) study of visual attention to faces and to a variety of control stimuli (inverted human face, monkey face, three-dimensional curvilinear forms, two-dimensional geometric patterns) among adolescents with HFASD and adolescents with TYP (mean CA = 14.5 years). Despite lower functioning on measures of facial recognition and social-emotional functioning, the adolescents with HFASD exhibited similar patterns of visual attention to human faces.

A different study analyzed adolescents' (CA = 11–16 years) verbal descriptions of photographs of everyday indoor and outdoor scenes, each of which contained at least one person (i.e., a picture of three people sit-ting and talking in a cafeteria), and recorded their eye movements while viewing these scenes to provide a window into understanding how these social situations are perceived (Freeth, Ropar, Mitchell, Chapman, & Loher, 2011). Interestingly, both the HFASD and TYP groups displayed general interest in the person(s) in these scenes, mentioning people in the vast majority of their descriptions and spending a large portion of viewing time fixating on people. In addition, participants in both groups spent a similar amount of time fixating on human faces. Furthermore, eye fixation on people emerged even for those adolescents who did not frequently men-tion the people in their verbal descriptions. Analysis of the verbal descrip-tions also showed no group differences in the described people's frequency or type of emotions (basic, complex). Thus adolescents with HFASD could articulate what a person in a scene was looking at without prompts to look toward the eyes or to follow the direction of the person's gaze. However, adolescents with HFASD were less likely to elaborate verbally on the person and were initially slower to fixate on the person compared with their peers with TYP. Saliency of the human in the social scene thus appeared to be more pronounced for the adolescents with TYP, but all in all, this research corroborates the conclusion that social attention in HFASD is surely not an all-or-nothing phenomenon.

Attention to Dynamic versus Static Stimuli

Researchers have suggested that social attention in HFASD is dependent on the type of stimuli being explored, with more intact visual attention emerging for static social stimuli and more severe deficits in attention emerging for dynamic social stimuli of social interaction (e.g., Klin et al., 2003; Klin, Jones, Schultz, Volkmar, & Cohen, 2002; Speer, Cook, McMahon, & Clark, 2007; van der Geest, Kemner, Camfferman, Verbaten, & van Engeland, 2002; van der Geest, Kemner, Verbaten, & van Engeland, 2002).

Indeed, van der Geest, Kemner, Camfferman, et al. (2002) and van der Geest, Kemner, Verbaten, et al. (2002) reported no impairment in processing of static facial or emotional stimuli among children with HFASD (mean CA = 10.6 years) compared with age-matched peers with TYP. In the van der Geest, Kemner, Camfferman, et al. (2002) study, the two groups revealed similar gaze behaviors when viewing cartoon-like static scenes that included human figures. In the van der Geest, Kemner, Verbaten, et al. (2002) study, the HFASD group resembled the TYP group when viewing still photos of human faces displaying emotional states. Different findings were presented by Klin et al. (2002) for dynamic social interaction scenarios. Klin et al. (2002) asked adolescent and young adult participants (mean CA = 15.4 years for HFASD and 17.9 years for TYP) to view video clips from Lehman and Nichols's 1966 film version of Edward Albee's *Who's Afraid of Virginia Woolf?*, a film that portrays four individuals involved in intense social interactions and complex social situations. Using eye-tracking technology, Klin et al. (2002) recorded participants' eye fixation durations for four regions: eyes, mouth, body, and object. Individuals with autism fixated less on the eye region and more on the mouth, body, and object regions than did those with TYP. The authors concluded that when viewing a stimulus that closely resembles a naturalistic social situation, individuals with HFASD demonstrate abnormal patterns of social visual pursuit consistent with reduced salience of eyes and increased salience of mouth, body, and objects. Likewise, Speer et al. (2007) compared the visual fixation patterns of children and adolescents (CA = 9–18 years) with HFASD and with TYP when viewing video clips containing dynamic emotional interactions based on the *Virginia Woolf* film clips from Klin et al.'s (2002) study versus viewing still photographs based on the same film. Group differences in gaze duration emerged only for the dynamic stimuli, not for the static stimuli, and only for two regions: The HFASD group spent significantly less time than the TYP group fixating on the eye region and significantly more time fixating on the body region only for the emotionally laden video clips. Group differences did not emerge for fixation on any other region (mouth, face/other, object) for either condition.

Summary of Social-Attention Research

Taken altogether, the literature to date suggests the importance of further exploration concerning social attention in HFASD, particularly in more naturalistic social interaction scenarios (e.g., Ames & Fletcher-Watson, 2010). In such situations as on the playground, children yell, jump, laugh, play, fight, and talk all at the same time and while shifting physical positions and locations. Thus children with HFASD must process an abundance of dynamic, rapidly changing verbal and nonverbal social stimuli, which requires the application of executive function skills such as mental flexibility to shift attention between stimuli. Even if subtle group differences (HFASD/TYP) appeared among the studies that compared static social versus nonsocial stimuli, they do not provide support for a fixation preference for objects over social stimuli in HFASD. It remains unclear whether indeed social stimuli are less salient for these children versus children with TYP, whether this plethora of simultaneous dynamic social stimuli is too demanding a challenge for these children's attention, or whether their deficits stem from a combination of both. It may be very interesting in future research to explore children's own qualitative reflections on their attention processes during such complex and dynamic social situations.

One other issue that has not yet been sufficiently explored is the relevance of the particular social situation to the child. Research has clearly shown that very early in life, children with TYP begin to orient toward human faces, even unfamiliar ones (e.g., see review in Nation & Penny, 2008). However, for children with ASD, and more specifically with HFASD, it may be that the meaningfulness or familiarity of different people will determine children's selective attention. For example, in a recent study (Bauminger & Shoham Kugelmas, 2012) we compared the social attention of preschoolers (CA = 3–6 years) with HFASD in two jealousy situations— one in which the child's mother provided selective affectionate attention to another child, and the second in which an adult stranger provided the rival child with selective affectionate attention. The HFASD children were as attentive to the situation as their agemates with TYP and reacted similarly, but only in the mother condition. Thus it may be valuable to investigate social attention to familiar peers or significant adults versus unfamiliar ones. To date, studies that used eye-tracking procedures to explore visual attention in ASD mainly focused on unfamiliar individuals. Although researchers continue to explore the boundaries of the social attention deficit in HFASD, it is already clear that social interventions for this population should certainly include training to increase children's attention to social and emotional stimuli within diverse social situations.

Attending to social stimuli enables its encoding, but after attending to stimuli the child with HFASD needs to continue processing until reaching a meaningful understanding. This occurs through social information processing, as described in the next section.

Social Information Processing in HFASD

Social information processing (SIP) is a major component of children's social competence that enables them to make sense of their social world, specifically regarding their social interactions within this world (Dodge, 1986; Gifford-Smith & Rabiner, 2004; Lemerise & Arsenio, 2000). Dodge and his colleagues (Crick & Dodge, 1994; Dodge, 1986) proposed a model to conceptualize the mental processes that underlie the processing of social interactions in children, detailing how children process and interpret cues in social situations and arrive at a behavioral or emotional decision regarding these cues. The six steps in this model are (1) encoding social cues (i.e., attending to appropriate cues, chunking and storing information); (2) mentally representing and interpreting the cues (i.e., integrating the cues with past experience and arriving at a meaningful understanding of them, considering one's own and others' perspectives on the situation); (3) clarifying social goals (e.g., to join a group game or to maintain on ongoing conversation); (4) searching for possible social responses; (5) making a response decision (i.e., behavioral, emotional, or no response) after evaluating the consequences of the various responses and estimating the probability of favorable outcomes; and (6) acting out the selected response while monitoring its effects on the environment and regulating behavior accordingly (e.g., Crick & Dodge, 1994; Dodge, 1986; Gifford-Smith & Rabiner, 2004; Lemerise & Arsenio, 2000). Overall, the SIP patterns of socially competent children reflect their priority for maintaining harmonious relationships with peers (Gifford-Smith & Rabiner, 2004).

Despite major difficulties in processing social information in HFASD, the six steps of the SIP model have not been extensively examined in this population. Three studies on SIP have compared children and adolescents with HFASD and children with TYP using video vignettes of social interactions involving various themes such as group entry, peer rebuff, and provocation (e.g., Channon, Charman, Heap, Crawford, & Rios, 2001; Embregts & van Nieuwenhuijzen, 2009; Meyer, Mundy, van Hecke, & Durocher, 2006). In Meyer et al. (2006), only a few differences emerged between the groups: Children with Asperger syndrome (mean CA = 10.1 years) made more encoding errors (added information that was not in the vignettes) and suggested more passive responses and fewer assertive responses than the children with TYP (mean CA = 10.2 years). Similarly, in Embregts and van Nieuwenhuijzen (2009), differences between HFASD and TYP (CA = 10–14 years) emerged on encoding, in which children with HFASD focused more on negative information in the scenario than did children with TYP. Group differences were also found on assertive responses; children with HFASD evaluated this type of response less positively and considered themselves less capable of acting assertively compared with the TYP group. As in the Meyer et al. study, both groups understood that aggressive and submissive responses were inadequate.

Channon et al. (2001) examined SIP through exposure to real-life types of problem solving that included social relationships in the family and in workplaces. Adolescents and young adults with Asperger syndrome (CA = 11–19 years, mean = 13.89 years) showed poorer SIP than their peers with TYP (CA = 10–17 years, mean = 14.38 years) in several ways: They required more prompts to recount the story's factual details (encoding); the quality of their suggested solutions was lower (i.e., less relevant to important aspects of the problem), although the solutions' total number did not differ; the social appropriateness, effectiveness, and practicality of their suggested solutions were all lower; and the quality of their final selected solution was also poorer, especially for social appropriateness.

Another study comparing children with Asperger syndrome (CA = 11–15 years, mean = 13.5 years) and same-age peers with TYP used an SIP interview that included four stories that depicted negative peer social interactions, such as peer-entry rejection and peer provocation (Flood, Hare, & Wallis, 2011). Similar to former findings, not all SIP steps were deficient. For the interpretation SIP stage, participants with Asperger syndrome were no more likely than the comparison group to attribute malevolent intent to the protagonists in the SIP scenarios, but the quality of their attribution style differed from TYP. That is, participants with Asperger syndrome provided more global attributions (e.g., "You get in kids' way all the time" for the provocation scenario) than participants with TYP rather than providing specific attributions (e.g., "You're getting in that kid's way"). This attribution style may provide support for the "cognitive hypotheses" often postulated concerning these children, upholding the idea that they employ cognitive strategies to cope with social scenarios rather than responding to specific, authentic social experiences. Interestingly, global attribution style was found to correlate with depressive symptoms, which characterize children with Asperger syndrome more often than children with TYP (Barnhill & Smith-Myles, 2001; see also Chapter 6). Participants with Asperger syndrome also showed greater difficulties in the response-generation step of SIP than participants with TYP, generating more nonsocial withdrawal responses (withdrawing from situations or doing nothing) and fewer prosocial-withdrawal responses (seeking out different people or social activities). Also, in line with former SIP research outcomes, the Asperger syndrome group evaluated assertiveness as a less effective response to the provocation scenario, compared with the TYP group's evaluations. They also rated withdrawal as a better quality response in entry scenarios compared with TYP. Thus, overall, in line with prior results, response generation and response evaluation were not intact in these children.

Difficulties in judging the social appropriateness of videotaped social behaviors also emerged in a study conducted by Loveland, Pearson, Tunali-Kotoski, Ortegon, and Gibbs (2001). These researchers exposed children and young adolescents (CA = 6–14 years, mean = 9.12 years) to four types of video scenarios: verbally appropriate (e.g., admiring a picture that someone offers to show), nonverbally appropriate (e.g., cooperating in making a sandwich), verbally inappropriate (e.g., when introduced, saying "Is your father dead?"), and nonverbally inappropriate (e.g., hitting someone). Children and adolescents with HFASD were less accurate at identifying examples of inappropriate social behavior than were their peers with TYP, particularly for verbal inappropriateness. However, this group difference did not emerge when identifying appropriate behavior. Also, the HFASD group had more difficulty providing explanations of the inappropriateness of verbal social behaviors than of nonverbal ones. Nah and Poon (2011) presented similar results when showing children with HFASD and children with TYP (CA = 9–13 years) a series of socially inappropriate events in a comic strip (i.e., putting a leg on a table in public to see what was causing an itch). No group differences emerged in rating socially inappropriate behaviors, but children with HFASD exhibited a specific difficulty in providing justifications for their responses. They provided inappropriate, bizarre, or inadequate ("I don't know") justifications instead of appropriate social justifications that would reflect social awareness.

One final study yielding deficits in response generation examined SIP in adults with HFASD (mean CA = 25.35 years) and adults with TYP (Goddard, Howlin, Dritschel, & Patel, 2007) by presenting five means–end social problem-solving scenarios such as girlfriend–boyfriend troubles or moving into a new neighborhood. In line with the former studies for younger participants, deficits emerged for adults, too, in generating responses. The HFASD group's solutions were less detailed, less effective, and more focused on the here and now than those of the TYP group. Moreover, autobiographical memories as a basis for solving the problems were found to be relevant only for the adults with TYP, not for the adults with HFASD. In HFASD, autobiographical memory performance was impaired, with significantly longer latencies to retrieve specific memories while solving a social problem and fewer specific memories retrieved in comparison with the TYP group.

Another social processing difficulty that children with HFASD show, which relates more closely to the encoding of social cues, consists of their tendency to describe peripheral details of a social situation, particularly physical characteristics, rather than describing the social meanings of the social stimuli. For example, in Bauminger, Shulman, and Agam (2004), preadolescents and adolescents with HFASD tended to describe physical details of a picture depicting two friends sharing secrets together (e.g., close proximity, children's activities, the color of the children's clothing) rather than describing these children as close friends. In another study, Klin (2000) also demonstrated less social sophistication in the understanding of cartoon figures among children with HFASD compared with their peers with TYP. The HFASD group was less sensitive to social elements, used considerably fewer affective terms, and was less able to derive personality features from characters' actions. It remains unclear as to whether this problem stems from a lack of social understanding and knowledge related to social norms and conventions, from problems in information processing that require taking the whole gestalt into consideration rather than its particular elements (i.e., the central coherence hypotheses; Happé, 2005; see Chapter 1, this volume, or both).

Summary of SIP

Taken altogether, research thus far indicates that even if not all SIP steps are impaired in children with HFASD, this population does demonstrate a major deficit in providing appropriate solutions to different social situations, as well as in their ability to evaluate the social appropriateness of solutions. In line with the findings for social attention in the preceding section, these children's ability to encode social cues was also shown to be distorted. This highlights a core deficit in social understanding, which may, at least in part, be due to limited peer interaction experiences and involvement. Full understanding of social situations requires understanding of the emotions within them. As stated at the beginning of this chapter, whereas cognitive information processes provide the structure for understanding social behavior, emotions cast their communicative meaning. The next section discusses the role of emotions in social behaviors.

EMOTIONAL COMPETENCIES

Understanding of Emotions in HFASD

Emotional understanding constitutes insight into one's own emotional state as well as into other people's feelings (Harris, 1989). Specifically, this ability encompasses a wide range of competencies, including: awareness of one's own affective state; use of a broad vocabulary of emotions when composing a narrative for emotional experience; identification of others' emotions; linking between emotions and social situations; identification of emotional clues and emotion-eliciting situations; comprehension of the possible gaps between inner and outer expression—the rules for displaying emotion; grasp of the simultaneous mixed and multiple emotions when reacting to a situation, even when these emotions conflict; and understanding of the more complex social self-conscious emotions (e.g., emotions in which the child expresses awareness or concern for others' evaluations), such as pride, guilt, shame, and embarrassment (e.g., Denham, 1998; Saarni, 1999).

Emotional Understanding in TYP

Emotional understanding gradually increases in complexity over development, necessitating ever-growing cognitive and social-emotional competencies. A case in point is that only in middle childhood does the ability develop in TYP to understand such complex emotions as pride or to label such complex emotions when they are experienced or observed in social situations. This understanding of complex emotions occurs much later than the ability to merely express such feelings (around 2 years of age) or the ability to understand basic emotions (e.g., happiness, sadness, anger, fear), which develops during the preschool years (Denham, 1998). The understanding of complex emotions such as embarrassment or loneliness requires the consideration of an audience—meaning to take another person's perspective of oneself and one's behaviors, thoughts, and feelings. For instance, only if someone sees me slipping on a banana peel would I experience embarrassment, because I would take the other person's perspective of my behavior; but if nobody was watching the incident, I would probably feel sad or hurt. Understanding complex emotions also requires the understanding of social norms (e.g., for pride and guilt) and the development of personal responsibility for a situation's consequences (e.g., for pride; Lewis, 1993). Furthermore, understanding of emotions requires that children attend to a situation's social cues, but in the case of complex emotions such cues can rarely be detected solely from facial expressions as in the case of simple, basic emotions. Thus, the understanding of complex emotions requires deeper consideration of the social context in which the expression is manifested (Lewis, 1993).

Another higher emotional understanding capability that develops in TYP in middle childhood, in line with growing cognitive abilities, is the realization that individuals can concomitantly experience multiple and even mixed emotions toward the same situation or person (Harris, 1989). For example, children moving to a different neighborhood may feel sad to leave their friends yet excited to meet new ones.

In addition, by midchildhood, children with TYP can also understand that the gap between an inner feeling and its external expression is what underlies hidden emotions (Harris, 1989). Children with TYP at this age have already grasped the concept of privacy (Harris, 1989) and can understand that they may feel an emotion but not necessarily manifest it in their behavior. Children in midchildhood can also realize that concealing their inner feelings can protect them from getting hurt by others (e.g., when friends might tease them about their fears) or from hurting other people's feelings (e.g., when receiving an undesired gift from a beloved person). Based on this understanding, children with TYP can also comprehend the fact that other children may be hiding their feelings, too.

The acknowledgment of this gap between externally manifested and internally experienced emotion allows children to make inferences regarding others' emotional states during complex social interactions. Children need to take into consideration the social context and their former knowledge of and familiarity with the other children or adults involved in the situation in order to accurately conjecture about the others' emotional states. In line with this complexity, as children grow older, they require fewer concrete, external, physical clues to detect emotional states in themselves and in others (e.g., "I know he is happy because he is laughing"). Instead, they can relate to more internal, psychological clues (e.g., "I know that I am happy because I feel good inside"; Greenberg, Kusche, Cook, & Quamma, 1995). Thus children's complex emotional behavior during midchildhood in TYP requires attributions to the social context and to the people who are involved in the situation. Moreover, this emotional behavior involves higher social and cognitive capabilities than the earlier understanding of basic emotions.

Emotional Understanding in HFASD

Emotional understanding capabilities pose a specific difficulty for children with HFASD, due to their limited social-emotional awareness and ToM capabilities. Studies in this area targeting HFASD have focused on children's understanding of: (1) their own simple and complex emotions (e.g., Bauminger, 2004; Bauminger & Kasari, 2000; Bauminger, Shulman, & Agam, 2003; Capps et al., 1992; Losh & Capps, 2006; Rieffe, Terwogt, & Kotronopoulou, 2007; Williams & Happé, 2010); (2) simple and complex emotions in others and in observed social situations (e.g., Bauminger, 2004; Begeer, Terwogt, Rieffe, Stegge, & Koot, 2007; Capps et al., 1992; Golan, Baron-Cohen, & Golan, 2008; Heerey, Keltner, & Capps, 2003; Hillier & Allinson, 2002; Hobson et al., 2006; Tracy, Robins, Schriber, & Solomon, 2011; Williams & Happé, 2010; Yirmiya, Sigman, Kasari, & Mundy, 1992); (3) mixed emotions (e.g., Rieffe et al., 2007); (4) rules for displaying emotions and hiding emotions (e.g., Barbaro & Dissanayake, 2007; Dennis, Lockyer, & Lazenby, 2000); and (5) reasons that evoke emotional states and ways to cope with negative emotions (e.g., Bauminger, 2004; Jaedicke, Storoschuk, & Lord, 1994; Rieffe et al., 2007; Rieffe, Terwogt, & Stockmann, 2000). I next elaborate on each of these areas.

UNDERSTANDING ONE'S OWN SIMPLE AND COMPLEX EMOTIONS

Capps et al. (1992) asked children with HFASD (CA = 12.4 years) to tell about a time they experienced basic emotions (happiness, sadness, fear, anger) and complex emotions (embarrassment, pride). The HFASD group was as good as the TYP group in differentiating happiness from pride based on locus of control (internal and controllable for pride versus external and uncontrollable for happiness), but in their examples they did not differentiate sadness from embarrassment. Likewise, in their examples of embarrassment, the children with HFASD related less to an audience, either implicitly or explicitly, than did the children with TYP. Except for happiness and sadness, examples given by the HFASD group were more general, conveying factual rather than personal knowledge. They were also more likely to rely on cognitive strategies and terms ("I think," "I guess") in the process of recalling examples of both basic and complex emotions. These findings strengthened the notion that these children were providing rule-learned emotions and relying on cognitive efforts and strategies while recalling personal emotional experiences (i.e., the cognitive "compensation hypothesis"; Hermelin & O'Connor, 1985; Kasari et al., 2001). In addition, compared to the TYP group, the HFASD group demonstrated slower response time for the complex emotions and for anger, and a greater number of prompts was needed when recounting situations engendering pride and embarrassment. Altogether, a more pervasive difficulty appeared in children with HFASD regarding their self-knowledge of complex emotions.

Losh and Capps's (2006) analysis of personal narratives to uncover children's broader emotional repertoire presented similar patterns of differences between HFASD and TYP groups of preadolescents (CA = 8–14 years). Their analysis differentiated simple emotions (e.g., disgust), complex but nonsocial emotions (e.g., curiousity, disappointment, surprise), and complex self-conscious social emotions (e.g., pride, embarrassment, guilt, or shame, in which the child expressed awareness or concern for others' evaluations). They found that, overall, the HFASD group produced contextually appropriate accounts of simple emotions but significantly less appropriate accounts of both types of complex emotions, with a more pronounced difficulty in social self-consciousness, compared with the TYP group. Preadolescents with HFASD were more apt to produce narratives lacking details or explanations that would distinguish socially complex emotions from basic emotions; for example, they reported "pride" on receiving a video game, but their actual descriptions were coded as happiness. Also, when asked to furnish examples of disappointed, ashamed, guilty, and embarrassed feelings, these preadolescents provided examples coded as basic, such as sadness or anger. In addition, they more often needed prompting to access and describe memories of emotional experience. Altogether, across the entire range of emotions (basic and complex), the preadolescents with HFASD were less able to organize and convey their accounts of emotional experience in a specific, personalized, casual–explanatory narrative framework. Their inability to attribute causes to their own emotions casts doubt on their genuine self-understanding of emotion.

A study by Rieffe et al. (2007) specifically demonstrated children's less well-developed awareness of their own negative basic emotions (e.g., anger) in HFASD (mean CA = 10.2 years) compared to TYP (mean CA = 10.3 years). Children with HFASD more often denied that they had ever experienced one or more negative emotions (sadness, fear, anger). The contents of their given examples also differed, such that the HFASD group provided fewer social examples and more idiosyncratic examples for negative feelings. Whereas children with TYP more often included attributions to interpersonal peer relations in their examples, the HFASD group's examples more often included objects (e.g., a science book for happiness) or family members (e.g., for sadness). Rieffe et al.'s findings suggest that children with HFASD may not have acquired well-developed knowledge about their own negative emotions. This group's deficit in social examples and references to peers seems to pinpoint these children's specific lack of awareness about the links between peer relations and emotions.

To further this discussion of attributions to interpersonal relations in children's examples of their own emotions, two other complex emotions that we studied in my Behavioral Research Laboratory are highly relevant: loneliness and jealousy. Both loneliness and jealousy are social emotions and relate directly to interpersonal relationships. Loneliness is experienced when social relations are absent, and jealousy is experienced when social relations with a significant other are seen as endangered due to a third party. As may be expected, children with HFASD (CA = 7.11–14.8 years, mean = 10.74 years) in Bauminger and Kasari (2000) were less likely to tell about their experience of affective loneliness, which reflects the absence of a close friend or the lack of intimate relationships, than children with TYP (CA = 7.8–14.5 years, mean = 10.89 years). However, the two groups provided a similar number of personal examples of social-cognitive loneliness, which reflects a sense of boredom or emptiness due to the lack of an accessible social network or peer group. Social loneliness is more a cognitive interpretation of the emotion (comparing one's own and others' social status), whereas affective loneliness is inherently rooted in interpersonal relations. The better recognition of social-cognitive than of affective loneliness in HFASD attests to these children's more profound difficulty in understanding and acknowledging interpersonal engagement (Hobson, 2005; Hobson et al., 2006).

The same difficulty with the more interpersonal aspect of emotion also appeared for jealousy (Bauminger, 2004). Affective jealousy arises when children experience the fear of losing love or exclusive attention from a significant other (mother, friend), whereas social-cognitive jealousy arises mainly through comparison with another person, when the individual senses that another individual enjoys more success or possessions than he or she does, challenging his or her own superiority or equality. As found for loneliness, preadolescents with HFASD (mean CA= 11.14 years) were more likely to include social-cognitive examples of jealousy in their personal accounts of the emotions (e.g., "When kids in school can buy whatever they want whenever they want") than affective examples (e.g., "When a kid from class is going to play with another kid from class, and not with me, I feel sad"), whereas their counterparts with TYP included both types.

One study's findings using personal narratives (Williams & Happé, 2010) contradicted this general direction of research outcomes, failing to show group differences between social emotions (pride, guilt, embarrassment) and nonsocial emotions (happiness, sadness, fear, surprise, disgust, disappointment). Williams and Happé reported that both groups (mean CA = 12.35 years for HFASD and 12.59 years for TYP) encountered more difficulty defining and sharing personal accounts of socially complex emotions than of nonsocial emotions. Their dissimilar results may be due to that study's different coding system (Williams and Happé ranked the relevance of examples' contextual situations whereas prior studies used content analysis) or to the lower verbal IQ capabilities in Williams and Happé's control group compared with those of the former studies.

Taken altogether, narration of personal accounts of one's own emotions is not intact in children with HFASD, especially revealing deficits in relaying socially complex emotions, in relating emotions to interpersonal relationships, and even in genuinely understanding negative basic emotions.

UNDERSTANDING EMOTIONS IN OTHERS

In TYP, knowledge of one's own emotions is linked to the ability to identify emotions in others based on multiple cues such as facial expression, body gesture, intonation, action, and the social context (e.g., Saarni, 1999). Therefore, children with HFASD may be expected to exhibit difficulties in identifying others' feelings and emotions based on facial expressions, external bodily cues, and observed social scenarios.

Basic Emotions. Studies have documented that children with HFASD can recognize basic emotions from faces, such as happiness, anger, sadness, and fear (e.g., Farran, Branson, & King, 2011; Hileman, Henderson, Jaime, Newell, & Mundy, 2010). Such emotion recognition was examined across a broad range of social signals including not only faces but also gestures and vocal intonation (e.g., Jones, Pickles et al., 2011; Philip et al., 2010), as well as between competing cues, such as auditory versus visual (e.g., Boggs & Gross, 2010), and as linked to social interaction situations (e.g., Semrud-Clikeman, Walkowiak, Wilkinson, & Portman Minne, 2010). Yet subtle differences have been found in emotion recognition of basic emotions in HFASD versus TYP.

Findings based on children's processing of human faces in order to recognize others' emotions have yielded mixed results, with more vigorous evidence of a deficit for LFA than for HFASD (see review of behavioral and physiological studies in Jemel, Mottron, & Dawson, 2006). In Farran et al. (2011), the ability to search for a target face in a crowd based on six basic emotions (fear, anger, sadness, happiness, surprise, and disgust) was examined in children with HFASD (mean CA = 12 years) and children with TYP. Each stimulus included 9 faces: the target emotion, a distracter emotion, and 7 neutral distracter faces. The child heard the name of the target emotion and had to point to it among the 9 stimuli. Speed and accuracy of detection were examined. Performance of the HFASD group on surprise, happiness, and disgust was as accurate and fast as that of the TYP group. However, children with HFASD were slower to detect sad, fearful, and angry faces than peers with TYP matched on CA but not compared with participants with TYP who were matched on verbal and nonverbal MA. Thus the HFASD group demonstrated an impaired response speed and accuracy for anger, fear, and sadness relative to the levels expected for their CA but no impairment in these emotions' recognition compared with younger peers with TYP who had the same mental capacity level.

Similar findings emerged in Hileman et al. (2010) for children's and adolescents' (CA = 9–17 years) identification of the same six basic emotions from facial cues. The HFASD group was no less accurate but needed more time and more cues in order to make their judgments. In addition, children with HFASD and TYP did not show different developmental trajectories for facial processing, thus providing no evidence for a developmental lag in HFASD regarding processing of basic emotions' facial expressions. Likewise, Tracy et al. (2011) recently found that children and adolescents with HFASD (CA = 9–17.3 years, mean = 12.25 years) were as accurate as their peers with TYP (CA = 8.25–17.25 years, mean = 12.25 years) at recognizing simple emotions (and one complex emotion, pride) from pictures of males and females from the chest up, including mainly facial expressions but also arms, shoulders, and head postures. No significant differences emerged even when the emotional stimuli were presented for a very brief time.

While using the procedure of *competing cues* to examine emotion recognition in faces, Boggs and Gross's (2010) study lent support to the notion of a relatively intact emotion-recognition process for basic emotions (happiness, sadness, anger, fear, and surprise). They presented adolescents with competing auditory and visual word cues for recognizing emotions in faces. Adolescents with HFASD did as well as those with TYP in making determinations about emotions in faces when competing word cues were inconsistent with the emotion portrayed in the face. Also, like their peers with TYP, adolescents with HFASD were more proficient in recognizing basic emotions when the competing words were consistent with the emotions portrayed in the faces.

Emotion recognition was also examined in a *naturalistic social interaction* setting. Semrud-Clikeman and colleagues (2010) asked youngsters with Asperger syndrome (CA = 9.1–16.5 years) to recognize the emotions and the meaning of nonverbal child–child and child–adult interactions from viewing 10 videos played at low auditory volume. Thus the study participants had full visual access to the interactions but could only hear the intonation without hearing individual words. Children were asked to explain how the character feels and how they know this, yielding two scores: total number of emotions recognized and total number of nonverbal gestures described. Children with Asperger syndrome revealed difficulty in emotional recognition from social interaction; they differed from peers with TYP in recognizing emotions and in recognizing the nonverbal gestural behaviors that guided their social judgments. It should be noted that this study included mostly basic emotions but also two complex emotions (frustration, embarrassment); however, specific findings with regard to basic versus complex emotions were not reported.

Implementing a rather different procedure for emotion recognition, based only on *vocal intonation*, yielded different results. Baker, Montgomery, and Abramson (2010) exposed young adolescents (CA = 10–14 years) to a task of listening to happy, sad, angry, and neutral spoken nonsense passages. Thus emotions could be detected based only on intonation processing. The HFASD group was as good as the TYP group in detecting these four basic emotions. The findings of these two last studies are interesting. Children with HFASD could recognize emotions based merely on intonation (Baker et al., 2010), but they had difficulty in recognizing emotions as part of social interaction (despite the fact that the recognition was partially based on vocal intonation in Semrud-Clikeman et al. (2010). These outcomes should be examined in future research, but they may pinpoint a specific difficulty in emotion recognition based on nonverbal gestural behavior rather than based on intonation. This difficulty also seems to resemble the aforementioned findings on social attention, which identified a specific difficulty in social attention to dynamic social situations.

This book focuses mainly on school-age children and adolescents; however, an intriguing study on adults with HFASD (mean CA = 32.5 years) and their agemates with TYP yielded somewhat different results (Philip et al., 2010). That study showed a comprehensive deficit in the HFASD group's ability to recognize basic emotions (happiness, sadness, anger, disgust, and fear) across a broad range of social signals such as faces, body movements, and voices. More specifically, difficulties emerged for the adults with HFASD in recognizing sadness, anger, and fear from faces, happiness and fear from body movements, and anger and disgust from vocal stimuli.

Looking at the developmental trajectory for recognizing basic emotions among individuals with HFASD, Rump, Giovannelli, Minshew, and Strauss (2009) explored recognition of six emotions' (happiness, sadness, anger, fear, disgust, and surprise) in four age groups—young childhood (CA = 5–7 years), middle childhood (CA = 8–12 years), adolescence (CA = 13–17 years), and adulthood (CA = 18–53 years)—comparing HFASD to TYP matched on CA and cognitive-linguistic capabilities. Differently from other studies that used prototypical static facial expressions, Rump et al. (2009) briefly presented dynamic expressions and also controlled for the emotions' subtlety, exposing participants to emotional stimuli that varied from the least to the most subtle facial expressions for each emotion. Findings demonstrated that the young children and the adults with HFASD performed more poorly than their TYP counterparts, with young children showing major difficulties in recognizing fear and anger and adults showing difficulties recognizing disgust, anger, and surprise. Moreover, for the TYP group, emotion recognition improved with age, but not for the HFASD group. Interestingly, when emotions were presented prototypically, no group differences emerged in either of these age groups. Thus young children and adults with HFASD revealed greater difficulty in emotion-recognition processes than their TYP counterparts only when the emotional stimulus was less clear-cut or less prototypical. Smith, Montagne, Perrett, Gill, and Gallagher (2010) demonstrated this same difficulty for the adolescent age group with HFASD (CA = 12–19 years, mean = 15.33 years). Using a procedure that exposed adolescents with HFASD and adolescents with TYP to different emotional intensities (low, medium, and high) via videotaped facial expressions of basic emotions, participants with HFASD revealed a major difficulty in recognizing disgust at every intensity level, including the highest. They were also less proficient at recognizing anger and surprise at low intensity levels, although they performed just as well as the TYP group at high intensity levels for these emotions. In contrast, Jones, Pickles, et al. (2011), like Rump et al. (2009), found no support for the notion of a specific impairment in the recognition of basic prototypical emotions among adolescents with HFASD (mean CA = 15.6 years).

Taken altogether, overall accuracy in recognizing others' basic emotions (most likely prototypical emotional expressions) was not shown to be impaired in HFASD. However, processing of basic emotions such as happiness, sadness, anger, and disgust was slower in HFASD than in TYP, and more cues were needed, especially when social interactions or emotional stimuli were less straightforward.

Complex Emotions. Research requiring children to infer complex emotions, especially emotions from a social situation, may seem to pose a much more demanding task. Williams and Happé (2010) recently found that regardless of grouping (HFASD or TYP), children (mean CA = 12.35 years) had more difficulty recognizing socially complex emotions (pride, guilt, embarrassment) than simple nonsocial emotions (happiness, sadness, fear, surprise, disgust, and disappointment) from video clips of actor-expressed emotions (including facial expressions, intonation, and body posture). Likewise, using a slightly different distinction between emotion types, Heerey et al. (2003) presented nine color photos of a male actor expressing self-conscious emotions (embarrassment and shame) and non-self-conscious emotions (anger, contempt, disgust, happiness, fear, sadness, and surprise) to children with HFASD (mean CA = 10.70 years) and children with TYP (mean CA = 10.51 years). Poorer performance in HFASD versus TYP emerged only for the understanding of self-conscious emotions, with significant results for embarrassment and near-significant results for shame. Interestingly, controlling for ToM capabilities eliminated the group differences in the recognition of self-conscious emotions.

Golan et al. (2008) used the "Reading the Mind in Films" task, which assessed recognition of complex emotions (e.g., guilt, loneliness) and mental states (e.g., bothered, friendly) based on cues from the social context, including facial expression, body language, and actions, as well as auditory input (prosody, verbal content). The presented emotions varied in valence, intensity, and complexity, thus designing an ecological measure that better approximated real-life emotion recognition from daily social situations.

The HFASD group (CA = 8.3–11.8 years, mean = 10.0 years) performed less well overall than the TYP group (CA = 8.2–12.1 years, mean = 10.1 years), but results for the specific emotions or mental states were not provided.

Another study examining the ability among HFASD and TYP groups to recognize others' complex emotions in social situations was conducted by Hillier and Allinson (2002). Their in-depth study of embarrassment investigated children's ratings of protagonists' degree of embarrassment and children's justifications for those ratings regarding a series of written embarrassing situations displayed on a computer and read by the experimenter, which differed in presence of an audience (large audience vs. none); type of audience present (best friend vs. authority figure); and whether or not the protagonist thought someone had seen him or her commit the embarrassing act. It also included one empathic scenario in which something potentially embarrassing happened to the protagonist's friend (he dropped his drink, which spilled all over the floor). Surprisingly, in contrast to research outcomes analyzing children's personal examples of embarrassment (Capps et al., 1992), children with HFASD at ages 10–14 years (mean = 12.3 years) in Hillier and Allinson's (2002) study could recognize the importance of the presence of an audience to the protagonist's embarrassment experience and rated this situation as more embarrassing than one with no audience. Furthermore, they showed the same level of understanding about audience types (that the presence of an authority figure is more embarrassing than that of a friend), as did younger children with TYP at ages 7–11 years (mean CA = 9.07 years), although their understanding level was lower than that of older children with TYP at ages 12–16 years (mean CA = 14.00 years).

Nevertheless, a major difficulty did emerge in Hillier and Allinson's (2002) study regarding the HFASD group's ability to provide justification for the empathic–embarrassing scenario by describing the effect of the friend's emotion on the protagonist's own subsequent emotion. This finding coincided with the specific difficulty in empathy found for children with HFASD (CA = 9–16 years) in Yirmiya et al.'s (1992) study of reactions to videos presenting empathy-provoking social scenarios (e.g., a boy is sad because he lost his dog). In Yirmiya et al.'s study, children with HFASD reported less empathetic responses to the protagonist and fewer justifications for why empathic responses should be enacted, implying that they could not take others' perspectives. In Yirmiya et al. (1992), children with HFASD who had higher Full Scale IQ scores did better on this task, suggesting a cognitive compensatory mechanism. Altogether, a marked deficit in emotional understanding of complex emotions seemed to appear when children with HFASD needed to integrate multifaceted stimuli in a social situation and to take the perspectives of the situation's participants in order to understand it; however, the deficit in identifying complex emotions in others may possibly be mediated by and related to other capabilities, such as ToM and IQ.

The ability to recognize others' basic and complex emotions utilizing external bodily cues, especially facial expression, as well as social context, is indeed important, but it makes up only one aspect of a broader capability for emotional understanding, as discussed next. Difficulties in HFASD also appear regarding the capability for understanding higher emotions, such as hidden or mixed emotions, as well as in the higher-level cognitive ability of providing explanations for the causes of emotions in social situations.

HIGHER EMOTION-UNDERSTANDING CAPABILITIES

Social situations and interactions are complex and dynamic, and multiple emotional reactions to the same situation often occur simultaneously. Few studies have investigated the understanding of multiple emotional reactions to a single situation in HFASD. In one rare study conducted by Rieffe et al. (2007) presenting stories entailing several concurrent emotions (sadness and happiness, anger and fear), the children with HFASD (mean CA = 10.2 years) detected fewer different emotions per story than their peers with TYP (mean CA = 10.3 years). More specifically, all of the children with TYP were able to identify more than one simultaneous emotion in at least two of the four stories, whereas 31% of the children from the autism group ($n = 7$) were unable to identify any pairs of concurrent emotions in any story. Furthermore, the children with HFASD revealed a specific difficulty in recognizing the presence of two negative emotions per story (anger and sadness), whereas they detected two opposing emotions (happiness and fear) more easily. Altogether, in Rieffe et al.'s study, children with HFASD showed a capacity to understand simpler, single emotions but difficulties in understanding a multiple-emotion perspective, especially in the negative domain.

Begeer et al. (2007) also found that children with HFASD revealed less sophisticated emotional understanding capabilities in terms of the link between mood and behavior. Compared with their peers with TYP, they less often referred to the influence of mood on behavior or to mood-related explanations, particularly when relying solely on implicit emotional information. In another study (Jaedicke et al., 1994), looking specifically at children's understanding of the causes of emotions, children with HFASD could provide descriptions of basic emotions (e.g., happy, sad, afraid, angry) but demonstrated qualitative differences from the TYP group when providing explanations for the causes of those emotions. They emphasized material causes for emotions, such as food, toys, and activities; they deemphasized social interactions; and their explanations exhibited idiosyncrasies and preoccupations.

Lastly, high-order emotional understanding encompasses children's ability to grasp the discrepancy between inner and outer emotional expression, referring to the phenomenon of hiding emotions and to the social rules for displaying emotions. Hidden emotions in autism were examined in two studies that yielded somewhat different results (Barbaro & Dissanayake, 2007; Dennis et al., 2000). In Dennis et al. (2000), children with HFASD (mean CA = 9.6 years) and children with TYP (mean CA = 9.4 years) were asked to try to understand the protagonist's actual emotion and deceptive emotion and to explain the reason for hiding the actual emotion. For example, Terry had a tummy ache but wanted to go to the playground, so she did not tell her mother about her tummy ache, and children were expected to reason that she was feeling sadness inside but outwardly showed happiness. Children with HFASD were less skilled than children with TYP in identifying the actual emotion in the context, in identifying the deceptive emotion (which involved an intersection of emotion with belief), and in explaining the reasons for the deception (which required awareness of mental states).

In contrast, in Barbaro and Dissanayake's (2007) study, children with HFASD (CA = 4–11 years) demonstrated good understanding of emotional "display rules"—the understanding of whether an emotion should be expressed or concealed in a particular situation. Children viewed three vignettes enacted by the experimenter using hand puppets and were told that a puppet really feels one way but does not want to show anyone how he feels, so he hides how he really feels. Children were asked to say how the puppet really felt (hidden emotion), how he tried to look on his face (deceptive external emotion), and how other characters in the story thought the puppet felt (understanding mental states). After controlling for verbal MA, no group (HFASD/TYP) differences appeared. This study's outcomes may differ from Dennis et al.'s (2000) findings due to methodological differences; in particular, Dennis et al. performed content analysis of children's reasons for the protagonist's deception, whereas Barbaro and Dissanayake (2007) mainly asked children to name emotions without providing explanations for their choices.

Children's understanding of irony and sarcasm can also testify to their grasp of the discrepancies between inner and outer emotional or social expressions. In irony and sarcasm, the speaker's real intention may only be conceived based on indirect social cues (the tone of voice, gesture, or situation) because it differs from the speaker's literal, spoken words. Children and adolescents with HFASD (mean CA = 10.9 years and 16.4 years, respectively) revealed major difficulties in understanding irony (e.g., Pexman et al., 2011) and sarcasm (e.g., Adachi et al., 2004), thereby capturing these children's deficits, both in attending to social and emotional cues and in social understanding. As seen throughout this section on emotional understanding, children with HFASD reveal a major difficulty in providing explanations for emotional behavior, which holds important implications for empirical methodology and for interpreting study outcomes, thus requiring researchers to differentiate between rote knowledge of emotional labels and higher-order understanding of emotional valences.

SUMMARY OF EMOTIONAL UNDERSTANDING IN HFASD

Overall, the great difficulty that children with HFASD showed in giving personal, specific examples of their own socially complex emotions and negative basic emotions calls into question the authenticity of their emotional understanding, especially for emotions related to interpersonal relationships and social interactions (Chapter 1). Also clearly evident were problems in identifying emotions in other people based on verbal, auditory, facial, or other nonverbal cues and in providing explanations for emotional behavior. In particular, these children revealed a profound difficulty in understanding others' emotions that arose in complex social situations, especially multiple emotional reactions to the same situation occurring simultaneously, which requires integration of information from multiple sources. Instead, these children showed only a simplistic understanding of the causes of emotions and a single rather than multiple perspectives of emotions.

Higher-order emotional understanding capabilities (e.g., hiding emotions, complex emotions) probably pose a special difficulty for these children because they are compounded with social understanding of norms, conventions, and rules of behavior and the ability to reflect on the self vis-à-vis others, which are all impaired in HFASD (e.g., Kasari et al., 2001; Lombardo & Baron-Cohen, 2011). Deficits in social understanding, especially regarding the understanding of interpersonal relationships, have indeed been found for children with HFASD. For example, the understanding of the concept of friendship is lacking in this population. In this regard, Bauminger and Kasari (2000) reported that in preadolescents with TYP, a friend is perceived as someone with whom to play, to be intimate as in sharing secrets, and to develop closeness. In contrast, a friend for preadolescents with HFASD was most often perceived as someone with whom to play, with far fewer attributions of affective closeness or intimacy to the concept (see Chapter 3 for elaboration). Emotional understanding is only one aspect of emotional functioning, and any discussion of emotions is incomplete without describing these children's capacities for emotional expressiveness and responsiveness.

Emotional Expressiveness and Responsiveness

In children with TYP, social interaction is based on an emotional dialogue, which provides the interaction with meaning and oftentimes steers its paths and duration (e.g., Halberstadt, Denham, & Dunsmore, 2001). When one child is smiling and looking at another child, the latter will most likely invite the former to interact. If this initiation is met with a positive response, whether verbal or nonverbal, an interaction may evolve. If this initiation is ignored, the interaction will be terminated before it even begins. Thus children's capacities for emotional expressiveness and responsiveness that create an emotional dialogue are important ingredients of every peer relationship. Unfortunately, despite its importance, this area has not been extensively explored specifically in HFASD.

Spontaneous emotions are probably expressed at a similar frequency in HFASD and TYP, but they are manifested differently and probably differ in quality (e.g., see review in Begeer, Koot, Rieffe, Terwogt, & Stegge, 2008). For example, whereas basic emotions of happiness, sadness, and anger appear at comparable levels between preschoolers with TYP and HFASD (mean IQ = 70), marked differences appear in the situational contexts in which the two groups display various facial expressions. Preschoolers with TYP were observed showing happy facial expressions at preschool, mostly directed toward peers and teachers during regular daily activities, but preschoolers with HFASD mostly directed their happy facial expressions to themselves during solitary play (e.g., McGee, Feldman, & Chernin, 1991). In a like manner, children with HFASD (mean CA = 14.5 years) revealed, as expected, differences in intonation between various basic emotions (happy, sad, angry) during spontaneous speech (Hubbard & Trauner, 2007). The way these children manifested intonation differed from their counterparts with TYP; for example, the HFASD group misplaced pitch peaks in sentences, used a larger pitch range, produced longer utterances, and tended to name the emotions to be expressed (e.g., Hubbard & Trauner, 2007). Looking differently at vocal emotional expression, Hudenko, Stone, and Bachorowski (2009) examined expressions of laughter during playful social interaction with an examiner, such as a surprise tickle game, popping bubbles, or hitting balloons. Unexpectedly, the children with HFASD (mean CA = 9.1 years) did not differ from those with TYP on the laughter's acoustic aspects (e.g., duration, number of laughs per turn), but the quality of laughter did differ between the groups. Children with HFASD revealed only "voiced laughter" (a prototypical laugh), whereas those with TYP revealed both "voiced" and "unvoiced" laughter (acoustically atonal and noisier, without involving vibration of the vocal folds). The distinction between these two laughter types is important for social interaction. Voiced laughter is strongly associated with one's spontaneous experience of positive affect, whereas unvoiced laughter seems to serve communicative functions during an interaction, such as affirming others during conversation or reinforcing aspects of social interaction. Unvoiced laughter is less related to personal experience and more related to the nonverbal emotional dialogue in the interaction. These findings seem to confirm that laughter in HFASD is primarily evident in response to positive internal states, rather than used to negotiate social interaction. This may be related to the social-cognitive difficulties described in this chapter.

Further support for difficulties in emotional expression that may possibly link with social-cognitive deficits emerged in Barbaro and Dissanayake's (2007) experimental situation, in which an experimenter shared a secret (relocation of a ball) with participants (CA = 4–11 years) and asked them to hide the secret from another experimenter. The children with HFASD used less effective emotion display rules for deceiving or hiding their emotions (e.g., regulating emotions via externally visible means like "hand to mouth"), whereas most of the children with TYP were able to use the most effective strategy for enacting the deception (i.e., "neutralization"; internal regulation whereby the child's affect was completely neutralized, without any external cues available to the experimenter). Also, children with HFASD showed more positive affect than children with TYP during the situation. Similarly, Capps, Kasari, Yirmiya, and Sigman (1993) found that, while watching "empathy videos," children with HFASD showed a higher frequency of positive affect, whereas children with TYP showed more natural facial expressions. Thus a lack of understanding of rules for displaying emotions in social interaction may mediate such atypicalities in emotion expression.

Physiological measures also support the existence of a gap between experiencing and understanding emotions among individuals with HFASD. Skin conductance responses taken from participants' fingers while they watched pictures of pleasant, unpleasant, and neutral events revealed that children and adolescents with HFASD (CA = 9–18 years) were similar to their peers with TYP regarding the physiological markers of emotions; however, the two groups differed on their self-reflection about their experienced emotions (Ben Shalom et al., 2006). Despite their intact physiological indices of the experienced emotions, the participants with HFASD demonstrated abnormal reflections about these experiences.

A number of studies have explored the ability to express social emotions (emotions that are inherently linked with social interaction), such as jealousy, loneliness, and empathy, in HFASD. This body of research is described next.

Jealousy in HFASD

Jealousy is an unpleasant social emotion that acquires meaning from the interpersonal context in which individuals interact. By definition, social-relation jealousy is experienced in the triadic context, when a potential threat exists that a valued relationship will be lost to a rival (e.g., Volling, McElwain, & Miller, 2002). Thus jealousy may be an indicator of children's ability to develop social relations with a significant other. In three studies executed by my Behavioral Research Laboratory, we explored jealousy in preschoolers and in preadolescents with HFASD (i.e., Bauminger, 2004; Bauminger, Chomsky-Smolkin, Orbach-Caspi, Zachor, & Levy-Shiff, 2008; Bauminger & Shoham Kugelmas, 2012). In a study of jealousy in preadolescents with HFASD (CA = 8–12 years), the majority displayed clear indications of jealousy, with no group differences from TYP controls during either of two different jealousy-provoking situations—one in which the child's parent praised another child's picture while ignoring his or her own child's and another in which the parent engaged in affectionate play exclusively with the other child (Bauminger, 2004). Group differences did emerge, though, on the kinds of jealousy expressions manifested; for example, children with TYP gazed more at the parent, whereas children with HFASD exhibited more actions.

In a study of preschoolers with ASD who had IQ levels ranging from low to high (Bauminger, Chomsky-Smolkin, et al., 2008), jealousy expressions were examined within a triadic interpersonal context, in which the child's main caregiver placed a familiar child (rival) on her or his lap, embraced the rival child, and read a story aloud to that child, while ignoring her or his own child. Two-thirds (68.75%) of the children with ASD, compared with 94.5% in the TYP group, expressed clear indices of jealousy. Importantly, IQ correlated positively with jealousy explicitness only for the ASD group, indicating that children with ASD who had higher IQs revealed more explicit expressions of jealousy. In addition, as with the preadolescents with HFASD, the preschoolers' ASD group manifested their jealousy differently than did the matched controls. Compared with the TYP group, preschoolers with ASD gazed less at the rival peer and more diffusedly at the interaction in general (i.e., a less focused gaze whose exact point of reference could not be determined). The preschoolers in the ASD group also performed fewer actions that attracted parental attention, and they required a longer response time before exhibiting jealousy behaviors compared with the TYP group.

Inasmuch as the participants in the ASD sample in Bauminger, Chomsky-Smolkin, et al. (2008) were of mixed capabilities (high and low functioning), we conducted a third study to explore jealousy using the same system but including only preschoolers with HFASD (Bauminger & Shoham Kugelmas, 2012). Unlike the prior study, here we found no group differences between HFASD and TYP in their expressions of jealousy. We also expanded our research on these preschoolers with HFASD in two areas to further investigate the links between emotion and affective bonds with parents. Our findings indicated two important areas of similarity between the HFASD and TYP groups. First, in both groups, we uncovered a significant difference between preschoolers' jealous behaviors directed toward the mother versus directed toward a stranger. As expected, children in both groups displayed more direct and intensive jealousy reactions in the mother situation than in the stranger situation. Second, we found that preschoolers classified as having higher levels of attachment security showed lower levels of jealousy in both the HFASD and TYP groups. Thus a secure attachment to the mother provided a sense of "safe haven" just as much for the HFASD group as for the TYP group. Overall, the results of this series of jealousy studies substantiate other data gleaned by attachment studies (see Chapter 3), indicating that the ability to form an affective bond (even if via different behaviors) does lie within the capacity of individuals with HFASD. However, again, like findings presented earlier in this section, the body of research on jealousy corroborates the fact that individuals' expression of emotions does differ qualitatively for HFASD.

Loneliness in HFASD

The experience of loneliness in HFASD can reveal these individuals' social desires and motivations, especially in light of Kanner's (1943, p. 249) statement that ASD is a disorder with "a powerful desire for aloneness." Self-reports of loneliness in preadolescents, adolescents, and young adults with HFASD did not provide support for Kanner's statement, because they reported consistently higher loneliness levels than those reported by individuals with TYP (e.g., Bauminger & Kasari, 2000; Bauminger et al., 2003, 2004; Jobe & White, 2007; Lasgaard, Nielsen, Eriksen, & Goossens, 2010; Locke, Ishijima, Kasari, & London, 2010). Moreover, loneliness and anxiety were found to correlate positively among youngsters with HFASD (CA = 7–14 years); those who reported higher anxiety experienced higher degrees of loneliness (White & Roberson-Nay, 2009). Different results emerged for somewhat younger children (CA = 7–11 years), whereby the HFASD group did not differ significantly from the TYP group on loneliness reports, despite poorer acceptance rates by the peer group (Chamberlain, Kasari, & Rotheram-Fuller, 2007). Loneliness is linked to acknowledgement of one's social isolation. This acknowledgement may evolve later in HFASD, toward adolescence; thus older youngsters with HFASD may show higher awareness of their social isolation. Indeed, higher risk for depression has been noted in adolescents with HFASD (e.g., Attwood, 2004). All told, a powerful desire for aloneness was not proved to correctly describe HFASD from middle childhood and up.

Empathy and Emotional Responsiveness in HFASD

The ability for emotional responsiveness—manifestations of a sense of concern or empathy—was examined in a series of studies on ASD (not limited to HFASD) in which an experimenter or the parent enacted distressing situations such as bumping a knee, hand, or elbow, pretending to be ill, or pretending to lose a pen. Preschoolers with ASD demonstrated impairment in emotional responsiveness capabilities (e.g., fewer eye gazes, lower concern responses) compared with children with TYP or compared with children with mental retardation (e.g., Bacon, Fein, Morris, Waterhouse, & Allen, 1998; Charman et al., 1997; Corona, Dissanayake, Arbelle, Wellington, & Sigman, 1998; Dawson et al., 2004; Dissanayake & Sigman, 2001; Dissnayake, Sigman, & Kasari, 1996; Sigman, Kasari, Kwon, & Yirmiya, 1992). Difficulties in empathy and in emotional responsiveness were also found for adults with HFASD (Baron-Cohen & Wheelwright, 2004), substantiating the deficits of individuals with HFASD in intersubjective sharing, identification, and ToM (see Chapter 1 for elaboration on theories).

However, it seems that higher cognitive functioning is linked to better emotional responsiveness capabilities in children with ASD. For example, in Bacon et al. (1998), IQ correlated with gaze toward the examiner in a hurt-knee procedure and verbal MA correlated with prosocial behaviors for the LFA group. Also, in Dissanayake et al.'s (1996) hurt-knee study, children's prosocial behavior and emotional responsiveness correlated with their MA. The link with IQ also emerged in Yirmiya et al.'s (1992) study of children's empathy while watching video segments that focused on a protagonist experiencing different events (i.e., a boy is sad because he lost his dog) and different emotions (i.e., happiness, anger, pride, sadness, fear). The children with HFASD (CA = 9–16 years) showed less empathetic responses than the controls with TYP. However, only for the HFASD group, those with higher Full Scale IQ scores showed higher empathy responses. Altogether, it seems that higher IQ may be a marker for better and higher empathy and responsiveness capabilities, thus supporting the cognitive compensation hypothesis for HFASD (e.g., Hermelin & O'Connor, 1985; for elaboration, see Chapter 1, this volume).

SUMMARY AND CONCLUSIONS

Social cognition encompasses the processes that enable social functioning. These are the mechanisms that help individuals make sense of the social world, including the people and the situations within this world. Emotions are important as well because they cast the communicative meaning of social behaviors and situations. All in all, the current review of available research outcomes for social cognition yields a mixture of capabilities and difficulties for individuals with HFASD. With regard to social-attention competencies, although researchers still need to more fully explore these children's attention during real-life social situations, from what we know now it seems that the preference for animate over inanimate stimuli is fairly intact in children with HFASD. Also, these youngsters' capacity to orient attention toward dynamic social stimuli is hampered. During SIP, these children show difficulties in encoding social cues, and they provide less assertive solutions. They also reveal difficulties in furnishing socially appropriate solutions to various social situations, as well as in detecting inappropriate social responses. Nonetheless, they understand that aggressive and hostile solutions are inadequate.

With regard to emotional competencies in HFASD, these individuals show relatively good capabilities for recognizing basic prototypical emotions, even though their processing is slower and they require more cues, especially with regard to less clear-cut stimuli. However, it seems that the ability to provide personal accounts of their own emotions is impaired in children with HFASD, especially with regard to socially complex emotions and negative basic emotions. When identifying emotions in others, they also show difficulties, especially in understanding emotions that arise in social situations that require processing of information from multiple sources. Moreover, these children reveal a deficit in understanding higher emotions such as complex or hidden feelings, which require social understanding. Alongside their difficulties in emotional expressivity and responsiveness, there is also evidence that individuals with HFASD do indeed experience various emotions, even including such social emotions as loneliness, jealousy, and empathy. Their difficulties in expressing emotions appear more in the emotions' quality and communicative use, which may be linked to their deficits in social and emotional understanding. Furthermore, IQ seems to be a protective factor contributing to better emotional responsiveness, which supports the cognitive compensation hypothesis. On the whole, social cognition and emotional competence are areas in great need of social intervention because they form the basis on which adequate social interactions are built.

Chapter 3

Peer Relations

Throughout development in the case of TYP, "peers are necessities, not luxuries" (Hartup, 2009, p. 3), both for well-being and for children's ample growth of cognitive, linguistic, and social skills. Children with ASD were first described by Kanner (1943) as having an essential and unchanged "powerful desire for aloneness" (p. 249) and also as "self-sufficient," "like in a shell," and "happiest when left alone" (p. 242). Kanner characterized the play behaviors of children with autism as mainly solitary, with very limited peer involvement, with children playing alongside but not with the peer group:

> He plays alone while they are around, maintaining no bodily, physiognomic, or verbal contact with them. He doesn't take part in competitive games. He just is there . . . but at the same time he quickly becomes familiar with the names of all the children in the group, may know the color of each child's hair, and other details about each child. . . . (p. 247)

Was Kanner's description accurate? Do children on the spectrum indeed powerfully desire aloneness? Based on empirical research reporting a higher degree of loneliness feelings among children with HFASD compared with children with TYP, which express a desire to be involved in peer relations (e.g., Bauminger & Kasari, 2000; Locke et al., 2010), the interpersonal picture for children on the spectrum appears to be much more complicated than originally thought, especially for those with higher cognitive and linguistic capabilities.

Indeed, peer relations constitute one of the major known deficits for children with ASD. The leading classification of mental disorders used by mental health professionals in the United States over the last decade, the DSM-IV-TR (APA, 2000), specifies a failure to develop developmentally appropriate peer relationships as a diagnostic characteristic for the disorder. The same diagnostic characteristic for ASD also appears in DSM-5 (APA, 2013), again specifying difficulties in peer relations rather than in parent–child relations. However, according to the DSM-5 definition of ASD, peer relations lie on a continuum ranging from a compelling lack of awareness of others (for individuals with the most severe social impairment and probably for some of the younger children) to lesser abnormalities in peer relations (for individuals who are less impaired and have higher cognitive-linguistic capabilities).

This chapter focuses mainly on children's actual social behavior with their peers, rather than on their social-cognitive understanding of such interactions (as elaborated in Chapter 2) and rather than on their interactions with adults. Peer relations pose a much more complex social challenge for children with HFASD than do adult–child interactions. Adults can more easily scaffold the interaction and the social setting for the child with HFASD compared with peers of the same age or developmental level. The term "peer relation" is used here to denote all types of peer involvement, which can roughly be divided into social "interactions" and social "relationships," although of course the two are interconnected. Whereas social interactions can be sporadic and include various children, social relationships inherently denote a mutual process of continuous exclusive interactions with a specific individual over a long time period that enable the evolvement of affective bonding and closeness (e.g., Booth-LaForce & Kerns, 2009; Bukowski, Motzoi, & Meyer, 2009).

Thus the description of peer relations in HFASD entails interactions and relationships. This chapter first discusses the ability of children with HFASD to establish and maintain social interactions with peers. Social interaction is defined as a reciprocal process in which children effectively initiate and respond to social stimuli presented by their peers in diverse social settings and situations (Shores, 1987). Second, the chapter focuses on children's ability to form social relationships with peers in the form of friendship. However, due to the fact that in TYP attachment with a caregiver is considered a precursor for friendship with peers (Booth-LaForce & Kerns, 2009), I first review attachment with a main caregiver and only then discuss peer friendship. Friendship and attachment are both considered to be forms of social relationships. The chapter closes with some integrative thoughts on peer relations in HFASD.

SOCIAL INTERACTION IN HFASD

Few studies have examined unmediated, spontaneous, authentic peer interactions in natural settings for children with ASD, and even fewer have focused on HFASD. Nonetheless, as seen next, five main themes concerning social interaction may be extracted from research thus far: (1) children's level of social involvement and participation in social interaction; (2) the nature and profile of children's social interaction (initiation and response, social play, conversation and cooperation); (3) the role of the partner

(HFASD/TYP, dyad/group); (4) the role of the social environment (level of structure, inclusive vs. special education setting); and (5) components that contribute to individual differences in social interaction.

Social Involvement and Participation in Social Interaction

Observational studies have consistently reported low rates of naturally occurring social involvement in daily peer interactions for children and adolescents with ASD during unstructured social situations such as school recess, lunch time, school playground, leisure time in classes, and physical education. These low rates of social involvement were observed not only in studies of special education settings, which usually compared children with LFA with children with developmental delay (e.g., Hauck, Fein, Waterhouse, & Feinstein, 1995; Sigman & Ruskin, 1999; Stone & Caro-Martinez, 1990), but also in research on inclusive regular education settings or day camps, which mostly compared children with HFASD with agemates with TYP (e.g., Bauminger et al., 2003; Kasari, Locke, Gulsrud, & Rotheram-Fuller, 2011; Lord & Magill-Evans, 1995; Macintosh & Dissanayake, 2006). The rates of social participation in peer interaction found for children with ASD appear to range between one-third and one-half of the rates found for children with developmental delay or TYP (e.g., Bauminger et al., 2003; Hauck et al., 1995; Humphrey & Symes, 2011; Lord & Magill-Evans, 1995; Sigman & Ruskin, 1999). A recent study (Humphrey & Symes, 2011) corroborated these low social participation rates for adolescents with ASD (mean CA = 13.8 years) from 12 mainstreamed secondary schools in the United Kingdom, in comparison with children with dyslexia and with children with TYP (IQ was not provided by the authors). Observations of social interactions revealed that children with ASD spent more time engaged in solitary behaviors, less time engaged in cooperative interactions with peers, and more time engaging in reactive aggression toward peers than either comparison group.

In ASD, higher levels of social participation and social play were found to be associated with higher cognitive capabilities such as IQ (above 50 vs. below 50, in Stone & Caro-Martinez, 1990), as well as MA and language age (Sigman & Ruskin, 1999), and also language skills such as the ability to use language functionally and maintain a good vocabulary (Hauck et al., 1995). Interestingly, time and probably familiarity were also found to be related to children's degree of social involvement. Lord and Magill-Evans (1995) examined social interactions during a 2-week day camp and found that children with HFASD (mainly older, with mean CA of 14.8 years) showed fewer purposeless social behaviors and more constructive play during the second week as compared with the first week of camp.

Beyond utilizing observational studies as a source of data on the social participation of children with ASD, recent research has examined social involvement in HFASD through the social network paradigm and sociometric evaluations, mainly by collecting target children's and peers' reports in inclusive settings (e.g., Chamberlain et al., 2007; Kasari et al., 2011; Locke et al., 2010; Rotheram-Fuller, Kasari, Chamberlain, & Locke, 2010). Findings using these methodologies supported the former observational outcomes, indicating across the board that even if children with HFASD were not rejected by their peers, they were more likely to be considered as peripheral to social relationships with peers (i.e., having only tenuous connections to one or two peers) or as secondary (i.e., involved in the classroom social network, but not the most nominated students in the class), and they received fewer reciprocal friendship nominations (i.e., in which they nominated a specific peer as a friend and vice versa). Interestingly, only a minority of children with HFASD were found to be socially isolated (i.e., no connections at all; 13% in Kasari et al., 2011) or to be socially nuclear (i.e., the children most frequently nominated by peers; 8% in Kasari et al., 2011). Thus, corroborating the observation studies, children with HFASD indeed tend to become involved in peer interactions, but to a much lesser degree and centrality compared to children with TYP.

So far, this section has examined the rates of participation in social interactions among children with HFASD. Part of the reason for the low social participation rates could be a poor quality of social interaction as performed by these children. In a recent study of children and adolescents with HFASD (CA = 6.4–18.9 years, mean = 13.4 years), Scheeren, Koot, and Begeer (2012) indeed found that an active-but-odd style of social interaction (in which participants actively sought interactions with others but in unusual ways such as conversing with friends in a monologue style on a preoccupied topic of interest) was positively linked with autism severity, attention and hyperactivity difficulties, and executive function (inhibitory) difficulties. Other social interaction styles, such as aloofness (e.g., no social involvement with peers at all) or passivity (e.g., no initiations of interaction but appropriate responses to peer initiations, according to Wing & Gould, 1979) did not yield such correlations. Thus this active-but-odd social interaction profile seems to pose a risk for social exclusion by peers. Also Meek, Robinson, and Jahromi (2012) found that young children with HFASD (CA = 2.75–6.5 years) were rated by their parents as more hyperactive and distractible with peers and as more socially excluded than their agemates with TYP. It seems that the level of comorbid ADHD may be considered to pose a risk to peer involvement.

A rather concerning recent finding has emerged regarding participation in negative peer interactions among children with HFASD, suggesting that they may be at risk for victimization at school. In Humphrey and Symes (2011), adolescents with ASD (mean CA = 13.8 years, IQ unspecified) were subject to more instances of instrumental verbal aggression by peers than were agemates with dyslexia or with TYP. Several studies have shown high rates of bullying and victimization in HFASD (e.g., Carter, 2009; Little, 2002; van Roekel, Scholte, & Didden, 2010; Wainscot, Naylor, Sutcliffe,

Tantam, & Williams, 2008). Based on teacher reports, van Roekel et al. (2010) found that 46% of the 230 adolescents with HFASD attending special education schools in the Netherlands had been bullied or victimized at school (CA = 12–19 years, mean = 14.97 years; mean IQ = 97.07). Also, it was found that those children with HFASD who were often bullied tended to misinterpret bullying situations as nonbullying and evidenced less developed ToM skills, thereby implying a connection between social understanding deficits and quality of social interactions with peers. However, it should be noted that peer reports and self-reports on the prevalence of bullying and victimization in this study reported significantly lower rates than teacher reports (7%, 19%, and 46%, respectively).

In Little (2002), middle-class mothers reported that bullying experiences by peers and siblings were over four times more likely among their children with Asperger syndrome than in a U.S. national sample of youth (55% vs. 13%, respectively). Other studies have reported that over two-thirds of children with HFASD experience bullying at school (Cappadocia, Weiss, & Pepler, 2012; Carter, 2009; Wainscot et al., 2008). Cappadocia et al. (2012) found that social difficulties in making and maintaining friendships were linked with higher levels of victimization in HFASD. Likewise, victimization was linked with mental health problems among children with HFASD, such as anxiety, hyperactivity, self-injurious and stereotypical behaviors, and oversensitivity. Thus, even if numbers are not absolute regarding the percentages of children with HFASD who suffer from bullying, cumulative findings suggest that these children's social difficulties in peer interaction place them at risk for bullying and victimization by their peers, a circumstance that holds significant implications for their quality of life and well-being.

The level of bullying toward children and youth with HFASD and the extent of their social participation seem to be highly related with the quality of their interactive behaviors. The nature and profile of these youngsters' social-interactive behaviors are described next.

Nature and Profile of Social Interactions in HFASD

To determine the quality of social interactions in HFASD, researchers have focused on initiation and response behaviors, as well as play and social conversation.

Initiations and Responses

Social interaction cannot take place unless children initiate social contact and respond to another's initiations (Shores, 1987). Such initiations and responses may be divided into three types: positive–adaptive, negative–nonadaptive, and low-level interactions (e.g., Fabes, Martin, & Hanish, 2009). Positive-adaptive interactions comprise verbal and nonverbal prosocial behaviors such as sharing, helping, cooperating, comforting, providing help, showing empathy, expressing positive affect, and sharing fun. Negative-nonadaptive interactions are characterized by high levels of conflict, negative affect, and/or verbal and nonverbal aggression. Low-level interactions comprise verbal and nonverbal behaviors that denote communicative intent to participate in an interaction; however, the child only makes it halfway to participation, as when he or she gains close proximity to a group of children on the playground without making a direct initiation with the hope that other children will notice and will take the lead and invite him or her to participate (e.g., Bauminger et al., 2003; Hauck et al., 1995). Other behaviors considered of a low level include vague looking without eye contact or imitating children's games or verbalizations with no addition of spontaneous social behaviors.

These three types of initiations and responses (positive, negative, and low-level) were examined among children with HFASD (mean CA = 11 years) in comparison with agemates with TYP in regular schools during recess and lunch times (Bauminger et al., 2003). Interestingly, the global profile of the two groups' social interactions (initiations and responses) was identical, although the HFASD showed a much lower frequency. In both groups, most social behaviors were positive, followed by low-level behaviors and, to a much lesser extent, negative behaviors, which were rarely observed in either group. Group differences appeared only for positive and low-level interactions: The HFASD group showed a significantly lower frequency of all positive-adaptive behaviors (e.g., eye contact with a smile, smile without eye contact, affection, object sharing, experience sharing, social communication, talk that reflected interest in another, and helping) except for eye contact (which occurred at a similar frequency between groups). However, significantly more instances of low-level, merely functional communication appeared in the HFASD group than in the TYP group. A deeper look at the specific behavioral profile for each group revealed that children with HFASD mainly showed passive low-level social behaviors such as eye contact (not combined with a smile) and close proximity, whereas children with TYP used a broader repertoire of more active and communicative behaviors such as eye contact and smiles, affection, object sharing, experience sharing, social communication, talk that reflects interest in another, and helping. Hence social interactions in HFASD appear to occur not only less frequently but also differently in quality compared with TYP.

This profile characterizing the children in Bauminger et al. (2003)—fewer complex interactive prosocial behaviors (sharing, expressing positive affect, shared fun) and more passive behaviors (mere close proximity)—was a consistent finding across other studies. Several researchers showed a high frequency of additional low-level functional behaviors in children with HFASD, such as giving and requesting information and fulfilling one's own needs (e.g., Kasari et al., 2011; Lord & Magill-Evans, 1995; Macintosh & Dissanayake, 2006; Stone & Caro-Martinez, 1990). The more passive social-behavioral profile observed for children with HFASD coincides with their more severe deficit in initiating social interaction than in responding to an interaction, which was observed in several studies (e.g., Kasari et al., 2011; Lord & Magill-Evans, 1995; Sigman & Ruskin, 1999).

Indeed, lower initiation rates and greater passivity may provide meaningful explanations for these children's low social participation rates; however, special attention should also be directed toward the possible implications of this population's low-level behaviors. Such unproductive social behaviors, like mere close proximity, have a high risk of remaining at the level of communicative intent only, without developing into productive ongoing interactions. However, from the children's point of view, they may believe that they made an initiation that was not reciprocated by peers; therefore, they may experience rejection, regardless of whether the initiation was actually seen or heard by the peer group. This sense of rejection may lead to further passivity or reluctance to initiate future social interactions. In all, identification of each child's social interaction profile, comprising initiations and responses, is a key factor for social interventionists.

Social Conversation and Social Play

Social conversation and social and cooperative play constitute the building blocks of children's social interactions. Hence deficits in these capabilities, which characterize children with HFASD, can affect both the frequency and the quality of their interactions. Cumulative research has pinpointed a specific deficit in social conversation among children with HFASD, rather than in functional-informational conversation (see reviews in Landa, 2000; Rubin & Lennon, 2004; Stefanatos & Baron, 2011; and also Capps, Kehres, & Sigman, 1998; Jones & Schwartz, 2009; Lord & Magill-Evans, 1995; Nadig, Lee, Singh, Bosshart, & Ozonoff, 2010; Paul, Orlovski, Marcinko, & Volkmar, 2009; Sigman & Ruskin, 1999). Social conversation is talk that aims to "be a friend with X" or to "get to know X better," whereas functional-informational conversation aims to extract information on an issue or topic for functional purposes. Social conversation involves children's sharing of experiences, feelings, and thoughts rather than sharing of information. For example, in informational talk children may describe the details about a movie they saw in terms of the movie's main characters, director, and plot; however, in social talk they may share their experience while watching the movie ("Like it? Dislike it? What was the most exciting/scary/funny part of the movie?"). The main goal of social conversation, then, is to be socially involved with peers.

Social conversational style in HFASD has been widely shown to be remarkably deficient. Due to the fact that most often the topics of interest for children with HFASD differ from those of their peers (e.g., Nadig et al., 2010) and due to their low rates of participation in peers' conversations, as shown earlier (e.g., Lord & Magill-Evans, 1995; Sigman & Ruskin, 1999), children with HFASD tend to limit conversations to their own areas of interest, experience difficulties in choosing topics appropriate to the setting and conversational partner, and find it hard to choose what to say and to decide what is relevant or irrelevant during a conversation. In a recent study, Nadig et al. (2010) showed that when children with HFASD (mean CA = 11 years) talked about their own peculiar areas of interest with an adult, the discourse was less reciprocal, including fewer contingent utterances and more monologue-style speech than the talk of agemates with TYP (CA = 10.10 years). Also, Sigman and Ruskin (1999) found that children with ASD (mean CA = 12.10 years) spent equal time in monologues and in conversation, whereas among children with developmental delay the duration of conversations was three times longer than that of monologues.

Based on their difficulties in intuitive reading of social situations and of social partners' mental states (Klin et al., 2003; see also Chapter 1 and 2, this volume), children with HFASD also exhibit problems in initiating and maintaining conversations that are sensitive to the social context and to others' interests and previous knowledge. Especially limited are their abilities to develop or expand an interaction by taking turns within an ongoing conversation or by switching between topics to accommodate the conversational partner's perspective. In Jones and Schwartz's (2009) study of a family dinner, young children with HFASD (CA = 3.5–7.0 years) initiated fewer bids for interaction, commented less often, continued ongoing interactions through fewer conversational turns, and responded less often to family members' communications. In addition, Capps et al. (1998) reported that children with LFA (CA = 11.9 years) provided fewer narratives of personal experience in a semistructured conversation with a familiar adult. Finally, children with HFASD more frequently walked away from a conversation without coherently ending the conversation by making a friendly closure that accounted for the other person's perspective (e.g., Rubin & Lennon, 2004).

Overall, it is important to note that most HFASD research in this area has been conducted on conversations with adults, using discourse analysis (e.g., Capps et al., 1998; Jones & Schwartz, 2009; Nadig et al., 2010; Paul et al., 2009). Few studies have systematically analyzed the spontaneous conversations of children with HFASD with peers (e.g., Lord & Magill-Evans, 1995; Macintosh & Dissanayake, 2006), despite such conversations' noted importance for peer interaction across development, especially from middle childhood up (Parker & Gottman, 1989). The major pragmatic deficit in conversational ability found in HFASD, as consistently presented by the research available thus far on discourse with adults, seems likely to render a tremendous impact on these children's ability to take part in productive peer interactions.

Similarly to their conversational difficulties, children with HFASD encounter problems in spontaneous social play (e.g., Humphrey & Symes, 2011; Kasari et al., 2011; Lord & Magill-Evans, 1995; Macintosh &

Dissanayake, 2006; Sigman & Ruskin, 1999). On the playground, these children were most often found to be involved in solitary nonsocial play or in low-level social engagements such as looking at other children's activities or playing in a similar activity and in proximity to others with or without awareness of them. Compared with their peers with TYP, children with HFASD were also less often involved in simple social play (comprising mainly turn-taking activities), and they engaged in fewer instances of rough and vigorous play. During simple social play, children engage in the same or similar activities while talking, smiling, and offering and receiving objects.

However, despite this tendency for aloneness on the playground, children with HFASD do demonstrate social play capabilities. For example, participation rates in games with rules (e.g., ball games, hopscotch) during unstructured free time were similar for HFASD and TYP groups (Macintosh & Dissanayake, 2006; Sigman & Ruskin, 1999). Likewise, Kasari et al. (2011) found that children with HFASD participated in structured games with rules (e.g., organized sports such as 4-square, basketball, or handball) for 20.0% of the observed free-play time and in joint engaged activities such as having a conversation for 18.6% of the time. Thus, even if social play is less frequent in these children, it is not absent. Moreover, when the rules of the social games are clearer, these children show higher participation rates. "Joint engagement" with peers, which requires the coregulation of thoughts, plans, and actions with another peer to form joint play, is indeed deficient in these children, but it is not absent.

Summary of Social-Interaction Profile

All in all, children with HFASD reveal a more passive and less interactive profile of initiations and responses, pragmatic deficits in conversation and social play, and a more profound difficulty in initiating social interaction than in responding. This behavioral pattern seems to provide an explanation for these children's low rates of social involvement that goes beyond the notion of a "desire" to be alone. Watching the peer group and maintaining close proximity to peers' social activities on the playground may in fact signal the opposite, a sign of social desire, but also may suggest an incapability to fulfill this desire. If this holds true, then social interventions are greatly needed to help these children shift their low-level social interaction capabilities into more fully developed, positive, interactive-communicative behaviors.

The Role of the Partner in Social Interaction

The child with HFASD contributes significantly to a social interaction's quality but only constitutes one side of the equation; the other side involves the partner's contribution to the interaction. Partners may differ in type (HFASD or TYP) and in number (group or dyadic).

Social interactions by children with HFASD generally occur with one of two peer partner types: another child with HFASD or a child with TYP. The role of the partner in the interaction is especially significant considering that most efforts to include children with HFASD in regular schools stem from the primary goal of providing opportunities for interacting with agemates with TYP. Indeed, Lord and Magill-Evans (1995) showed that all of the groups they examined (children with HFASD, with behavioral disorders, and with TYP) performed the most initiations toward children with TYP. Unfortunately, not many studies have specifically compared interactions with the two types of peer partners.

In Bauminger et al. (2003), we did examine peer interactions during recess in an inclusive school setting, where children with HFASD could spontaneously interact with partners of either type—other children with HFASD or those with TYP. Our main findings demonstrated higher frequencies of interaction with peers with TYP compared with peers with HFASD, although group differences between interactions with these two partner types were not statistically significant for the majority of the specific behaviors tested. Nevertheless, these children with HFASD revealed a clear tendency to prefer partners with TYP over partners with HFASD as follows: The target children with HFASD both initiated and responded using a higher frequency of complex positive behaviors (e.g., eye contact with a smile) toward partners with TYP, and they more often initiated low-level behaviors such as close proximity and functional communication toward partners with TYP.

It is important to emphasize that children with HFASD did interact with both types of partners. This may imply that these children gain from exposure to peers with TYP, but proximity to other children with autism continues to hold importance. Perhaps each type of partner satisfies different needs of the child with autism, such as the need to learn about normative social interaction from partners with TYP and the need to feel belonging from partners with HFASD. For example, peers with autism or other disabilities may offer a sense of familiarity or may enable identification with someone similar to oneself, thereby holding conceivable implications for children's self-esteem. Partners with TYP, on the other hand, may provide a role model for well-adjusted social behavior, offering possible implications for children's social competence.

Further support for the facilitation of social competence that may be inherent in exposure to social partners with TYP was obtained by Macintosh and Dissanayake (2006). Children with HFASD in inclusive settings who had exposure to peers with TYP evidenced involvement in a full range of simple to complex forms of social play and conversation, comparable to that of children with TYP (although at a lower frequency and quality). Also, Sigman and Ruskin (1999) found that children with ASD who had access to peers with TYP compared with those who did not have such access showed higher levels of social interaction and less nonsocial play. These studies suggest that exposure to interaction partners with TYP may indeed be important for enhancing more complex social behaviors in HFASD.

Not only does partner type influence interaction quality but also the number of partners participating in the interaction can also render an effect on the social interactions of children with HFASD. Ongoing group interactions and group entry (joining into group activities or conversation) constitute the highest social challenge in HFASD (Lord & Magill-Evans, 1995; Sigman & Ruskin, 1999). Indeed, children with ASD have been found to cooperate with relatively more ease in dyadic interactions (most preferably with a familiar child) than in a group of children (Bauminger, 2007a; Hauck et al., 1995; Macintosh & Dissanayake, 2006). Taking into consideration the difficulties found among children with HFASD in understanding others' minds, as well as their executive functioning deficiencies—mainly in shifting attention and flexibility (e.g., Frith, 2004; Liss et al., 2001; see also Chapter 1, this volume)—these children's social demands gradually increase with greater social stimuli. Thus group situations—compared with one-on-one interactions—comprise their highest social challenge.

The Role of the Social Environment and the Type of Social Situation

Any understanding of social interactions in HFASD must thoroughly address the social setting (regular or special education school) and the type of social situation (free play vs. rule-governed, more structured setting). As just described, exposure to potential social partners both with TYP and with HFASD seems to be important for peer interaction, and the two types of partners may serve different functions. Thus an optimal social setting seems to be placement in a school setting that enables exposure to both. Most preferably, this entails a regular education school with special classes for HFASD or individual inclusion in a regular class. The major benefits of such an educational setting are the opportunities it offers to engage socially with peers with TYP and, correspondingly, its lack of the disadvantages associated with exposure only to playmates with handicaps and similar social difficulties (e.g., Sigman & Ruskin, 1999). However, as demonstrated earlier, mere exposure to peers is insufficient; children with HFASD require assistance to develop and maintain such interactions with both types of social partners: those with HFASD and with TYP.

The optimal social situations for increasing social interaction in HFASD have yet to be determined. However, social interactions in the schoolyard or during free-play hours pose the highest demands for these children. In such situations, children must extract social and emotional display rules, as well as sufficient creativity to suggest activities to peers, to plan them, and to work them out as an ongoing social endeavor—which are all deficient competencies in HFASD (e.g., Barbaro & Dissanayake, 2007; Travis & Sigman, 1998). In fact, most of the purposeless behaviors observed among children with HFASD were seen during recess time; in addition, participation rates for children with HFASD resembled those of children with TYP during rule-governed games but differed during less structured situations such as simple social play (e.g., Macintosh & Dissanayake, 2006; Sigman & Ruskin, 1999). Also, even after a social-skills intervention (Bauminger, 2007a), children with HFASD were able to increase their spontaneous social behaviors toward peers in a shared group cooperative-drawing situation, but not during recess time in the schoolyard.

Taken altogether, spontaneous interactions during nonstructured social situations are clearly the most challenging situations for these children. However, it is also important to keep in mind that an overly structured social interaction, such as an academic lesson, is unlikely to elicit spontaneous social behaviors. For instance, in an unpublished study of social-interaction behavior frequencies for preadolescents with HFASD conducted by my Behavioral Research Laboratory team in inclusive schools (Bauminger & Cohen, 2000), we found that the fewest social behaviors appeared during academic lessons, more appeared in unstructured situations such as school recess, and the most appeared in semistructured situations such as lunchtime and nonacademic lessons, such as art or physical education.

Individual Differences in Social Interaction

Unsurprisingly, consistent findings across many studies have indicated that children who exhibit less social impairment—who participate in more social interactions with peers, show higher levels of social behaviors, reveal more social play, and initiate more toward peers—are those children who demonstrate higher cognitive and language capabilities (e.g., Hauck et al., 1995; Orsmond, Krauss, & Seltzer, 2004; Sigman & Ruskin, 1999; Stone & Caro-Martinez, 1990). For example, in Stone and Caro-Martinez (1990), those children who had speech utilized more gestures, more varied communicative functions, more commenting, and more information giving than those children who lacked speech (CA = 4–13 years, mean = 8.4 years).

Interestingly, studies have shown stability across social profile components for those children who demonstrated higher capabilities. For instance, in Sigman and Ruskin (1999), children who revealed a higher level of social play also showed more initiation behavior toward peers, longer interaction durations, and fewer initiations that were rejected. In Hauck et al. (1995), children who showed more initiation behavior toward peers also scored higher on the socialization and communication scales of the Vineland Adaptive Behavior Scales (VABS; Sparrow, Balla, & Cicchetti, 1984) and showed a higher level of comprehension of emotional situations and affects. In a like manner, in Kasari et al. (2011), those elementary school children with HFASD (CA = 6–11 years) who were observed participating in relatively more joint engagements and games on the playground were also seen initiating behavior more frequently toward other children on the playground and responding more often to peers' initiations. Also, teachers rated these children with HFASD who were more engaged on the playground as possessing higher social skills. Altogether, these recurrent associations seem to imply that the rates and quality of social interactions derive strongly from children's level of social impairment and cognitive-language skills and therefore go beyond mere social interest or "desire" or lack thereof.

Other factors appear to be linked with individual differences in social interactions in this population. For one, Orsmond et al. (2004) reported that higher rates of participation in social and recreational activities among adolescents and adults with HFASD (CA = 10–21 years and 22–47 years, respectively) were a function not only of these individuals' social impairments but also of reports by mothers that the mothers had participated at higher rates in similar activities. Thus more socially oriented mothers had more socially involved children. Additionally, larger number of services received and greater extent of inclusion in the school environment (full rather than partial) were both associated with more participation in social and recreational activities. The latter finding may suggest that fuller inclusion in a regular school setting may possibly provide more opportunities for children with HFASD to participate in a variety of non-school-based activities. In a related vein, Kasari et al. (2011) found that children with HFASD who were more often engaged with peers on the playground were significantly less likely to have one-on-one aides; likewise, children who had aides were most often unengaged on the playground. We cannot untangle the cause-and-effect relations underlying this correlation; however, this finding suggests that aides' mediations should be carefully designed to eliminate the risk of disengagement in children. Altogether, the study of individual and environmental contributors to social interaction has provided important initial information that should be further explored.

Summary of Social Interactions

All in all, compared with their peers with TYP, children with HFASD demonstrate lower participation in spontaneous social interactions, as well as a poorer quality of social initiations and responses, alongside difficulties in cooperative capabilities and social conversation. Exposure to multiple partner types seems to be important for social interaction: Availability of partners with TYP most likely results in the development of more complex cooperative social behaviors; yet children with HFASD in inclusive settings do continue to seek out peers with HFASD, suggesting that such interactions may potentially enhance emotional needs such as self-esteem and identification. Thus regular education frameworks that offer dual exposure to peers with HFASD and with TYP appear to be the optimal setting for social interaction. Likewise, semistructured social situations reveal the highest potential for eliciting a better quantity and quality of social interaction behaviors in this population. To obtain a more comprehensive view of peer relations in HFASD, we next discuss the capabilities to form social relationships in the form of attachments and friendships.

SOCIAL RELATIONSHIPS: ATTACHMENT AND FRIENDSHIP IN HFASD

Ever since Kanner's (1943, p. 250) conceptualization of autism as a disorder of "affective contact," researchers have focused their investigations on these children's capacity to develop social relationships. The affective nature of human attachment and friendship requires that children intersubjectively share with others as well as understand others' minds (ToM). In children with ASD, neither intersubjective sharing nor representational capabilities develop normally, a fact that may limit these children's ability to develop social relationships (e.g., Baron-Cohen, 2000; Hobson, 2005; Rogers & Pennington, 1991; Tager-Flusberg, 2001a). Despite these pessimistic conceptual predictions about children's ability to form social relationships in ASD, empirical findings have shown evidence not only of attachment security with adults (e.g., Rutgers, Bakermans-Kranenburg, van IJzendoorn, & van Berckelaer-Onnes, 2004) but also of reciprocal friendships with peers (e.g., Bauminger, Solomon, Aviezer, Heung, Brown, et al., 2008; Bauminger, Solomon, Aviezer, Heung, Gazit, et al., 2008) Indeed, in order to review the existing literature on children's ability to form social relationships (friendships) with peers, I first review studies on children's security of attachment with a main adult caregiver, which is considered a precursor for friendship with peers in TYP (Booth-LaForce & Kerns, 2009).

Attachment in ASD

The study of attachment in children with ASD encompasses three main themes: (1) attachments to a stranger versus a caregiver and rates of secure, insecure, and disorganized attachment quality; (2) identification of individual differences in security of attachment; and (3) caregiver characteristics that are linked to attachment security.

Caregiver–Stranger Differentiation and Attachment Quality

According to Bowlby (1969/1982), attachment constitutes the first affective bond that an infant forms with the primary caregiver. The perception of attachment as an affective bond means that the child forms a tie with an exclusive "significant other" (Ainsworth, 1989). Thus the infant's initial ability to differentiate between people and inanimate objects and then the capacity to distinguish the primary caregiver from other individuals are precursors to the ability to form attachment in TYP. On the basis of these differentiations, the child directs increasingly more proximity-seeking behaviors (e.g., approaching, following, clinging) and signaling behaviors (e.g., smiling, crying, calling) toward the primary caregiver than to other people, shows distress in the caregiver's absence, and calms down in the caregiver's presence (Buitelaar, 1995). Earlier research on attachment in ASD showed that children (mostly preschoolers) with ASD were able to develop exclusive interest in the main caregiver that surpassed their interest in a stranger during the Strange Situation, most notably during the reunion stage of the experiment but also after the separation stage (e.g., Dissanayake & Crossley, 1996, 1997; Sigman & Mundy, 1989; Sigman & Ungerer, 1984). This pattern emerged despite the lower number of proximity-seeking behaviors (e.g., showing, looking, smiling, touching) shown by the HFASD samples compared with their TYP counterparts.

As young children with TYP develop further, they construct internal working models of secure or insecure attachment, reflecting the extent to which they feel able to use the main caregiver as a "secure base" that enables exploration of the environment. Securely attached children show distress at separation from the caregiver and attempt to reestablish interaction when reunited. In contrast, insecurely attached children can be coded as one of three classifications (Ainsworth, Blehar, Waters, & Wall, 1978): "avoidant" (e.g., showing indifference at separation and actively avoiding the caregiver at reunion); "resistant/ambivalent" (e.g., presenting high distress at separation and responding to reunion with mixed rejection and approach); or, as later identified by Main and Solomon (1986, 1990), "insecure/disorganized" (e.g., lacking observable goals, intentions, or explanations in the caregiver's presence, such as stereotypical movements or misdirected and incomplete expressions).

Consistent findings emerged regarding rates of secure and insecure attachment in ASD, showing that 40–50% of children with ASD (vs. two-thirds in the typical population) were able to form a secure attachment with their main caregivers, albeit through behaviors that differed in quality compared to those with TYP. These percentages characterized toddlers (e.g., Naber, Swinkels, Buitelaar, Bakermans-Kranenburg, et al., 2007); preschoolers and kindergartners (e.g., Capps, Sigman, & Mundy, 1994; Marcu, Oppenheim, Koren-Karie, Dolev, & Yirmiya, 2009; Rogers, Ozonoff, & Maslin-Cole, 1991, 1993; Shapiro, Sherman, Calamari, & Koch, 1987; Willemsen-Swinkels, Bakermans-Kranenburg, Buitelaar, van IJzendoorn, & van Engeland, 2000); and preadolescents (e.g., Bauminger, Solomon, & Rogers, 2010). Often researchers had difficulty using TYP classification systems for attachment in ASD, attesting to differences in the two groups' expression of relationships. For example, in Capps et al.'s (1994) sample, all children except 3 obtained a first classification of disorganized attachment, and only in a second screening were 40% rated as securely attached to the mother. Similarly, Rogers et al. (1993) developed a customized rating scale to tap the attachment behaviors of children with autism in their sample, because these children's behaviors were too subtle to fit the classic ABC classification (e.g., Ainsworth et al., 1978). Interestingly, a recent study that looked at disorganized attachment in a clinical sample of children with ASD, mental retardation, or language development disorder found an overrepresentation of the disorganized attachment type in the clinical sample versus the TYP sample but a similar rate of disorganized attachment in ASD and the other two clinical groups (Naber, Swinkels, Buitelaar, Bakermans-Kranenburg, et al., 2007). According to these authors, disorganized attachment type seems to be related more to lower developmental level than specifically to ASD symptoms. Additional support for this assumption was also found by Willemsen-Swinkels et al. (2000), who identified higher rates of disorganized attachment in children with ASD whose intellectual functioning was at the mental retardation level (IQ < 70) compared with those children with higher IQs (> 70).

Individual Differences in Attachment Security

Attachment studies have also focused on the understanding of individual differences between securely and insecurely attached children with ASD. Hence research has examined the roles played by severity of the disorder, MA, CA, receptive and expressive language, and representational skills (joint attention, symbolic play) in security of attachment. Although an early study (Rogers et al., 1993) asserted that severity of ASD was not related to secure attachment, a more recent meta-analysis (Rutgers et al., 2004) identified severity of autism and mental retardation as risk factors for the development of insecure attachment in ASD. Altogether, data are accumulating to support the link between disorder severity and insecure attachment (e.g., Naber, Swinkels, Buitelaar, Bakermans-Kranenburg, et al., 2007; van IJzendoorn et al., 2007). Higher receptive language capabilities were also found to significantly correlate with secure attachment, and expressive language neared significance (Capps et al., 1994). Thus children with ASD who possessed higher cognitive and language skills and fewer autism symptoms were shown to form more secure attachments with their main caregivers. Intellectual functioning at the mental retardation level probably increases the chances of disorganized attachment in ASD (Naber, Swinkels, Buitelaar, Bakermans-Kranenburg, et al., 2007). Rutgers et al. (2004) did not find a link between CA and attachment security, but the associations between attachment security and representational skills such as joint attention and symbolic play were somewhat mixed with age.

In terms of symbolic play, securely attached toddlers with ASD (mean CA = 2.4 years) spent more time engaged in symbolic play, showed higher levels of play, and spent more time actually playing compared with insecurely attached toddlers with ASD (Naber et al., 2008). Such correlations did not emerge for older children with ASD (mean CA = 4.11 years; Marcu et al., 2009). Adding to this complexity, studies on the association of attachment with joint attention yielded mixed results but in the opposite age direction. Attachment security for toddlers with ASD (mean CA = 30 months) was not significantly related to joint attention (Naber, Swinkels, Buitelaar, Dietz, et al., 2007). In contrast, Capps et al. (1994) reported that among older children (mean CA = 48 months), the securely attached group more frequently used requesting behaviors such as looking, pointing, and giving to obtain assistance from their mothers than did children in the insecure group, but no group differences emerged for initiating joint attention. In sum, the link between joint attention and attachment may reflect a developmental trajectory in which older children show more complex internal working models and better joint-attention skills than younger children, even if those skills remain limited to only requesting and responding. However, the results for symbolic play—in which older securely attached children did not show higher symbolic skills than older insecurely attached children—are hard to interpret and should be further examined longitudinally with larger groups.

Caregiver Characteristics

There has been some question about whether attachment constructs in ASD reflect similar underlying mechanisms to those seen in TYP. Capps et al. (1994) and Koren-Karie, Oppenheim, Dolev, and Yirmiya (2009) reported that mothers of securely attached children with ASD revealed greater sensitivity (parent's attunement and responsiveness to the child's signals while expressing warmth and emotional connectedness to the child during play interaction) to their children compared with mothers of insecurely attached children. However, van IJzendoorn et al. (2007) found that sensitivity among mothers of children with ASD did not differ from sensitivity among mothers of children in other clinical groups (mental retardation, language development disorders); moreover, maternal sensitivity did not correlate with children's attachment security for their autism sample. Inasmuch as Bowlby (1969/1982) considered maternal sensitivity to be the main contributor to children's sense of security, this finding raises the question: What actually contributes to security of attachment in ASD if not the mother's responsiveness to her child's signals?

Two recent studies shed light on parental antecedents of secure attachment in ASD. Oppenheim, Koren-Karie, Dolev, and Yirmiya (2009) demonstrated the importance of two parental processes in combination for the attachment security of children with ASD—namely, maternal insightfulness (attunement of responsiveness and openness toward the child's inner world) and maternal resolution (effective coping with painful feelings related to the child's ASD diagnosis). Children of insightful and resolved mothers were more likely to develop secure attachment. In Seskin et al. (2010), parents' own internal working models of attachment were correlated with children's capacity to engage in developmentally appropriate social interactions with the parent and with children's social-emotional development. Children with ASD whose parents were securely attached were better able to initiate communication with their parents by using gestures such as reciprocal smiles and turn-taking vocalizations, compared with children of insecurely attached parents. The children of securely attached parents were also better able to integrate their perceptions of self and other into social problem solving with their parents and to engage in imaginative thinking, symbolic play, and verbal communication. Thus secure attachment in parents contributed to better communicative skills in their children with ASD.

Summary of Attachment

All told, we still need to travel a long road in order to fully understand how children with ASD develop secure internal working models of attachment and how the parents of these children contribute to such models. However, it seems that autism symptoms do not preclude a child from forming attachments. Most children with ASD across the different studies, from toddlerhood up to preadolescence, were classified as securely or insecurely attached to their main caregivers, like their peers with TYP. But rates of secure versus insecure attachment and the specific behavioral manifestations of attachment do differentiate autism from TYP, and this finding seems due to the significant social deficit of children with autism. Those children who demonstrated more severe autism symptoms and lower cognitive capabilities also exhibited a poorer ability to form secure attachment (e.g., Rutgers et al., 2004). Moreover, the same parental characteristics (e.g., sensitivity and attunement to children's needs) contributed to security of attachment in both HFASD and TYP. This may imply that formation of attachment security may follow similar trajectories in both HFASD and TYP, thus calling for further empirical examination.

Friendship in HFASD

Friendships are another, but different, type of affective tie that children develop throughout life. Friendship is more symmetrical than attachment because it occurs between peer agemates who share similar developmental capabilities (e.g., Bukowski et al., 2009). In the more asymmetrical relationships with adults, the mature adult can take on more of the responsibility for the reciprocal social interaction, thereby easing the social and communicative load for the child. Thus friendships with peers place higher requirements on the child to coregulate another person's perspectives and behaviors in order to develop the ongoing reciprocal interactions that qualify as friendship (for a minimum of 6 months; Howes, 1996) and that result in affective closeness and intimate bonding. Indeed, research has reported that children with ASD were more likely to engage in social activities with their parents and other adults than with their peers (e.g., Solish, Perry, & Minnes, 2010). Orsmond and Kuo (2011) have shown this finding for adolescents with ASD too. Nevertheless, reciprocal friendships do exist in HFASD despite several caveats—specifically, that friendships are not observed frequently in HFASD (e.g., Howlin, Goode, Hutton, & Rutter, 2004; Koning & Magill-Evans, 2001; Orsmond et al., 2004), that friendships are less reciprocal in HFASD than in TYP (e.g., Chamberlain et al., 2007; Church, Alinsanski, & Amanullah, 2000; Kasari et al., 2011; Rotheram-Fuller et al., 2010), and that children with HFASD evidence major difficulties in the social-emotional-representational capabilities related to friendship formation (e.g., Baron-Cohen, 2000; Hobson, 2005; Rogers & Pennington, 1991; Tager-Flusberg, 2001a).

This section zooms into friendship processes in HFASD by describing several key aspects: (1) the nature and quality of friendship for those children with HFASD who do have at least one reciprocal friendship; (2) the characteristics of those partners who form friendships with children with HFASD; and (3) the individual, familial, and environmental components that may contribute to friendship formation in HFASD.

Friendship Nature and Quality in HFASD

In TYP, friendship functions as an important source of emotional support and as a marker for social adjustment, but the consequences of friendship for children's psychosocial development are highly dependent on the friendship's nature and quality (e.g., Vitaro, Boivin, & Bukowski, 2009). The nature of friendship with peers in HFASD can best be explored through observation of an ongoing interaction with a friend. Such observations of 164 preadolescents with HFASD and TYP were executed in a recent binational project (Bauminger, Solomon, Aviezer, Heung, Brown, et al., 2008; Bauminger, Solomon, Aviezer, Heung, Gazit, et al., 2008) that I led on the Israeli side (with 47 Israeli recruited participants; 24 HFASD and 23 TYP) and that Sally Rogers and Marjorie Solomon led on the United States side (with 35 recruited U.S. participants; 20 HFASD and 15 TYP). Each target child (HFASD or TYP) was invited to visit the laboratory with an identified close friend; thus the study included each of these target children's best friends ($n = 82$ altogether for both sites). All four groups of target children (HFASD and TYP in each nation) were matched according to maternal education, verbal performance, CA, and sex.

Each friendship dyad was observed and videotaped during a 40-minute session while they participated in two different noncompetitive tasks: the "construction game" scenario and the "drawing" scenario. In the construction game, children were instructed to construct a shared design (a marble maze) while using ramps, connectors, funnels, and tunnels. After completion, children could roll the marbles down and through the maze. In the drawing scenario, children were given a box of colored markers, magazines, scissors, glue, stencils, and a large blank sheet of paper and were asked to draw a shared design. Overall, TYP dyads outperformed HFASD dyads in the behavioral manifestations of friendship and in the dyadic qualities of interaction, as follows: The children with HFASD showed poorer cooperative skills, less positive affect, and less skillful conversational skills, as well as a more rigid conversation style. With regard to play complexity, the children with HFASD exhibited a higher frequency of mere parallel play and a lower frequency of constructive play. The qualities of the dyadic interactions containing a child with HFASD were less socially oriented, cohesive, harmonious, and responsive, as well as less enjoyable and close. All these differences support clinical as well as theoretical perspectives on friendship as a challenging social relationship for the child with HFASD.

However, interesting similarities also emerged between the HFASD and TYP friendship dyads on several complex social behaviors, such as the incidence of prosocial behaviors, sharing, and eye contact with a smile, possibly suggesting that friendship may nonetheless offer an advantageous framework for enhancing social skills among children with HFASD. If indeed interactions with friends are advantageous for these children, then their interactions with a friend should surpass their interactions with a nonfriend in terms of social complexity and dyadic affective closeness. My Behavioral Research Laboratory team recently examined this question among preschoolers with HFASD (Bauminger-Zviely & Agam Ben-Artzi, 2012). Each child was videotaped separately interacting with a friend and with a nonfriend during a construction game, a drawing scenario, and snack time. As expected, results indicated that, when interacting with a friend compared with a nonfriend, children with HFASD showed more positive affect, more complex forms of social and collaborative pretend play, more shared fun, and more reciprocity (see a more extensive description of this study in Chapter 4). These recent findings corroborate the notion that interaction with a friend may indeed serve an important function in the enhancement of social skills in HFASD and should be given serious weight when designing social interventions that aim to facilitate peer friendship among children with HFASD. Also, according to Kuo, Orsmond, Cohn, and Coster (2012), those adolescents with ASD (CA = 12–18 years, mean = 14.8 years) who reported having more friends also reported more positive friendship quality with the listed "best friend" and a greater sense of companionship in that friendship. Thus social experience with friends is important for growth in social competence for HFASD.

Self-reports offer another window into friendship quality. According to such reports, friendships of younger children up to preadolescents with HFASD were not seen as more conflictual than those of their agemates with TYP, but group differences favoring the TYP group did emerge in self-reports of important friendship functions such as intimacy, help, and companionship (e.g., Bauminger & Kasari, 2000; Bauminger et al., 2004;

Bauminger, Solomon, Aviezer, Heung, Gazit, et al., 2008; Chamberlain et al., 2007), as well as affective closeness for preadolescents (e.g., Bauminger, Solomon, Aviezer, Heung, Gazit, et al., 2008; Kasari et al., 2011). Adults with HFASD also reported less closeness, empathy, and support in their friendships compared with adults with TYP (e.g., Baron-Cohen & Wheelwright, 2003; Jobe & White, 2007).

Friendship, by definition, is an ongoing meaningful relationship lasting 6 months or more with a developmentally similar partner. Several studies have documented that only 20–40% of individuals along the autism spectrum develop meaningful friendships (e.g., Howlin et al., 2004; Koning & Magill-Evans, 2001; Orsmond et al., 2004). Despite the well-documented difficulties in forming friendships in ASD, friendships in HFASD were found to be similar to those reported in TYP regarding length and partner's sex and age. Friendships in HFASD were found to be relatively long, ranging from about 6 months to 4 years, and comprised mainly same-age, same-sex pairs (e.g., Bauminger-Zviely & Agam Ben-Artzi, 2012; Bauminger & Shulman, 2003; Bauminger, Solomon, Aviezer, Heung, Gazit, et al., 2008; Howlin et al., 2004 ; Kasari et al., 2011; Kuo et al., 2012; Locke et al., 2010; Orsmond et al., 2004).

However, the frequency of meetings with friends and the types of activities they shared seemed to differ between the HFASD and TYP groups. Play dates outside the school were reported at about once per week for children with HFASD, which was lower than for children with TYP. Activities preferred by children with HFASD and their friends were the more structured ones that provided clear, explicitly stated rules (e.g., board games) or activities that did not require high levels of social exchange (e.g., watching TV or playing on the computer). In contrast, children with TYP and their friends preferred activities with a high level of social engagement, such as ball games (basketball, football) or hanging out together (e.g., Bauminger & Shulman, 2003). However, in Kuo et al. (2012), differences in activities among adolescents with ASD were found to be associated with sex. Male adolescents with ASD frequently played video games with friends (60%), whereas none of the females did; likewise, 37% of the male adolescents but only 4% of the females were involved in physical activities with their friends, such as swimming and playing basketball. In contrast, 71% of the female adolescents engaged in conversations with friends, compared with only 16% of the males. Thus further inquiry into activities with friends, in relation to the proband's sex, seems important.

Friendship Partners: The Friends of Children with HFASD

One key factor to understanding friendship in HFASD is to recognize the unique characteristics of those children who choose to form friendships with children with HFASD. Friends of children with HFASD can be children with TYP, thus forming a "mixed" friendship, and/or children who themselves have a disability, most likely another child with HFASD but also other disabilities such as ADHD, learning disabilities, or Down syndrome, thus forming a "nonmixed" friendship (e.g., Bauminger, Solomon, Aviezer, Heung, Brown, et al., 2008; Bauminger-Zviely & Agam Ben-Artzi, 2012; Bauminger & Shulman, 2003; Kuo et al., 2012).

According to peer reports describing children who were chosen to serve as peer buddies for a potentially unfamiliar child with autism, such chosen buddies with TYP were evaluated by their TYP classmates as helpful and smart but also as less popular in their classrooms (Campbell & Marino, 2009). According to reports by mothers of preadolescents with HFASD (CA = 8.25–17.10 years, mean = 10.45 years), a possible partner's ability to form a friendship with a child with HFASD depends on several factors, which differ according to whether the partner has a disability or not (Bauminger & Shulman, 2003). For friendship partners with TYP (mixed friendships), mothers emphasized the importance of these children's kindheartedness, sensitivity, responsiveness, and openness, whereas for friendship partners with a disability (nonmixed friendships), mothers accentuated the importance of the partner's social expressiveness and similarity in level of functioning to the child with HFASD. Shared areas of interest seemed important to mothers for both friendship types.

In Bauminger, Solomon, Aviezer, Heung, Brown, et al., (2008), we also investigated qualitative differences that may distinguish nonmixed friendships (two children with HFASD) from mixed friendships (HFASD together with TYP) and from TYP friendships (two children with TYP). Mixed friendship was found to resemble TYP friendship and to differ from nonmixed friendship on many observed friendship qualities. Nonmixed dyads showed the poorest qualities, such as the highest frequency of mere parallel play and the lowest levels of engagement in goal-directed activity, sharing, and positive affect. Also, compared with mixed dyads, nonmixed dyads were less responsive and cohesive, exhibited a lower level of positive social orientation, and showed less complex levels of play. Nevertheless, despite these lower qualities observed for nonmixed dyads when interacting with a friend, the nonmixed friendships appeared more symmetric in the degree to which each partner assumed dominant or subordinate roles, such as leader and follower, whereas children with HFASD in mixed friendships had fewer leadership opportunities. Although only little research has thus far been conducted on the contribution of the partners to friendship quality in HFASD, the available data indicate that children with HFASD may benefit from both types of friendship partners—children with TYP and children with HFASD—just as found for social interaction partners (see earlier discussion). Again, in friendship, each partner may offer different benefits; for example, friends with TYP may help children with HFASD extract higher levels of social interaction behaviors and play, whereas friends with HFASD may provide children with HFASD with easier, less energy-consuming interactions and the opportunity to act as leader instead of follower, whereas in mixed dyads the friend with TYP may consistently lead.

In addition, clinical reports from teachers, parents, and the children themselves that we collected in my Behavioral Research Laboratory suggest that each type of friendship partner may also pose certain risks for children with HFASD. One risk of friendship with a partner who also has HFASD is that the two friends may each persist in very restricted activities deriving from peculiar interests. Another difficulty may be that one child develops an unusual dependency on this rare friendship relationship and, possessively, does not let the other child become involved in social activities with other children. On the other hand, the risk of friendship with children with TYP is the excessive pressure experienced by the child with HFASD due to the amount of effort required to maintain such a friendship, which increases as the children grow older and face new developmental exigencies. Overall, it seems that whether the friend is a child with TYP or with HFASD, both friendship types may require intensive support from significant others in the child's social environment, such as teachers and parents, as described next.

Individual, Familial, and Environmental Contributors to the Formation of Friendship in HFASD

Considering that friendship is a real challenge for children with ASD and that those who do develop meaningful friendship struggle with its quality, two crucial questions emerge: (1) Who are those children along the spectrum who form the subgroup that is able to develop friendship? (2) What are the familial and environmental conditions that can support the development of friendship in HFASD? Hence this section discusses friendship formation processes, as well as supportive individual, familial, and environmental components for friendship in HFASD.

Not many studies have examined predictors of friendship in HFASD; therefore, current knowledge of friendship formation processes remains quite limited. With regard to individual-level contributors to friendship formation, it seems that cognitive and verbal functioning are crucial components. Only recently, Mazurek and Kanne (2010) investigated the feasibility of reciprocal friendship in children with ASD (CA = 4–17 years, mean = 9.1 years), comparing those with IQs below 85 (LFA) and those with IQs equal to or above 85 (HFASD). They found that the presence of reciprocal friendship (i.e., sharing personal activities and meeting outside of prearranged groups) differed significantly according to IQ, with only 8% of the LFA group having reciprocal friendships compared with 20% of the HFASD group.

Additionally, verbal IQ based on the Peabody Picture Vocabulary Test (PPVT; Dunn & Dunn, 1997) was also linked to better friendship qualities (Bauminger, Solomon, Aviezer, Heung, Gazit, et al., 2008; Bauminger et al., 2010). In our binational study (Bauminger, Solomon, Aviezer, Heung, Gazit, et al., 2008), higher verbal IQ was correlated with higher frequencies of positive affect and coordinated play and lower frequency of parallel play. Furthermore, dyadic qualities (cohesiveness, harmony, responsiveness, coordinated play, shared fun, and affective closeness) were all related to higher verbal IQ only in the pairs with HFASD and not in the pairs with TYP. Moreover, only verbal IQ was found to differentiate between children who formed mixed versus nonmixed friendships; the children with HFASD whose friends had TYP showed higher verbal IQs compared with those whose friends had HFASD (Bauminger, Solomon, Aviezer, Heung, et al., 2008).

Interestingly, older age appears to be a risk factor for developing lower rates of reciprocal friendship in ASD (e.g., Orsmond et al., 2004; Rotheram-Fuller et al., 2010). For example, Orsmond et al. (2004) showed that adolescents with ASD had more reciprocal friendships than adults. In a like manner, in Rotheram-Fuller et al.'s (2010) study, in kindergarten through first grade children with ASD and children with TYP revealed similar rates of reciprocal best friendships, whereas in the middle to late grades (second to fifth grades) children with ASD showed significantly lower rates of reciprocal best friendships than their TYP peers. However, other research has shown that older preadolescents of approximately the same age as in the latter study (8–12 years) who had reciprocal friendships demonstrated more prosocial behaviors, less parallel play, more coordinated play, and higher levels of conversational flow when interacting with their friends than younger preadolescents (Bauminger, Solomon, Aviezer, Heung, Gazit, et al., 2008). Additionally, dyads consisting of older preadolescents with HFASD showed more affective closeness, responsiveness, and cohesiveness than younger preadolescents (Bauminger, Solomon, Aviezer, Heung, Gazit, et al., 2008; Bauminger et al., 2010). Thus it may be that for the whole spectrum an increase in age is linked to difficulties in forming reciprocal friendships but for the more cognitively able HFASD group, as age increases, friendship qualities also increase. Hence the role of age in friendship formation merits further in-depth research.

The contribution of children's social-emotional capabilities to their friendship formation was also a focus of empirical interest in several studies. Not surprisingly, higher rates of reciprocal friendships correlated with fewer autistic social symptoms, based on prominent diagnostic tools such as Rutter et al.'s (2003) ADI-R (e.g., Orsmond et al., 2004) or Lord et al.'s (2000) ADOS-G (e.g., Mazurek & Kanne, 2010). In contrast, unexpectedly, the contribution of ToM and of attachment security to friendship was similar in HFASD and TYP (Bauminger et al., 2010). More specifically, ToM and attachment security were each found to contribute to the explanation of friendship qualities only indirectly, through their interrelations with other predictors and among themselves, thereby providing support for a moderator model. Thus higher ToM skills appeared to compensate for lower verbal IQ in the observed dyadic friendship qualities of responsiveness and coordinated play. For coordinated play, higher ToM skills and a higher sense of attachment security enhanced children's ability to coordinate play with a friend. The interrelations of ToM and attachment security attest to the complexity of friendship formation and may provide some explanation for the low rates of such friendship experience among children with ASD in light of their documented difficulties in ToM and low rates of attachment security (Tager-Flusberg, 2001a; Rutgers et al., 2004). Indeed, in Daniel and Billingsley's (2010) study, 10- to 14-year-old boys with HFASD described the establishment of friendship as the most difficult aspect of their social lives.

Familial and environmental contributors to friendship in HFASD have seldom been examined. In one rare study, Orsmond et al. (2004) found that, surprisingly, none of the environmental factors examined was a significant predictor of having peer relationships. These factors included mother's level of participation in social activities, the number of services received by her child, and the child's regular versus special educational setting. In a different study (Bauminger & Shulman, 2003), all of the interviewed mothers of children with HFASD (CA = 8.25–17.10 years) said that their children's development and maintenance of friendship greatly depended on their (the mothers') ongoing support. They also provided suggestions to parents for furnishing such support: helping their child to arrange continuous ongoing meetings after school; helping their children to choose friends; contacting the parents of the chosen friends; physically bringing the children or friends to each other's homes; and helping their children plan social activities with the friends. Mothers also emphasized the importance of the link between the parents and the children's teachers; for example, teachers can identify potential pairs who share common areas of interest or who demonstrate mutual interest in one another and can notify the parents in order to achieve continuity between school and home. According to mothers' reports, teachers can also support friendships in other ways, such as arranging shared activities for the identified pairs to experience; for example, working together on a shared project; incorporating conversations about friendship into discourse for children with special needs; and providing help in contacting parents of potential friends with HFASD and TYP. Based on this preliminary study, the role of the environment—parents and teachers—is crucial to the development and maintenance of friendship in HFASD.

Summary of Friendship

Overall, the ability to form and maintain reciprocal friendships is a cardinal aspect of the social deficit for children with HFASD, yet researchers have primarily focused on providing data about its low prevalence rather than describing its process of formation and vital components. It is clear that durable and reciprocal friendship with a partner who is most likely of the same age and sex and who may have TYP, HFASD, or another disability is indeed within the capacity of some children. It appears that those children who reveal better chances of making friends possess higher verbal functioning and IQ capabilities and are less socially impaired. But even for this subgroup, the qualities of their friendships remain poor compared with the friendships of children with TYP. Thus children with HFASD not only struggle in forming friendships but also struggle in developing and maintaining friendships over time.

Children who remain without friends are at risk for experiencing higher degrees of loneliness, as reported by children with HFASD, compared with children with TYP (e.g., Bauminger & Kasari, 2000; Locke et al., 2010). Furthermore, a negative by-product of friendships that are characterized by lower quality is the experience of heightened anxiety, as found by Mazurek and Kanne (2010). These researchers showed that children with ASD who had one or more friends, but whose friendships were limited in reciprocity and responsiveness, were more likely to experience anxiety and depression compared with children who had one or more very good friendships with approximately same-age peers (that included sharing of personal activities and meetings outside prearranged groups). Children's awareness of their social difficulties in forming and maintaining relationships may be one of the reasons that affective disorders (e.g., anxiety, depression) increase more during adolescence and adulthood among individuals with HFASD versus TYP (e.g., Attwood, 2004). All in all, intervention studies that explore ways to support friendship formation and maintenance in HFASD are vital in the near future.

PEER RELATIONS IN HFASD: INTEGRATIVE THOUGHTS

There is little doubt, then, that ASD is a disorder involving severe deficits in peer relations, even for the more cognitively able children on the spectrum. However, we can also say unequivocally that friendship in HFASD is not an all-or-nothing phenomenon. Peer relations would probably best be described as a continuum of interpersonal resources, with some children doing better than others. The literature so far has provided some initial guidelines for understanding the individual and environmental contributors that lead to more active and successful peer relationship processes. Children with higher cognitive and language skills are more likely to be more active on the playground and to form reciprocal friendships. These phenomena support the "compensation hypothesis" for HFASD, which suggests that such children make cognitive efforts to learn and experience their social-emotional lives through their relatively high-functioning cognitive channels (e.g., Hermelin & O'Connor, 1985; Kasari et al., 2001). However, cognitive and verbal strategies, even if seemingly helpful to some degree, cannot fully compensate for the profound social deficits characterizing these children, which result in a challenging peer relations profile. It is not surprising that those children who are less socially impaired show better qualities of peer relations. Yet, in addition to individual factors in HFASD, participation in peer relations and the quality of this social involvement seem to depend highly on the child's social environment, such as the school setting and situational characteristics, as well as on significant others within this environment, such as parents, teachers, and peers, who all play crucial roles in increasing the child's likelihood of developing more productive peer relations. Thus a full understanding of peer relations in HFASD should adopt a multidimensional ecological perspective (e.g., Bronfenbrenner, 1992), which assumes an interplay between the child's characteristics and the characteristics of the social environment, including the child's main social agents within this environment (e.g., parents, teachers, and peers). Unfortunately, many elements within this ecological interplay have not yet been explored empirically; thus comprehensive future research is called for.

A case in point is the individual predictors of peer relations beyond general capabilities in social competence in HFASD, which remain relatively unmapped. We do know that joint-attention skills play an important part in predicting children's social competence in areas such as pretend play (e.g., Rutherford, Young, Hepburn, & Rogers, 2007), and recent research has indicated that children's initiation of joint engagement with parents was positively related to social competence with peers approximately 1 year later (e.g., Meek et al., 2012), but this link has not yet been examined for the development of peer friendships. In addition, interesting recent findings have identified children's atypical sensory profile (mainly oral sensory–olfactory and haptic characteristics) as the strongest predictor of greater social impairment in participants with HFASD and TYP (e.g., Hilton et al., 2010). Thus the role of sensory profile in friendship formation or in social interaction should be further explored. Likewise, children's individual differences in reactivity and self-regulation, as reflected in their temperament, was found to predict social skills in HFASD (Schwartz et al., 2009), calling for further inquiry with regard to peer relations.

Social-cognitive capabilities beyond ToM—such as abstract reasoning and other related executive functions, such as flexibility and planning—may also contribute to variability in peer relations and therefore deserve further empirical scrutiny. For example, performance on abstract reasoning, as demonstrated in concept identification (i.e., to recognize underlying category attributes so as to better understand them), was positively related with friendship quality (on a global dimension of friendship quality based on the dimensions of companionship, help, intimacy, and closeness), according to the friend's perception (Solomon, Bauminger, & Rogers, 2011).

Also, Lemerise and Arsenio (2000) proposed that the processing of social information with friends is more complex than with nonfriends, but this was not investigated in HFASD. Other social-cognitive correlates may include children's overall social and emotional knowledge and their understanding of social situations.

Studies that assess chains of interactions, rather than the individual children's social behaviors or their dyads' quality, are also lacking. The investigation of interaction chains can clarify ongoing dynamic processes— for instance, identifying which initiations support an interaction and which lead to its termination.

Current knowledge of environmental characteristics that support peer relations is also limited. Some initial suggestions for how parents and teachers may optimally support friendship in HFASD have been provided by mothers of such children, but this merits more extensive examination.

Social interventions should go beyond teaching social skills to help teach children the skills necessary to form friendships with their peers. Both peer interactions and peer friendships should be considered as integral aims of ASD social interventions across the lifespan, and future studies need to further explore the necessary skills leading to the formation of each type of peer relations. Only recently have studies started to include friendship as a target for intervention (e.g., Laugeson & Frankel, 2010; see also Chapter 7, this volume).

Altogether, it is important to keep in mind that not just differences but also similarities in peer relations emerged between HFASD and TYP groups, attesting to higher social capabilities in those children with higher cognitive capabilities. However, it was also clearly demonstrated that external support for such peer relations processes is crucial. Adding to this complexity, this population's interactions with friends clearly evidence higher qualities than their interactions with nonfriends, implying the potential advantages of friendship relations for developing children's social competence. Thus peer relationships, and even more specifically friendships with peers, are key factors for children's well-being. Consequently, efforts should be made to find ways to increase social participation and foster the growth of more productive, rewarding peer relationships in HFASD.

SUMMARY AND CONCLUSIONS

Returning to Kanner's observation that children with ASD have a "powerful desire for aloneness" (1943, p. 249), the findings presented here definitely do not support this statement. To the contrary, children with HFASD are at a greater risk of experiencing loneliness and anxiety as a result of fundamental, core difficulties in their social interactions and peer friendships, but this goes beyond a choice to be alone. These children are involved in social interactions but use fewer and less effective interactive and communicative play and conversational behaviors, and they employ more passive, low-level, and merely functional social behaviors with their peers, thus ending up with less productive social interactions. Likewise, some of these children are capable of developing reciprocal, durable friendships with children with both TYP and HFASD. Yet such friendships are not very frequent and also differ in quality from the friendships documented in TYP.

Chapter 4

Developmental Changes in Social Functioning

As children with TYP grow from the youngest ages through childhood, adolescence, and then young adulthood, their social and emotional functioning rapidly changes and transforms, both in frequency and quality. Yet children with HFASD reveal considerable difficulties in each and every skill required for competent social functioning. In previous chapters pertaining to social development, this book has focused primarily on school-age children, from elementary school through secondary school. To complement these chapters, the current chapter undertakes a developmental perspective in which a lifespan description of the social deficit is provided, starting from infancy up to young adulthood.

OVERVIEW OF THE SOCIAL CHALLENGES EXPERIENCED DURING TYP

As reviewed by Rubin, Bukowski, and Laursen (2009) in their handbook on peer interaction, as children grow and develop, they must cope with substantial, ever-increasing demands in order to function effectively as social human beings, whether in one-on-one interactions, small or large groups, or ongoing friendships. Rapid transformations occur in the frequency and quality of social experiences. Time spent with peers increases significantly from the early ages (preschool) to older ages (middle childhood, adolescence, and then young adulthood). Moreover, social behaviors become less straightforward, thereby demanding much more effort to decipher and perform. The spontaneous, authentic behaviors and emotions exhibited between peers at younger ages are gradually replaced by mediated or inhibited behaviors and hidden emotions, requiring children to acquire deeper social and emotional understanding and knowledge in order to comprehend interpersonal situations and participate in them effectually. To a great extent, as described in Chapter 1, these progressively demanding social interactions and relationships necessitate social-cognitive and social-communicative competencies, such as children's capacity for joint attention and for understanding their own and others' mental states (ToM).

Furthermore, as children grow, games and social activities are gradually replaced with verbal conversation, thereby emphasizing the importance of emerging conversational and self-disclosure skills. Such social communication efforts also require greater language proficiency on the part of the children. On the other hand, during preadolescence and middle childhood, many social encounters, especially for boys, involve outdoor ball games such as basketball and football, which involve social coordination in large groups, as well as good physical skills. Over the years, children's friendships with peers become more complex and intimate, and ongoing long-term reciprocal interactions result in affective closeness and intimate bonding (see Chapter 3). Moreover, toward puberty and young adulthood, romantic relationships evolve, with their unique social demands.

Adding to this complexity, the school transitions, from preschool to elementary school, from elementary to middle school, from middle to high school, and from high school to "real life" as a young adult, all entail mounting challenges regarding the social environment. From a more predictable, structured social environment with few teachers and peers and with one main figure who is responsible for the child's needs, children's experience shifts to much more chaotic, unstructured environments with many teachers and peers and frequent changes in daily routine. These shifts lead to rising demands in terms of children's executive functioning, such as flexible cognitive shifting and organizational and planning skills (see Chapter 1). Adolescents' transition from the high school setting into young adulthood poses another major challenge because, despite its complex interpersonal conditions, high school nonetheless offers a social framework. Young adults who do not proceed directly from their educational setting into another structured social group or network face possible exclusion from any social setting whatsoever, which likely escalates their risk of loneliness and depression.

SOCIAL FUNCTIONING ACROSS DEVELOPMENT IN HFASD

Individuals with HFASD, as described in the earlier chapters in this book, demonstrate deficits in all of the domains necessary for successful social functioning and for coping with the multiple social transitions from each developmental period to the next. These deficits pertain to social-cognitive skills (see Chapter 2), peer interactions, friendships, and language-conversational skills (see Chapter 3), and more. Because in the previous chapters of this book I described the major social difficulties experienced in HFASD during the school years (mostly middle childhood and adolescence), the current chapter describes the early markers of social deficits and the early development of social play and friendship, from infancy and toddlerhood and continuing into the preschool years, and also briefly presents social functioning issues during the transition to elementary school. The chapter also examines social trajectories and predictors and then concludes with social outcomes during young adulthood and adulthood.

THE BEGINNING OF THE SOCIAL-EMOTIONAL DEFICIT: EARLY MARKERS IN INFANCY THROUGH THE PRESCHOOL YEARS

Rapidly growing research efforts are working to identify the early markers for social deficits in ASD in order to explore the origin of social impairments. These studies derive from parents' retrospective recollections, from home videos, and from prospective longitudinal studies looking at young siblings of children with ASD (ages 4–6 months) who later develop ASD (at 24–36 months). However, to date, no clear developmental trajectory associated with ASD has been identified (see reviews in Tager-Flusberg, 2010, and in Yirmiya & Charman, 2010).

Interestingly, during the first few months of life, the clinical profile of infants with ASD does not portray a clear picture of deficits in social engagement. In one recent prospective study, infants with ASD could not be differentiated from low-risk infants who had normal outcomes, based on their social disinterest or disengagement; indeed, to the contrary, at age 6 months, infants with ASD showed more frequent social-communicative behaviors compared with low-risk, normal-outcome infants (Ozonoff et al., 2010). In another study, only a somewhat passive temperamental profile, showing relatively few initiations and less responsiveness to efforts to engage their attention, was found to characterize 6-month-old siblings of children with ASD who later received a diagnosis of ASD at 24 months (Zwaigenbaum et al., 2005).

At the age of 12 months, more deficits in social-communicative behaviors were identified among siblings diagnosed later with ASD (at 24 months). These markers included poor and atypical eye contact as well as limited social responsiveness skills, including reduced social smiling, orienting to name, social interest, expression of positive affect, reactivity, and response to bids for joint attention (Ozonoff et al., 2010; Zwaigenbaum et al., 2005). Decreased orienting to name among 12-month-old siblings of children with ASD demonstrated high specificity (but low sensitivity; .50 for ASD) for a 24-month diagnosis of ASD (also in Nadig et al., 2007). Delay in gestures for communication, such as pointing, giving, and head nodding, were also reported by parents of 12-month-old siblings who later received an ASD diagnosis at 24 months (Mitchell et al., 2006).

In Zwaigenbaum et al. (2005), 12-month-olds' play behaviors and use of play materials were found to be limited (lack of imitation, poor coordination of eye gaze and action) and were of a stereotyped self-stimulatory nature (e.g., swinging a string of beads and waving it in front of the eyes). Moreover, these toddlers showed atypical development of visual attention, including poor visual tracking and prolonged latency to disengage visual attention, as well as a tendency to fixate on nonsocial aspects of the visual environment combined with reduced responses to social approaches from others. Similar findings emerged in Ozonoff et al.'s (2008) study, which pinpointed atypical object exploration (with novel play materials) at 12 months as a predictor of subsequent ASD diagnosis (at 24 and 26 months). Their autism/ASD group was characterized by increased frequency of object spinning, rolling, and rotating and by unusually prolonged visual inspection, often associated with atypical features such as examining the object from odd angles. Furthermore, repetitive behaviors at 12 months were significantly associated with cognitive and symptomatic status at the 36-month outcome; yet some infants who showed these behaviors did not receive an ASD diagnosis later on. Thus Ozonoff et al. (2008) concluded that repetitive or stereotyped behaviors may be early risk markers in the development of some but not all children with ASD.

Temperamental profile at 12 months differed from that at 6 months; the older toddlers showed increasing irritability and intense responses to sensory input (often associated with distress; Zwaigenbaum et al., 2005). Lastly, these siblings also showed delayed early language, both in expressive and receptive capabilities (Zwaigenbaum et al., 2005). Interestingly, Young, Merin, Rogers, and Ozonoff (2009) showed that diminished gaze toward the mother's eyes relative to her mouth at 6 months predicted higher expressive language scores at 24 months. The authors concluded that gaze toward the mouth may play an important role in language development.

The aforementioned markers found in prospective studies corroborate other research on the first year of life using parents' retrospective reports, home videos, and symptoms based on the ADOS–G (Lord et al., 2000). These retrospective studies showed abnormalities in social orienting, poor quality of social overture, impaired early joint-attention behaviors (lack of pointing/showing, gestures), poor social interest, and emotional expression delays, as well as abnormalities in play behaviors (see review in Yirmiya & Charman, 2010).

Early Social-Deficit Markers for Children at Different Levels of Cognitive Functioning

Despite the fact that cumulative data have demonstrated early markers for social deficits as early as 12 months, the inclusiveness of these markers for the more cognitively able children on the spectrum is not clear. For example, in Zwaigenbaum et al. (2005), siblings who received a diagnosis of ASD at

24 months exhibited lower language scores (expressive and receptive) on the Mullen Scales of Early Learning (Mullen, 1995) compared with non-diagnosed siblings and with low-risk controls. These low language scores may hint that at least some of those ASD-diagnosed siblings did not have HFASD, because the latter would have probably received a diagnosis only after these prospective studies' 24- or 36-month follow-up. Considering that some of the more able children on the spectrum (those with Asperger syndrome or PDD-NOS) are not diagnosed by those ages, the early markers that were identified in such research may possibly be unrepresentative of siblings with HFASD.

Indeed, in Chawarska, Klin, Paul, and Volkmar's (2007) study examining ASD symptoms in the second year of life (between 14 and 25 months), differences emerged between children classified with autism and children classified with PDD-NOS at that time. Although these two groups of 14- to 25-month-olds showed similar verbal and nonverbal capabilities (Mullen, 1995), the PDD-NOS group later showed higher verbal and nonverbal capabilities at age 36 months. In addition, although their ADOS-G (Lord et al., 2000) evaluation at ages 14–25 months indicated highly pathological behaviors in both groups (e.g., limited response to name, poor eye contact, limited response to joint attention, lack of pointing, delays in functional and symbolic play), marked differences also emerged between the autism and PDD-NOS groups at both time points (14–25 months and 3 years).

Specifically, Chawarska et al. (2007) found that although both groups were socially impaired, the children diagnosed with PDD-NOS in their second year were more likely to engage in dyadic exchanges and to show emerging intentional communication skills. The PDD-NOS group directed vocalizations and facial expressions toward others, smiled socially, and shared enjoyment more frequently (based on the ADOS evaluation). Despite poor eye contact, children with PDD-NOS integrated gaze into social overtures more frequently. In a like manner, even without language at 14–25 months, they were more likely to engage in spontaneous initiation of joint attention and showing behaviors. Also, motor mannerisms and unusual sensory interests were less frequent in the PDD-NOS group than in the autism group.

As mentioned, at the age of 3 years children who were diagnosed earlier with PDD-NOS showed higher verbal and nonverbal skills compared with children diagnosed earlier with autism (Chawarska et al., 2007). Interestingly, acquisition of verbal and nonverbal skills in the entire sample was associated with a decline in the level of stereotypical behaviors and the severity of social and communicative symptoms and with an increase in the level of play skills over time, highlighting the importance of IQ capabilities for social-communicative functioning in ASD. Key symptoms, though, remained stable in both the autism and PDD-NOS groups at age 3, such as limited coordination of social-communicative behaviors, impaired eye contact, low initiation of joint attention, inability to direct facial expression to others, and limited responsiveness to name.

Summary of Early Social-Deficit Markers

Overall, the cumulative research literature indicates that early social-communicative impairment is indeed noticeable in children with ASD as young as 12 months of age: however, its distinctive profile regarding the more able children on the spectrum, such as the Asperger syndrome and PDD-NOS groups, has yet to be adequately explored. Altogether, it seems that up to the first 6 months, no clear signs of the socio-communicative deficit in ASD appear; however, at 12 months a set of social-communicative repetitive behaviors and attention deformations appears, which can predict later diagnosis of ASD. Thus the beginning of the atypical social-communicative deficit defining ASD seems to emerge sometime during the second half of the first year of life, and it varies considerably among infants, with no clear understanding of individual differences that may explain this heterogeneity in social-development trajectories, such as the role played by high cognitive abilities in scaffolding for some of the early social deficits (e.g., Tager-Flusberg, 2010). The social deficit of children with HFASD continues into their preschool years, manifesting itself mainly in difficulties in early peer relations, as discussed in the next section.

EARLY PEER RELATIONS: SOCIAL PLAY AND FRIENDSHIP IN THE TODDLER AND PRESCHOOL YEARS

Peer relations in TYP are considered cardinal for the development of ample cognitive, linguistic, and social skills (e.g., Coplan & Arbeau, 2009). During toddlerhood and preschool, adequate social play is key for efficient peer interaction and friendship with peers. Inasmuch as social play does not develop typically in HFASD, these young children gain only limited early interpersonal peer experiences, which in turn sets the stage for reduced peer engagement in the school years, as described in Chapter 3 on peer relations (Manning & Wainwright, 2010). This section, then, presents the characteristics of social play in toddlers and preschoolers with HFASD, as well as the ability to form peer relations.

Social Play in HFASD

Social play is hard to define, but certain components seem to be important in the definition of play: It involves active, pleasurable, and enjoyable engagement by at least two players; it is spontaneous and voluntary; it is free from means–end directiveness (the play activity is an end in itself); and it should be flexible and dynamic (e.g., Garvey, 1977; Jordan, 2003). Social play, which requires joint action and attention, provides children with opportunities for peer interaction, as well as a context for constructing representations of intentional states and knowledge, such as ToM (e.g., Toth,

Munson, Meltzoff, & Dawson, 2006). Thus it significantly contributes to toddlers' and preschoolers' cognitive development, social-cognitive development (e.g., learning to share symbolic meaning, attention, and intentions with a partner through pretend play; executive functions such as shifting attention, planning, and generativity), and social-emotional development (e.g., moving from isolated play to joint play), which involves fundamental social and prosocial skills such as collaboration, negotiation, empathy, interrelatedness, and intimacy (e.g., Jordan, 2003; Schuler, 2003; Toth et al., 2006). Social play also provides an essential social context in which early friendships can emerge (Guralnick, Neville, Hammond, & Connor, 2007; Jordan, 2003), as well as intersubjective capabilities such as joint attention and social referencing.

Social play differs in quality and quantity in children with HFASD as compared with agemates with TYP, acting as both the cause and the consequence of their social isolation (Schuler & Wolfberg, 2000). The underlying mechanisms that enable creative joint play with peers are hampered in toddlers and preschoolers with HFASD (Jordan, 2003). These impaired mechanisms include representational skills (e.g., joint attention, ToM), creativity and imagination (e.g., executive functions such as attention shifting, generativity in pretend play, and flexibility rather than repetitive and obsessive interests and actions), social understanding of "play culture" (e.g., game rules and norms), and spontaneous peer interaction (Schuler & Wolfberg, 2000).

The specific characteristics of social play in HFASD are not well defined due to a paucity of studies focusing on spontaneous social play in the more cognitively able young children with ASD; most of what we know is based on participants of mixed cognitive levels. For example, Rutherford et al. (2007) demonstrated that joint-attention ability significantly predicted pretend play performance in preschoolers with ASD of mixed cognitive capabilities (mean CA = 57.6 months, mean MA = 12.25–56.25 months). In addition, executive-function generativity was found to be most predictive of pretend play performance in very young children with ASD of mixed cognitive functioning levels (mean CA = 33.93 months, mean MA range: 11.5–41.75 months; e.g., Rutherford & Rogers, 2003). Furthermore, ToM was found to correlate with pretend play (Lam & Yeung, 2012) among young children with ASD (mean CA = 6.11 years; PPVT score = 70; Dunn & Dunn, 1997). Notably, though, these studies examined pretend play solely in the child–adult context (when mother or experimenter played with the child), not the peer pretend play context. In addition, based on parental reports, repetitive behaviors were associated with child–adult play in the more cognitively able children with ASD between 2 and 8 years; those who demonstrated few repetitive behaviors engaged in more play activities than those who demonstrated frequent repetitive behaviors (e.g., Honey, Leekam, Turner, & McConachie, 2007).

In research on children with ASD, social play was found to be highly structured, rigid, and stereotyped, most often taking the form of learned routine rather than a genuinely playful engaging experience (Hobson, Lee, & Hobson, 2009; Jordan, 2003). Play activities in ASD ranged from manipulating objects and enacting elaborate routines to pursuing obsessive and narrowly focused interests, including high rates of inappropriate and inflexible toy use. Free-play situations involving peers were shown to pose particular difficulties for children with ASD, who may avoid or resist social overtures, passively enter play with little or no self-initiation, or approach peers in an obscure and one-sided fashion (e.g., Wolfberg, 1999). Greater structure in a social environment involving adults' scaffolding was found to elicit higher rates of responsive communication acts, such as more responsiveness or compliance behaviors and increased following of pointing gestures and gaze in young preschoolers between 2 and 5 years (mean CA = 45 months, mean nonverbal MA = 27.5 months) compared with free-play situations with peers that involved various games (e.g., jack-in-the-box, modeling clay, birthday cake and associated materials such as candles and a knife, bubble gun with soapy liquid), but these were preschoolers with LFA (Clifford, Hudry, Brown, Pasco, & Charman, 2010). Manning and Wainwright (2010) demonstrated similar results for older children with HFASD, too (mean CA = 8.25 years).

In sharp contrast to the rich thematic variations of play in children with TYP, the restricted range of interests and the obsessive insistence on sameness in children with ASD often result in pretend play that is highly repetitive and seems almost obsessive in its literal repetition of identical acts (e.g., Bass & Mulick, 2007). Play in ASD is sometimes defined as *echoplalaiya*—immediate or delayed literal repetition of others' play behaviors and unimaginative repetitions of play acts—which is analogous to echolalia, stereotyped repetitions of utterances (e.g., Schuler & Wolfberg, 2000; Wolfberg, 1999). Likewise, social play in children with ASD includes fewer novel play acts and less elaboration and diversity compared with agemates with TYP (e.g., Murdock & Hobbs, 2011). Jordan (2003) asserted that after accounting for general cognitive difficulties, what seems to hinder the development of creative playful acts in children with ASD is their lack of joint play with others, which is important to create variety and flexibility in the play interaction. According to Hobson et al. (2009), these children's impairment in social play stems from their deficit in the understanding of self as creating symbolic and functional meaning for and with others. Jordan summarized the evidence that play patterns of children with ASD are not just delayed or deficient in cognitive complexity but also are deficient in social competencies, mainly in coregulating play behaviors with others. Friendship in young children with TYP evolves mostly from the context of social play. Likewise, deficits in social play will probably predict difficulties in friendship formation among young children with HFASD. In the next section, friendship in HFASD is described.

Friendship and Peer Interaction in Preschoolers with HFASD

Stable friendships that are based on mutual affection and provide emotional support have been well documented for preschoolers with TYP (Howes, 1996). Also, in TYP, interactions with friends reveal greater social complexity than interactions with acquaintances. Friend versus nonfriend comparisons revealed that social play with friends is characterized by more positive affect, higher levels of social interaction, and more effective forms of conflict management (Newcomb & Bagwell, 1995). However, we know very little about friendship in young children with HFASD. Likewise, friendship development is a neglected aim in early interventions.

In light of the scarcity of research on friendship in preschoolers with HFASD, we recently undertook two comprehensive studies in my Behavioral Research Laboratory on this population of young children ages 3–6 years. The first study compared preschoolers with HFASD and with TYP (Bauminger-Zviely & Agam Ben-Artzi, 2012) with the following aims: (1) identifying the two groups' friendship characteristics, (2) exploring group differences in the quality of those friendships, (3) examining within-group differences on friendship type for the HFASD group—nonmixed friendships (of two children with HFASD) versus mixed friendships (of a child with HFASD and a child with TYP), and (4) investigating within-group differences on interaction partner type for both HFASD and TYP—a friend versus a nonfriend. The study included 177 preschoolers in three groups: (1) 59 recruited (target) research participants (HFASD: n = 29, mean IQ = 103.52; TYP: n = 30, mean IQ=107.60); (2) 59 of these participants' friends, defined as friends by the following criteria: mutual preference during spontaneous interaction along different activities (i.e., playground), mutual interest, close proximity, showing affection (touch), and sharing objects during play (Howes, 1996); and (3) 59 preschool classmates who were not participants' friends according to the same criteria and who were matched to the friends by age and diagnostic status.

In the Bauminger-Zviely and Agam Ben-Artzi study (2012), friendship was explored based on semistructured observations of children's interactions with a friend versus a nonfriend partner (classmates) during three main dyadic social situations in their preschool. The social situations comprised the following:

1. Free play during snack time. Pairs were provided with snacks and drinks and with age-appropriate toys such as means–end games, toys for pretend play, and fine-motor games.
2. Shared construction game. Pairs constructed a shared design using ramps, connectors, and blocks. After completion, they rolled balls down their design structure.
3. Shared drawing. Pairs created a shared design on a large blank sheet of paper using a box of colored markers, magazines, scissors, glue, and stencils.

Parents also reported about their children's friendships.

With regard to identifying preschoolers' friendship characteristics, we found that most of the friends of the target children with HFSAD held the same diagnostic status—HFASD (62%, n = 18 pairs)—that is, they were nonmixed friendships. However, a significant number had mixed friendships with a peer with TYP (38%, n = 11 pairs). In both groups, most friends were of a similar age as the target children, and most friendships were fairly durable and stable according to parental reports (duration of 4–60 months; mean = 13.00 months for HFASD; mean = 18.60 months for TYP; stability of 79.3% in HFASD and 83% in TYP). Most of the friends met both at home and at the preschool (69% HFASD; 76.7% TYP).

The exploration of group differences between HFASD and TYP in their quality of friendships revealed that the preschoolers with TYP shared and conversed more with their peer partners (friends and nonfriends) during the three social situations than did the preschoolers with HFASD. The children with TYP also showed a higher frequency of positive affect while interacting with a peer and a higher level of social play, as in collaborative pretend play. The preschoolers with TYP also outperformed their HFASD counterparts in the quality of their dyadic interactions; they had more shared fun, revealed more interrelatedness while playing, and were more responsive to each other.

These group differences were unsurprising in light of the major difficulties in intersubjective sharing and the social deficits in play and conversation characterizing young children with HFASD (American Psychiatric Association, 2000); however, the results for the friend-versus-nonfriend comparison were intriguing. Both in HFASD and TYP, interactions with friends showed a higher dyadic quality (shared fun, closeness, and reciprocity) than did interactions with a nonfriend, and the interactions with friends included a higher level of social collaborative play and collaborative pretend play than did the interactions with nonfriends. These findings for the HFASD group suggest that friendship is a feasible and meaningful experience in these young children and that friendship may offer a valuable context contributing to the evolvement of important capabilities in complex social play and intersubjectivity (sharing, interrelatedness). Finally, in line with this study's last aim of exploring the interactions of mixed versus nonmixed friendships within the HFASD group (Bauminger-Zviely & Agam Ben-Artzi, 2012), findings demonstrated that the mixed dyads (a child with HFASD and a friend with TYP) exhibited a higher level of social complexity in their interactions, were more reciprocal, collaborated at a higher level, and showed a higher level of collaborative pretend play than did the nonmixed dyads (a child with HFASD and a friend of the same diagnosis).

The second study examining preschoolers' friendships in my Behavioral Research Laboratory (Kimhi & Bauminger-Zviely, 2012) focused on the context of collaborative problem solving (CPS)—the ability of partners to work together to solve a problem leading to a joint outcome (e.g., Fawcett & Garton, 2005; Kumpulainen & Kaartinen, 2003). CPS requires children to cooperate with one another and coordinate their behaviors. As two children collaborate to solve a problem, they must share their goals, attention, and intentions (e.g., Liebal et al., 2008). Considering that the social and cognitive underpinnings of CPS are deficient in ASD (e.g., executive functions, ToM, social interaction), research on CPS offers a unique opportunity to complement other empirical studies on social play and conversation and to highlight the role of cognitive deficits in hampering social interaction.

Research showed that in children with TYP, CPS is more effective when the partner is a friend than when the partner is not a friend (e.g., Cooper, 1980). However, prior to the Kimhi and Bauminger-Zviely (2012) study, no research had yet compared friend versus nonfriend dyads in preschoolers with HFASD. Thus, using the same sample of 177 preschoolers from the Bauminger-Zviely and Agam Ben-Artzi (2012) study (59 target children with HFASD or TYP, 59 friends, and 59 nonfriends), Kimhi and Bauminger-Zviely (2012) aimed to examine: (1) the differences and similarities in CPS between preschoolers with HFASD and preschoolers with TYP; (2) the differences in CPS with a friend versus with a nonfriend; (3) the group differences in ToM (e.g., false belief) and executive functioning (planning and cognitive flexibility); and (4) the links between CPS, ToM, and executive functioning. CPS was examined by exposing each dyad to balancing scales and blocks that varied in color and in weight. Dyads' task was to locate pairs of blocks that would balance the scales. Each target child solved the problem twice, once with a friend and once with a nonfriend, in counterbalanced order.

As expected, Kimhi and Bauminger-Zviely's (2012) findings revealed group differences in CPS; dyads in the HFASD group solved the block-balancing problem slower and showed more irrelevant behaviors while solving it, in comparison to the dyads with TYP. In addition, the dyads with HFASD used fewer sharing comments and demonstrated fewer attempts to coordinate their actions with their partners' actions by aid of gestures in comparison with the dyads with TYP. However, surprisingly, the HFASD preschoolers were more responsive to their partners than were the TYP preschoolers.

Regarding CPS with a friend versus a nonfriend, the study outcomes demonstrated advantages to the interaction with a friend over the interaction with a nonfriend. Beyond the effect of HFASD–TYP group differences, when target children in both groups solved the block-balancing problem with a friend, they were more responsive to the friend's suggestions and comments, had more shared fun, and exhibited a higher level of reciprocity than when solving the problem with a nonfriend. Also, more focus on object manipulation rather than on the interaction emerged when working with a nonfriend partner.

Group differences were also found with regard to these young children's ToM and executive function capacities, whereby children with HFASD showed lower capabilities on ToM and on executive function: cognitive flexibility and planning. Yet examination of the link between ToM and CPS yielded informative data. Target preschoolers with TYP and with HFASD who had higher ToM capabilities surpassed their counterparts with lower ToM on their understanding of the block-balancing problem (i.e., understanding that color and weight were key to solving the problem), despite the fact that these ToM subgroups showed no significant differences in IQ. Interestingly, ToM levels correlated differently with preschoolers' speed of processing the problem, yielding a positive correlation in the HFASD group and a negative correlation in the TYP group: Those children with TYP who had higher ToM capabilities solved the problem quickly, whereas those children with HFASD who had higher ToM capabilities solved it slowly. This finding seems to indicate that for young children with HFASD, taking another's perspective into account is a very demanding task, requiring cognitive efforts and slowing down processing time. Slower processing time during a collaborative interaction may reflect these children's difficulties in negotiating the dynamic, rapidly changing ongoing peer interaction. It also supports the hypothesis that children with HFASD compensate cognitively for their social-emotional deficits when dealing with social-cognitive tasks such as ToM (investing more cognitive efforts into deciphering the partner's mental state; Hermelin & O'Connor, 1985).

Fewer significant correlations emerged between CPS and executive functioning, but, overall, in both groups, better executive function skills were linked with preschoolers' better CPS skills. More specifically, better planning skills (as measured by the Tower of London; Shallice, 1982) were linked with a more efficient solution to the problem in the HFASD group, with faster problem solving in the TYP group, and with higher levels of understanding of the problem in both groups. Cognitive shifting, as measured by the Flexible Item Selection Task (Jacques & Zelazo, 2001), significantly correlated with only one CPS measure for each group: better understanding of the problem in HFASD and faster problem solving in TYP.

To sum up the overall results in both studies (Bauminger-Zviely & Agam Ben-Artzi, 2012; Kimhi & Bauminger-Zviely, 2012), interacting with a friend is an advantageous setting that can lead to cognitive growth of important social competencies as well as intersubjectivity. Hence, early intervention planners should seriously consider friendship as a valuable context not only for enhancing key social skills in young children with HFASD, such as social play, but also as a goal in itself, to promote such friendships' quality. Peer friendships at young ages may also contribute to a reduction in rates of depression and anxiety at older ages. Lack of play experience with peers influences the development and characteristics of later peer relations (Manning & Wainwright, 2010).

Indeed, our studies demonstrated the importance of such a context for peer relations in HFASD; however, it should be noted that our sample was biased in that it only included children who already did have friends.

Overall, friendship is an infrequent experience for these children; therefore, support from significant caregivers and professionals in the child's environment seems crucial for the development of friendship in HFASD (see Chapter 3 for expansion on peer friendship in HFASD).

Summary of Social Functioning in Toddlers and Preschoolers

Overall, during the early childhood period, children with HFASD show areas of possible strength alongside major difficulties in social-communicative functioning. They have difficulties in ToM and in major executive functions such as cognitive shifting and planning. The quality of their peer interactions and their social play skills are lower than those of their age-mates with TYP. However, some of these young children with HFASD are able to develop friendships with peers (with TYP and/or HFASD), thereby creating a context conducive to the development of complex play behaviors, despite their deficits in ToM and executive functioning. A review of the currently available research pinpoints the fact that the processes by which friendship is formed at early ages, as well as the identification of those children who are capable of developing early friendships, are areas still in great need of further exploration. At the same time, more efforts should be directed toward designing early interventions to help these young children develop fruitful friendships and social play experiences with peers.

SCHOOL TRANSITIONS: TRAJECTORIES AND PREDICTORS

School transitions pose a considerable challenge for children with HFASD. During school years, social functioning increases in complexity in children with TYP, requiring more advanced language and pragmatic skills to establish and maintain peer conversation, higher representational skills to observe and make sense of peer behavior, more sophisticated levels of social and emotional understanding, and greater executive function skills such as planning and cognitive flexibility in adapting to diverse social interactions and situations.

Longitudinal observational examinations of peer interaction processes for tracing the transition from preschool to school ages in HFASD do not yet exist. Most of what we know is based on prospective and retrospective studies that evaluated outcome results based mainly on quantitative interview-based scales such as Lord, Rutter, and Le Couteur's (1994) ADI-R (e.g., Charman et al., 2005; Fecteau, Mottron, Berthiaume, & Burack, 2003; Moss, Magiati, Charman, & Howlin, 2008; Starr, Szatmari, Bryson, & Zwaigenbaum, 2003; Szatmari, Bryson, Boyle, Streiner, & Duku, 2003) and Sparrow et al.'s (1984) VABS (e.g., Klin et al., 2007; Szatmari et al., 2003). These studies have presented mixed results with regard to the trajectories of the social deficits in ASD from early ages to the school-age period.

Starr et al. (2003) prospectively examined ADI-R (Lord et al., 1994) outcomes over a 2-year period (from ages 4–6 to 6–8 years) for two groups: 41 children diagnosed with HFASD (nonverbal IQ scores in the nonretarded range) and 17 children diagnosed with Asperger syndrome (IQ > 70). The ADI-R symptoms were based on the three main domains (social, communication, and repetitive behaviors) related to the increasing social demands and social complexity facing children along the spectrum in the early school years. Starr et al. (2003) found significant differences between the groups over time, with the Asperger Syndrome group showing fewer symptoms than the HFASD group in all three domains at both time periods. On the ADI-R communication and social domains summary scores, the results showed a greater decrease in communication symptom severity between preschool and early elementary school in the HFASD group than in the Asperger syndrome group, as well as a larger increase in social symptoms over time.

The profile of change on the specific symptoms helps delineate these children's social complexities as they enter the school years (Starr et al., 2003). Analysis of individual ADI-R items indicated that the HFASD group improved over time on six items in the communication domain (i.e., complexity of nonechoed utterances, immediate echolalia, use of neologisms, use of instrumental gestures, head shaking, and unusual preoccupations) and one item in the social domain (offering comfort). On the other hand, both groups (HFASD and Asperger syndrome) revealed a significant increase in symptom severity on three items from the social domain (i.e., greeting, range of facial expression, and use of inappropriate facial expression) when comparing their symptoms at ages 4–6 and at ages 6–8. Moreover, the Asperger syndrome group also deteriorated between the two time periods in three other social symptoms: vocal expression, sharing others' pleasure and excitement, and appropriateness of social response. The group of children with Asperger syndrome showed improvement on only two symptoms over time: use of immediate echolalia and unusual preoccupations. These declines in social functioning may stem from greater exposure to peers during the early school years and from the environment's higher expectations for appropriateness of social interaction among school-age children in both the HFASD and Asperger syndrome groups, thereby possibly making their social difficulties more noticeable and severe.

Using the same sample as in Starr et al.'s (2003) study but adding a follow-up period at ages 10–13 years, Szatmari et al. (2003) examined the contribution of early cognitive predictors (verbal and nonverbal IQ) and early language predictors (linguistic knowledge, mainly vocabulary and grammar) at ages 4–6 years to two later factors in middle school among these children with HFASD and Asperger syndrome: (1) the explanation of the social and communication deficits (based on the VABS; Sparrow et al., 1984); and (2) the clinical diagnosis based on a composite score as measured by the Autism Behavior Checklist (Krug, Arik, & Almond, 1980), including autistic symptoms such as abnormal language, abnormal body and object use, difficulties relating to others, sensory issues, and social and self-help difficulties. The advantage of the Asperger syndrome group over the HFASD group in the socialization domain at ages 10–13 years resembled the outcomes reported by Starr et al. (2003) for the first two time periods. The explanatory power of the cognitive and language predictor variables was most substantial for the VABS communication scores (60%), weaker for the VABS socialization scores (40%), and to a lesser extent explained the Autism Behavior Checklist autistic symptoms (22%). Also, the power of the cognitive and language predictors remained stable over time, at least until preadolescence (CA = 10–13 years). However, in general, early language skills were stronger predictors of middle-school outcomes for the HFASD group than for the Asperger syndrome group in three domains: communication, socialization, and autistic symptoms. Other studies highlighted the importance of intellectual functioning and early language in young children with ASD, with an emphasis on the development of meaningful speech by the age of 5–6 years, as predictors of positive social outcomes in later childhood (e.g., Sigman & Ruskin, 1999). Interestingly, several prospective (e.g., Charman et al., 2005; Moss et al., 2008) and retrospective (Fecteau et al., 2003) examinations of trajectories of the social deficit from early ages to school age in LFA (based on the ADI-R; Lord et al., 1994) showed a reduction in social symptoms.

To sum up the trajectories from early to later childhood, based mainly on the ADI-R and VABS results, it seems that young children who function below the normative IQ level (i.e., with LFA), who probably start at a more severe basic level of social functioning at early ages (compared with children with HFASD), make more significant progress in their social symptoms and functioning by later childhood, whereas the more cognitively able children on the spectrum appear to begin at a more advanced level of early social functioning and thereafter their progress on social symptoms is highly varied. Some of this variance may reflect the higher expectations of these children with HFASD and the more complex social milieu with which they must cope in inclusive settings (e.g., interactions with peers with TYP).

Support for this supposition comes from the discrepancy in results between IQ and the overall adaptive scores on the VABS (Sparrow et al., 1984). VABS scores are consistently lower than IQ scores in children with ASD; furthermore, the VABS socialization subdomain is the most delayed in comparison with the communication and daily living skills domains (e.g., see review in Charman, 2011). This gap between IQ and adaptive capabilities is most noticeable in HFASD; for example, Klin et al. (2007) found that the standard scores for the socialization domain were 2 to 3 standard deviations below the Full Scale IQ scores in two independent HFASD samples. This study also found that adaptive skills (in terms of standard scores) decreased with age, suggesting that the "lag" between measured intelligence and everyday coping widened with development for these children (Szatmari et al., 2003). It seems that school-age children who are more cognitively able show difficulties in coping with the increasingly complex demands of school age than they do at earlier ages, including developing peer interactions and relationships, managing the peer social environment, and coping with school's academic demands. At a later point in the lifespan, social demands do not become easier with the transition from school to young adulthood, as described in the following section.

THE TRANSITION FROM SCHOOL TO THE "REAL" WORLD: FROM ADOLESCENCE TO ADULTHOOD

Extensive work by Seltzer and her colleagues (e.g., Esbensen, Seltzer, Lam, & Bodfish, 2009; Seltzer et al., 2003; Shattuck et al., 2007) followed a large cohort of individuals with ASD from adolescence to adulthood, mainly using maternal reports about children's diagnoses based on the ADI-R (Lord et al., 1994) and about participants' repetitive and maladaptive behaviors. Among the different studies, 50–75% of participants had HFASD, and the remainder had LFA. A general trend emerged from this research series: As individuals with ASD aged from adolescence to adulthood, they showed poorer reciprocal social interactions but fewer repetitive behaviors and stereotyped interests based on the ADI-R (Seltzer et al., 2003; Shattuck et al., 2007; see also Gillespie-Lynch et al., 2012, for an increase in social interaction symptoms from adolescence to young adulthood). The ADI-R communication profile showed mixed results. Adults seemed more impaired than adolescents in their ability to communicate nonverbally, in their ability to engage in reciprocal conversations, and in their overall level of language; however, in verbal symptoms adolescents performed more poorly than adults, particularly regarding their likelihood of making inappropriate statements (Seltzer et al., 2003). When considering specific symptoms, the greatest improvement emerged for speaking in phrases of at least three words, and the least improvement emerged for having friendships. Overall, as age increased, greater impairment appeared in nonverbal communication and social reciprocity than in verbal communication and in repetitive behaviors and stereotypic interests in ASD. It seems that the social reciprocity deficit is a central and persistent deficit in ASD, more than in the communication or repetitive diagnostic domains.

An interesting differential age profile was identified for the various types of repetitive behaviors and stereotyped interests in a study that included follow-up on children from preschool up to adulthood (Esbensen et al., 2009). Restricted interests were the most prevalent symptom that persisted across development, and self-injuries were the least. Stereotyped movements were common among young children with ASD, more so than rituals and compulsions, but they became less prevalent than rituals and compulsions in adulthood. Thus repetitive behaviors and stereotyped interests seemed to be a heterogeneous phenomenon in ASD.

Cognitive functioning level in individuals with ASD seems to play an important role in the progress of symptoms with age. Individuals with autism who had IQs in the intellectual disability range (i.e., LFA) demonstrated more autism symptoms and maladaptive behaviors than those with IQs over 70, and they improved less over time (e.g., Esbensen et al., 2009; Shattuck et al., 2007). However, several recent studies by Taylor and Seltzer (2010, 2011a, 2011b) indicated that the period after high school exit seems to be a time of especially increased risk, surprisingly, for those individuals with HFASD, probably because their families are underresourced. Apparently, greater resources are directed toward adults with more severe cognitive impairments, who function below the intellectual disability level.

Overall, leaving school appears to be linked with a slowing rate of improvement across the whole spectrum, but high-functioning individuals seem to experience the greatest slowing of phenotypic improvement (Taylor & Seltzer, 2010). This may stem from a scarcity of structured settings and environmental supports available for young adults with ASD who are not diagnosed with LFA. For example, Taylor and Seltzer (2011b) found that young adults with HFASD were three times less likely to have day activities than their agemates with LFA. Moreover, only 18% of young adults with HFASD were receiving some sort of employment or vocational services (e.g., supported employment, sheltered workshop) compared with 86% of young adults with LFA (Taylor & Seltzer, 2011b).

In addition, mother–adolescent relationships (e.g., warmth) continued to improve in high school but slowed or stopped after the adolescents exited school, and indeed those young adults with HFASD who had more unmet service needs evidenced the least improvement in relationships with their mothers after exiting school (Taylor & Seltzer, 2011a). Furthermore, following school exit, maternal warmth toward young people with ASD decreased more for youth with HFASD than for youth with LFA. Interestingly, sex played a role in mother–youth relationships after school exit, whereby mothers of daughters with ASD reported greater increases in positive affect in the mother–child relationship over time relative to mothers of sons (Taylor & Seltzer, 2011a). One possible explanation for the HFASD group's greater deterioration in relationship qualities after school exit may be these parents' disappointment based on unmet expectations for their high-functioning youth to become independent—live independently, finish college, and attain jobs. Also, expectations for sons to be independent may likewise be higher than expectations for daughters. Notably, a mother–child relationship that becomes less positive over time, along with slowing of improvements in the behavioral phenotype and a scarcity of community supports, may place youth with HFASD at high risk for poor outcomes in the years immediately following their exit from the secondary school system, and possibly beyond.

Employment that leads to and is related to independence poses an enormous challenge and area of difficulty for individuals with HFASD. A substantial percentage of adults with HFASD are unemployed or under-employed. They make less money than their counterparts with TYP and hold less prestigious jobs that demand lower cognitive capabilities and offer fewer prospects for future advancement, even for those individuals who attain postsecondary educational experience (Howlin, 2000). Adults with HFASD also demonstrate difficulties in maintaining steady employment, switching jobs frequently. Adjusting to the workplace environment is difficult, especially with regard to managing interpersonal connections with coworkers and supervisors (e.g., Cederlund, Hagberg, Billstedt, Gillberg, & Gillberg, 2008; Hurlbutt & Chalmers, 2004; Jennes-Coussens, Magill-Evans, & Koning, 2006).

Some have emphasized the social-communication difficulties in interpersonal connections in HFASD as the primary obstacle to successful job performance (e.g., see review in Hendricks, 2010) in areas such as the inability to understand instructions and follow rules, social-cognitive deficits (e.g., understanding social norms and nonliteral language; emotional understanding; reading facial expressions, body gestures, and tone of voice), and difficulties in social interactive behaviors (e.g., making inappropriate comments, demonstrating odd behaviors, having difficulty working in cooperation with coworkers). A mixture of psychiatric difficulties (anxiety, depression) and rigid and stereotyped behaviors also hamper the ability of individuals with HFASD to function efficiently in the workplace; these difficulties presumably rise from major difficulties in executive functioning such as poor decision-making ability (e.g., Cederlund, Hagberg, & Gillberg, 2010). Taking it all together, adults with HFASD require specific supports in the work environment; however, it seems that a wider variety and quantity of services are available targeting the needs of the lower-functioning adults on the spectrum than of those with HFASD, thus leaving the more able individuals to face poor outcomes.

Educational outcomes may be somewhat more promising for adults with HFASD. Taylor and Seltzer (2011b) reported that nearly half of the adults in their sample (8 of 17) pursued postsecondary educational degrees, but Cederlund et al. (2008) found that only 10 out of the 66 adults with Asperger syndrome in their study completed some university studies (15%), and only two of those attained university degrees (in computer science and civil engineering). White, Ollendick, and Bray (2011) recently explored the prevalence of HFASD among 667 undergraduate students in a large technology-oriented public university in the southeastern United States. They found 13 students who met criteria for HFASD (1.9%), most of whom majored in engineering and computer science (54% of students with HFASD vs. 28% in students without HFASD). Interestingly, these adults with HFASD showed high academic excellence (according to grade point average) but less satisfaction with university life and with life overall and higher rates of social anxiety compared with the nonidentified students. Symptoms of HFASD correlated with scores on social anxiety, depression, and aggression. It seems that in the educational arena, as found for the work arena, the real challenge for these young adults with HFASD is to cope with the social-interpersonal demands of being university students, rather than with its cognitive and intellectual challenges. These young adults may experience social isolation, loneliness, and depression, based on their peculiar social behaviors and odd interests (e.g., White et al., 2011).

Individuals with ASD who do not function below the intellectual disability level (i.e., HFASD) are more likely to present better outcomes in terms of employment, social relationships, and postsecondary education relative to those with LFA (e.g., Cederlund et al., 2008; Eaves & Ho, 2008; Engström, Ekström, & Emilsson, 2003; Howlin et al., 2004). However, many adults with HFASD do not obtain these developmental milestones in a satisfactory way, and they reach suboptimal outcomes with respect to making friends, attaining decent jobs, and maintaining independent living; indeed, most continue to need extensive support (e.g., Cederlund et al., 2008; Eaves & Ho, 2008; Taylor & Seltzer, 2011b).

For example, Cederlund et al. (2008) compared outcomes for adults with Asperger syndrome (IQ > 70, mean CA = 21.5 years, CA range: 16–34 years) with those for adults with LFA (83% with IQ < 70) and found that 64% of those who were age 23 or older in the Asperger syndrome group (*n* = 22) lived independently versus only 8% in the LFA group (*n* = 40). However, all of those living away from their parents continued to remain dependent on the parents for some support. Of those adults with Asperger syndrome who were age 23 or older, 3 (14%) had long-term romantic relationships, and an additional 10 (43%) had maintained such relationships for varying periods of time in the past. In the group of LFA, all of those who lived independently continued to rely on their parents for intensive support. Only 2 adults (5%) with LFA had long-term relationships (1 currently, 1 in the past). Overall psychosocial adjustment was "good" for 27% of these adults with Asperger syndrome (i.e., either paid or voluntary employment with some degree of support in daily living and some friendships or acquaintances), "fair" for 47% of them (i.e., achieving some supported independence and having acquaintances but no close friendships), and "poor" for 23% of them (i.e., requiring a high level of support and having few social contacts); 3% led very restricted lives, had no friends, and had no occupation of any type. In contrast, in the LFA group, 76% showed "poor" psychosocial adjustment, only 7% showed "fair," and none showed "good" outcomes. All in all, the adult Asperger syndrome group, which evidenced the higher IQs, achieved better outcomes. Yet a significant portion of individuals in this group lagged far behind their peers with TYP.

In a like manner, Engström et al. (2003) examined psychosocial functioning in a group of Swedish adults with Asperger syndrome and HFASD (mean CA = 30.8). Only 12% obtained good results, 75% had fair out-comes, and 12% had poor outcomes. Although the majority lived independently, only one adult (6.25%) was employed, few had close relationships, none was married or had children, and only a few had some friends. Most of these cognitively high-functioning adults nevertheless required a great deal of public and/or private support.

In her review of older studies that included HFASD samples (from 1985 to 1999), Howlin (2000) reported that the various studies presented high variability in outcomes. The proportion of adults with HFASD who were employed ranged from 5 to 44%; those living independently ranged from 16 to 50%; assessment of "good" outcomes ranged from 16 to 44%; and rates of psychiatric disturbance ranged from 11 to 67%. Howlin attributed these wide ranges to the variability in the measures researchers used to assess outcomes, as well as in the amount of services provided in each geographical area. In a later longitudinal study, Howlin et al. (2004) examined individuals with IQs over 50 at two time points: in childhood (mean CA = 7 years, range: 3–15 years) and in adulthood (mean CA = 29 years, range: 21–48 years). They found that, overall, only 12% of the adults were rated as having "very good" outcomes (i.e., having residential and employment independence and some friendships); 10% were rated as "good"; 19% were rated as "fair"; and the majority (46%) was rated as "poor" (i.e., requiring a high level of support and having few social contacts). An additional 12% was even rated "very poor" (i.e., living in a hospital or institution). Altogether, a significant proportion of the adults with HFASD remained highly dependent on others for support. Individuals with childhood Performance IQs of at least 70 had significantly better outcomes than those with IQs below 70; however, within the normal IQ range, outcomes varied widely, and on an individual level neither Verbal nor Performance IQ proved to be a consistent prognostic indicator.

Summary of the Transition from Adolescence to Adulthood

Consideration of the existing literature suggests that the social deficit is the most persistent difficulty for adults with HFASD, hampering their ability to fully meet their cognitive-academic potential in work and educational settings. A substantial proportion of young adults do not have friends or social networks once they leave school. The period after school exit seems to be one of high risk for these more able adults on the spectrum; this situation calls for the design of appropriate external support services to meet their specific needs. Predictors for successful adult social functioning were examined in several studies; however, only a few predictors specifically investigated this question in HFASD. Full Scale IQ and Verbal IQ seem to contribute to a higher level of adult psychosocial adjustment, including employment status and independence level, in adults with Asperger syndrome (e.g., Cederlund et al., 2008).

Yet, in a different study on adults with LFA (mean CA = 26.6 years; Gillespie-Lynch et al., 2012), intellectual functioning did not contribute specifically to better social functioning, whereas early measures of childhood language level and responsiveness to joint attention (both collected at mean CA = 3.9 years) did contribute. Gillespie-Lynch et al. (2012) highlighted responsiveness to joint attention as an important predictor of adult social behavior because it reflects children's ability to learn from the environment. Although this study's participants mostly had LFA, its results may signify that IQ (Full Scale or Verbal) cannot fully compensate for the social deficit in adulthood, explaining the relatively high percentages of adults with normative IQ level who still show restricted social functioning, as reviewed earlier. It also may explain why these adults continue to have major difficulties in making friends and in having appropriate and satisfactory social networks. A deeper look at other characteristics beyond early language and IQ may yield a better understanding of those adults with HFASD who reach good social outcomes versus those who do not. Such characteristics may include social-cognitive capabilities such as ToM and joint attention, affective capabilities such as emotional understanding and regulation, and cognitive capabilities such as executive functions and central coherence (all overviewed in Chapter 1). This thorough examination should also include evaluation of the available community support services provided for adults with HFASD in the individuals' locale, as well as the characteristics of the interaction quality with the individuals' main caregivers.

SUMMARY AND CONCLUSIONS

The investigation of social development in HFASD to discern trajectories for the social-emotional deficit reveals a rather complicated profile, with no clear pattern of change across development. Overall, social-emotional functioning poses a great challenge for individuals with HFASD at various developmental periods, from very early ages up to adulthood. Early markers of the social deficit in ASD comprise major social-communication deficiencies that may already appear at the age of 12 months and possibly even start between 6 and 12 months. Such deficiencies may include, among others, reduced social responsiveness and reactivity, limited social interest, limited expression of positive affect, delay in gestures for communication, and distortions in play. At the toddlerhood and preschool ages, difficulties in social play are observed regarding ToM, executive functioning, and quality of friendship.

However, alongside these major difficulties, strengths can also be observed in some young children (e.g., preschoolers) who are able to develop friendships that qualitatively differ from interactions with acquaintances. Yet the processes by which such friendships form at early ages, as well as the individual differences among children who are and are not able to develop such friendships with peers, have not yet been uncovered.

When looking at older ages, we can see evidence that shows some degree of social advantage for adolescents over adults with HFASD, and it seems that the exit from school is a period of great risk, especially for the more able individuals on the spectrum, possibly because they have far fewer appropriate services to meet their needs. The social difficulty seems to be a key obstacle to successful adjustment in adult work and study environments. Thus individuals with higher IQs (i.e., those with HFASD) do indeed show better results as compared with individuals with LFA, but those who are high functioning nevertheless lag way behind adults with TYP in terms of achieving residential independence, education, and social life. Thus adults with HFASD are still in great need of support at the family and community levels in order to fully meet their high potential to become independent citizens in society.

Chapter 5

Cognitive Strengths
and Weaknesses

with Yael Kimhi

The cognitive and academic domain of children with HFASD has been less explored in the literature than the social-communication domain, perhaps because it is not considered to be a core deficit of the disorder. Nonetheless, children with HFASD exhibit many specific difficulties alongside areas of strengths in the cognitive and academic areas, which have attained increasing attention in recent years. Chapter 1 dealt extensively with the underlying social-cognitive, social-communicative, and cognitive mechanisms (such as ToM, central coherence weakness, and executive functioning) that may shed light on the cognitive and academic abilities and disabilities described in this chapter.

This chapter, written together with my colleague Yael Kimhi, first describes the cognitive strengths and weaknesses that make up the academic profile of children with HFASD. The major cognitive characteristics include uneven memory capabilities, varied imitation skills, and ineffective language and narrative abilities. We then focus on the academic profile that characterizes individuals with HFASD in the three major academic domains: reading, writing, and mathematics.

Yael Kimhi, PhD, is a lecturer at the School of Education in Bar-Ilan University and a special education inspector at the Israeli Ministry of Education. Prior to her position as inspector, she was the leading national ASD educational counselor in Israel. Dr. Kimhi's main field of interest is academic and cognitive development in ASD and HFASD.

COGNITIVE CHARACTERISTICS OF HFASD

Children with HFASD are said to show uneven intellectual abilities, as indicated by the cognitive strengths and weaknesses they present within IQ testing. The characteristic profile of children and adults with HFASD on intelligence tests depicts higher abilities in concrete tasks as opposed to abstract ones (Bolte, Dziobek, & Poustka, 2009; Kamio & Toichi, 2000; Minshew, Turner, & Goldstein, 2005); thus, abstract tasks are often beyond their grasp. For example, on Wechsler IQ tests (Wechsler Adult Intelligence Scale—Revised [WAIS-R], Wechsler, 1981; Wechsler Adult Intelligence Scale—Third Edition [WAIS-III], Wechsler, 1997; Wechsler Intelligence Scale for Children—Revised [WISC-R], Wechsler, 1974; Wechsler Intelligence Scale for Children—Third Edition [WISC-III], Wechsler, 1991; Wechsler Preschool and Primary Scale for Intelligence—Revised [WPPSI-R], Wechsler, 1989), individuals with HFASD score high on visual-spatial subtests such as Block Design (on which one arranges blocks of different colors according to a given pattern, thus measuring visual-spatial and motor skills), and they score low on verbal subtests such as Comprehension (on which the child answers oral questions concerning social and practical understanding). It is important to note that, in line with the defining characteristics of ASD, scores on the latter social comprehension measure are low even in children with HFASD who score normally on other aspects of intelligence (Goldstein et al., 2008).

Kuschner, Bennetto, and Yost (2007) examined the relative strengths and weaknesses in nonverbal cognitive functioning of young children with ASD (mean CA = 4.8 years) in comparison with children with developmental delays and children with TYP who were matched to the ASD group on nonverbal MA (mean = 3.8 years). Their cognitive performance was examined with the Brief IQ (BIQ) Screening Assessment from the Leiter International Performance Scale—Revised (Roid & Miller, 1997). As hypothesized, the results demonstrated an uneven profile of nonverbal abilities, in which the young children with ASD succeeded in tasks that demanded disembedding abilities (finding an individual item within a complex field) and also in detail-focused perceptual processing (mentally manipulating and synthesizing pieces of a pictured object), but they had difficulties in abstract reasoning and concept formation (completing patterns and sequences of items). On the one hand, the children showed intact perceptual processing skills, which were in the normal range when compared with those of their peers with TYP; yet, on the other hand, they showed nonverbal conceptual weaknesses. According to Kuschner et al. (2007), children's difficulties that arose in this study may be part of a wider deficit within ASD pertaining to concept formation and the formation of new ideas. Furthermore, the authors asserted that these difficulties may constitute part of a broader deficiency in the ability to create meaningful connections between multiple concepts.

The notion of concept formation is relevant to academic abilities, as students are expected to generate conceptual categories while processing information in class. Categorizing requires the ability to discriminate properties, objects, or events into groups on the basis of a principle or rule. The mental representation that exemplifies the relations of the objects within a category is termed a concept; therefore, categorization is a basic cognitive process that reduces the demands on memory storage and reasoning processes (Johnson & Rakison, 2006). In a study that examined toddlers' (mean CA = 38 months) ability to categorize animate and inanimate objects, the HFASD group (mean Verbal IQ = 74; mean Nonverbal IQ = 81) tended to attend selectively to specific features of the objects presented, and, according to the authors, this localizing attentional bias displayed at this young age may contribute to the later observed cognitive deficits in older individuals with HFASD (Johnson & Rakison, 2006).

Alderson-Day and McGonigle-Chalmers (2011) examined the utilization of categories during a problem-solving task among adolescents with HFASD (mean CA = 13 years) in comparison with agemates with TYP. The authors devised a novel game by adapting the classic "20 questions" game and constructing it with artificial items (robot-shaped characters varying in color, shape, and features). The adolescents in the HFASD group asked more concrete, functional questions and fewer abstract ones in comparison with the TYP group. Furthermore, the quality of their questions was lower; they eliminated fewer items or referred to fewer items at a time, using category grouping in a limited and concrete manner. Importantly, these authors emphasized caution in interpreting the results due to the small size of the study group and due to the fact that the groups were not matched on Verbal IQ. Verbal IQ is believed to be lower in individuals with ASD and is therefore an important factor in cognitive processes.

IQ testing within ASD generally leads to a profile of lower Verbal than Performance IQ in much of the autistic spectrum, whether high or low functioning (Joseph, Tager-Flusberg, & Lord, 2002; Mayes & Calhoun, 2003b), although not in all cases. Charman et al. (2010) found only weak support for a distinctive Performance > Verbal IQ profile. Within Charman et al.'s study group of 156 children, mean Performance IQ level was higher than mean Verbal IQ level by a few points, but when clinically meaningful discrepancies were examined, the most common profile revealed similarities in Performance and Verbal IQs. Depending on the child's ability, IQ was measured using the WISC-III U.K. edition (WISC-IIIUK; Wechsler, 1992) or Raven's Standard Progressive Matrices or Coloured Progressive Matrices (Raven, Court, & Raven, 1990a, 1990b). Furthermore, other researchers found that, in many cases, the gap between Performance and Verbal IQs diminished with age and was associated with improvement in language ability, especially among children with HFASD (Joseph et al., 2002; Sigman & McGovern, 2005).

The variability in cognitive profiles within the autistic spectrum holds implications for their learning styles—whether visual or auditory. Teaching according to the child's learning style is critical in order to enable the processing of the information presented. It is believed that many children with ASD are visual learners; therefore, visually based interventions are usually recommended (Broun, 2004; for visual strategies, see Chapter 8, this volume). A novel study that examined the auditory characteristics of children with ASD (mean CA = 5.7 years) found that physiological test results were equivalent to those of peers with TYP; yet behavioral observations revealed that, when a sound was presented, 41% of the ASD group responded in such a manner as to indicate that they did not hear normally. The authors explained that these behaviors may be due to weak attention processes rather than auditory deficits (Tharpe et al., 2006). Attention problems are also linked to academic underachievement in TYP (Nelson, Benner, Lane, & Smith, 2004), and many children within the spectrum are known to have comorbid attention deficits (Lecavalier, 2006; see also Chapter 6, this volume). Much of the variability in the cognitive profile is also memory related.

Memory

Memory functions of children with HFASD differ from those of children with TYP, yet the nature of these differences is not completely clear. Research indicates that the deficits found in memory functions are not universal but rather are specific to various functions within memory itself (Williams, Goldstein, & Minshew, 2006b). For example, these children generally have intact memory function on simple recall and recognition tasks (Bennetto et al., 1996; Hala et al., 2005), but they demonstrate impairments in or rarely use organizational or contextual strategies to support their memory (Minshew & Goldstein, 2001; Toichi & Kamio, 2002, 2003). Studies also show that children with HFASD tend not to use semantic or syntactic strategies to organize lists of words (Bowler, Limoges, & Mottron, 2009; Minshew & Goldstein, 2001; Smith, Gardiner, & Bowler, 2007). Furthermore, they usually reveal more difficulty recalling complex material, whether visual or semantic, compared with their peers with TYP (Minshew & Goldstein, 2001; Williams et al., 2006b). The abnormal memory functioning in autism can be explained in relation to more general cognitive impairments, such as executive function deficits (Bennetto et al., 1996) or central coherence weakness (Lopez & Leekam, 2003), as discussed in Chapter 1.

This section reviews research on the abilities of children with HFASD in the different aspects of memory, including working memory (comprising spatial, verbal, and temporal aspects) and autobiographical memory (comprising episodic, semantic, and everyday memory).

Working Memory

Working memory is different from either short-term or long-term memory in that it involves not only storage of information but also both the ability to store and maintain spatial and verbal information on the one hand and the ability to process that information on the other hand (Reed, 2002; Steele, Minshew, Luna, & Sweeney, 2007). Research on the working memory abilities of individuals with HFASD has yielded mixed results, as described next for studies that examined spatial and verbal working memory in HFASD.

SPATIAL WORKING MEMORY

Spatial working memory is the ability to remember over time where something is located once it is out of sight (Williams et al., 2006b). Studies that examined the ability to remember spatial location information under conditions of increasing memory load found impairment in individuals with HFASD compared with individuals with TYP. As the task demands increased, their spatial working memory became increasingly impaired (Minshew & Goldstein, 2001; Steele et al., 2007; Williams, Goldstein, Carpenter, & Minshew, 2005). For example, Williams et al. (2005) examined verbal and spatial working memory, asking participants with HFASD or with TYP to follow various sequences while increasing the stimulus load in each sequence. The spatial working memory tasks revealed deficits in HFASD in both of two age groups (CA = 17–48 years for adults and 8–16 years for children and adolescents), although their verbal working memory was found to be intact. According to the authors, further study is necessary to understand this discrepancy between intact verbal working memory and impaired spatial working memory across development.

In a study of increasing spatial working memory load conducted by Steele et al. (2007), the TYP group tended to use the same sequential search strategy to facilitate their performance, beginning each search sequence at a specific point and excluding irrelevant stimuli accordingly. The individuals with HFASD (CA = 8–29 years) failed to apply this organizing strategy, suggesting that ineffective strategy use, along with increased memory load, leads to deficits in spatial working memory. Thus working memory deficits may be related to tasks' complexity, especially those that demand larger memory loads.

TEMPORAL MEMORY

Gras-Vincendon, Mottron, Salame, Bursztejn, and Danion (2007) tested temporal memory for visual information in adolescents and young adults with HFASD and with TYP (mean CA = 20 years). In each of six visual recognition tasks, participants were shown 6 pictures and, after a short interval, had to find the 6 pictures out of an array of 30 pictures. The distracters became the target pictures of the following tests. Results showed that the HFASD group performed as well as the control group, recognizing the target items as asked. According to the authors, the participants with HFASD succeeded because they did not need to use organizational strategies in order to memorize the context information; apparently, the task demanded only automatic processing (Gras-Vincendon et al., 2007).

Reed (2002) examined the visual perspective-taking ability of 60 participants (ages 3.1–52.0 years) matched on sex and verbal age according to the PPVT (Dunn & Dunn, 1997): 25 participants with ASD (10 with LFA, mean verbal age = 8.2 years), 10 participants with mental retardation (mean verbal age = 5.7), and 25 participants with TYP (mean verbal age = 7.11). Participants were expected to find an appropriate hiding place for a doll, while taking into consideration the visual perspective of up to six imaginary observers. For each potential hiding place, the participants had to check the perspective of the first observer, hold that information online in their working memory, then check the perspective of the next imaginary observer, and so on, for an increasing number of perspectives. Participants then integrated all of these perspectives to decide whether the hiding place was "safe" or not. As predicted by the authors, only 56% of the participants with ASD completed the highest level of the task, whereas the vast majority of participants with mental retardation and with TYP (90% and 92%, respectively) achieved full success.

The reviewed studies show that spatial working memory and temporal memory in HFASD clearly decline as the task load on the memory increases. These findings were also seen for LFA and ASD (Reed, 2002). The findings regarding verbal working memory are less clear-cut, as seen next.

VERBAL WORKING MEMORY

This form of working memory stores and manipulates linguistic material. Deficits in verbal working memory can lead to academic and linguistic impairment. Individuals with HFASD may show poor performance on various measures related to verbal working memory, such as impairment in their recall of phonologically and semantically related lists (Smith, Gardiner, & Bowler, 2007), although no impairment was found in their ability to recall lists of random words (Smith et al., 2007; Williams et al., 2006b). According to Smith et al. (2007), the deficit in recalling phonologically and semantically related lists, as opposed to random word lists, coincides with the central coherence weakness theory (described in Chapter 1), supporting the notion that individuals with HFASD are less likely to use organizational strategies to enhance recall. It is important to note that this finding does not indicate that people with HFASD do better on random lists than on related lists, but rather that people with TYP make use of relatedness, whereas those with HFASD usually do not and consequently do relatively worse on related lists. Notwithstanding, Whitehouse, Maybery, and Durkin (2007) examined the semantic and phonological recall ability of children with HFASD (mean CA = 10.11 years) by aid of cued recall (see Chapter 8) in comparison with children with TYP (mean CA = 8.4 years) matched on verbal and nonverbal age and found no significant differences between the two groups. This difference between these studies' results presumably stems from the fact that Whitehouse et al. (2007) used cued recall, whereas Smith et al. (2007) used free recall. The cued-recall strategy apparently aided the children with HFASD to find the relational links between words that they could not provide for themselves, thereby facilitating unimpaired recall. This advantage of cued recall holds ramifications for teaching strategies and intervention planning, as discussed in Chapter 8.

Verbal working memory deficits are seen when children with HFASD are required to recall complex verbal stimuli, such as sentence repetition and story recall—tasks characterized by increasing complexity (Gabig, 2008). In a study that examined the ability to recall verbal stimuli among young school-age children (mean CA = 6.7 years), children with HFASD performed progressively worse as the task's cognitive linguistic demands became more complex, from word and sentence repetition to story recall (Gabig, 2008). However, in a study investigating verbal working memory without complex linguistic demands, adults with HFASD performed as well as the TYP group (Williams et al., 2005). These findings reinforce the concept that individuals with HFASD are at a disadvantage when complexity increases beyond their ability, whether dealing with visual or verbal stimuli.

Autobiographical Memory

Autobiographical memory is a higher-order cognitive process that includes episodic and semantic (generalized knowledge) memories (Willoughby, Desrocher, Levine, & Rovet, 2012). It is considered to be central to the psychological and social functioning of the individual and enables one to define oneself in relation to others and to the past (Bruck, London, Landa, & Goodman, 2007). This memory begins to develop as young as 2 years of age and continues to develop as children mature. Studies related to autobiographical memory within individuals with HFASD demonstrate impairments (Bruck et al., 2007; Goddard et al., 2007). The autobiographical memory of children with HFASD was compared with that of children with TYP (CA = 5–10 years) via two paradigms (Bruck et al., 2007). The first paradigm examined children's recall of salient personal events, confirming accuracy of the memory through the parents. In the second paradigm, the children participated in a staged event and were later given true and false reminders about that event. The intent of the false reminders was to examine the children's suggestibility. After an interval of time, the children were interviewed again about the staged event. Corresponding with Millward et al. (2000), Bruck et al.'s (2007) results revealed deficits in memory for personally experienced events within the HFASD group in comparison with the TYP group. The children with HFASD showed these deficits for events in their recent past as well as their far past, for which they even failed to recall events. According to the authors, their autobiographical memory was characterized by sparseness. Furthermore, contrary to the author's predictions, they did not exhibit more suggestibility.

EPISODIC MEMORY

Episodic memory refers to the ability to remember personally experienced events and is related to the ability to imagine one's possible future experiences, thus enabling one to fluctuate between past experiences and imagined future episodes (Lind, 2010). Episodic memory is related to one's source memory—the ability to recall the source of a memory (Lind & Bowler, 2010). In TYP, self-experienced events are recalled far better than observed events (Baker-Ward, Hess, & Flannagan, 1990); yet memory for specific episodes and personal events situated in specific places and times seems to be impaired in individuals with HFASD (Gras-Vincendon et al., 2007).

Lind and Bowler (2009) investigated the episodic and semantic memory of children with ASD and children with TYP who were matched for age (mean CA = 9 years) and verbal ability (mean verbal MA = 6.6 years). In this procedure, the experimenter showed the child pictures of items presented on cards; the experimenter named some items, and the child was asked to name others. Then the child was read a list of words and was expected to say whether that item had appeared on the cards and, if so, who had named the item. As predicted, the children with ASD succeeded on the semantic aspect of the study (general knowledge), accurately recognizing the items, yet were impaired in episodic memory—in recognizing which person had named the item. Interestingly, both the ASD and TYP groups showed better memory for items that they had named themselves than for items that were named by the experimenter. The authors suggested that this may be due to the motor component that accompanied their actions, during which they physically picked up the cards and named the items.

Millward et al. (2000) examined the ability to recall personally experienced events among children with ASD (mean CA = 13 years, mean verbal MA = 5.8 years) in comparison with children with TYP who were matched on verbal MA (mean CA = 6.3). The children went on two 25-minute walks, during which the experimenter pointed out various locations. Afterward, when children were asked about the walks, the children with ASD recalled fewer personal events than the TYP group; yet no group differences emerged regarding reports about what happened to other people during the walk. Similar results concerning impaired episodic memory were found among adults with HFASD (Crane & Goddard, 2008; Lind & Bowler, 2010).

EVERYDAY MEMORY

Everyday memory refers to memory use in routine, day-to-day events that occur in one's daily environment, such as remembering names, chores, grocery lists, and so forth. In one recent study of parent reports about adolescents' everyday memory (defined as the functional use of memory in day-to-day life that enables easy transitions throughout the day), Jones, Happé, et al. (2011) found that parents of adolescents in the HFASD group (*n* = 94; mean CA = 15.6 years) reported that their children showed significantly more difficulties in remembering everyday functional information both at home and at school compared with parents of adolescents in the TYP group (*n* = 55; mean CA = 15.6 years).

Summary of Memory

There is a growing body of literature demonstrating memory deficits within children, adolescents, and adults with HFASD. Most aspects of memory, whether verbal, nonverbal, or autobiographical, are more impaired individuals with HFASD than in their peers with TYP (Southwick et al., 2011). As task load increases, individuals with HFASD show decreasing verbal and spatial working memory abilities. Furthermore, these individuals do not tend to facilitate recall by considering the relatedness of items unless cued recall is supplied at the retrieval stage (as opposed to the storage stage). In addition, the various components of autobiographical memory and everyday memory are also impaired within individuals with HFASD.

Links between Memory Function and Information Processing

One possible explanation for the uneven memory function in ASD is a specific disorder in the ability to process information, which may be caused by a poor ability to store, retrieve, and transform concepts and schemas appropriately (Williams, Goldstein, & Minshew, 2006a). Williams et al. (2006a) claimed that deficits in the memory domain in ASD are caused by an information-processing disorder, not a sole cognitive deficit. They tested the abilities of children with HFASD (mean CA = 11.4 years) in comparison with agemates with TYP on simple and complex skills in different domains (sensory, motor, language, and memory). A pattern emerged of intact simple information processing and impaired complex information processing. Namely, the HFASD group showed greater difficulties than the TYP group on tasks that demanded the highest information-processing resources and the highest integration of information, such as memorizing a large amount of material or comprehending long and complex texts. Nevertheless, the two groups did not differ on simple cognitive skills within the same domains.

According to Reed (2002), working memory deficits have three main effects on how information is processed. Reed asserted that memory performance is better on: (1) tasks that provide concrete cues, permitting one to look at the cues, rather than those providing transient cues; (2) tasks involving fewer items, rather than many items; and (3) predictable situations, especially those requiring previously acquired strategies rather than novel situations that require novel strategies. Interestingly, Whitehouse et al.'s (2007) findings regarding cued memory recall coincide with Reed's explanation concerning the information-processing explanation for working memory. Likewise, Williams et al. (2006a) found that children with HFASD seem to acquire less information when processing complex stimuli such as composite pictorial scenes, verbal sentences, or stories.

Another influence on cognitive and academic achievement is imitation.

Imitation Skills

Imitation is the basic ability that enables learning—whether social or academic (McDuffie et al., 2007; Vivanti, Nadig, Ozonoff, & Rogers, 2008). The ability to imitate other people is known to be deficient in children with ASD (McDuffie et al., 2007; Shih et al., 2010). Williams, Whitten, and Singh's (2004) comprehensive literature review on imitation reported that individuals with ASD reveal specific difficulties in imitating others, when compared with individuals with other developmental disorders or with TYP. Nevertheless, considerable variability characterizes motor imitation performance within the ASD population (McDuffie et al., 2007). For example, imitation involving actions on objects (imitating an action that a person performed with an object) is impaired in autism, but imitation of gestures was found to be even more impaired (Ham et al., 2011; Vivanti et al., 2008).

To date, the majority of imitation studies examined motor imitation, which may be problematic because children along the spectrum are known to exhibit impairments in motor functioning, planning, and coordination. (For further reading on motor impairments, see relevant references in Subiaul et al., 2007.) Subiaul et al. (2007) examined the cognitive imitation ability of adolescents with ASD (mean CA = 15 years; mean verbal MA = 4.8 years) in comparison with 3- to 4-year-old children with TYP. They were shown a series of pictures on a computer screen in a specific order and then were told to point to the pictures in the correct serial order when the pictures appeared in varying spatial settings onscreen. Thus the task relied solely on cognitive imitation and could not be aided or facilitated by motor imitation. Their findings demonstrated no significant group differences, calling into question the notion of a global imitation learning deficit within ASD.

Imitation skills are said to have a prominent role in the development of spoken language, especially for children with ASD. Ingersoll and Lalonde (2010) demonstrated that gestural imitation training, together with training in imitation of actions with objects (such as imitation of opening a toy car's door), can lead to greater gains in the rate of language use by young children with ASD in comparison with training of imitation actions with objects alone.

Language and Narrative Abilities

Poor language and communication skills are a defining feature of ASD (APA, 2012). Between 25 and 40% of the children with ASD may fail to acquire verbal language, and many other individuals have early language delays (APA, 2012). Studies examining the language skills of children with ASD have shown diverse findings along with deficits in various areas, although overall the research indicated a clear, fundamental deficit in language in these children (Eigsti, de Marchena, Shuh, & Kelley, 2011). Their linguistic deficits include impairments in pragmatics (Tager-Flusberg, 2001b), syntax (Eigsti, Bennetto, & Dadlani, 2007), lexical functioning (Perkins, Dob-binson, Boucher, Bol, & Bloom, 2006; including qualitative differences in novel-word learning in comparison with TYP, see Norbury, Griffiths, & Nation, 2010), and prosody (Hesling et al., 2010; McCann, Peppe, Gibbon, O'Hare, & Rutherford, 2007). Notwithstanding these findings for children across the spectrum, in HFASD the deficits may be so subtle that they are not reflected in standardized language test scores (Tager-Flusberg, 2008; Tager-Flusberg, Paul, & Lord, 2005).

A comprehensive overview of language abilities in ASD is beyond this book's scope, yet these children's narrative ability is relevant because of its importance for communication, as well as for structuring thoughts (Eigsti et al., 2011), and mainly for academic and social functioning (Spencer & Slocum, 2010). Narrative abilities require the successful integration of cog-nitive skills, the use of world knowledge, and the awareness of the listener (Wetherell, Botting, & Conti-Ramsden, 2007). Children with poor narra-tive ability are at risk for poor reading development (Boudreau & Hedberg, 1999) and poor academic achievement (Wetherell et al., 2007).

To date, only a few studies have examined the narrative abilities of children and adolescents with HFASD. Narratives consisting of personal accounts were found to be limited among youngsters with HFASD and seemed to lack goals (Goldman, 2008). However, children with HFASD were able to introduce narratives into familiar settings (i.e., family dinners), even though they showed difficulty maintaining those narratives (Solomon, 2004).

Capps, Losh, and Thurber (2000) compared the narrative abilities of children with ASD, children with developmental delays, and children with TYP, all matched on language ability (mean verbal MA = 6.2 years). The children were asked to tell a story to the experimenter while following the pictures in a wordless picture book. The children with ASD (like the children with developmental delays) did not use complex syntax in their narratives, but their narratives were as long as those of the other two groups. The use of complex syntax in narrative telling is important as an aid for conveying causal ties, showing plot development, and amplifying general themes. The limited syntax use suggested a linear narrative typical of younger children, in which the narrator did not explain the characters' motives or the ties between events. Furthermore, although the children with ASD made the same amount of references to the characters' affective and cognitive states as the other two groups, the ASD group did not analyze or explain the reasons for characters' various internal states (again, similarly to the children with developmental delays). A further difference between the groups was in their use of attention-getting mannerisms (such as emphatic markers, repetition, and sound effects): Children with ASD mainly made use of concrete directives (e.g., "Look at that!"), whereas children with TYP used a variety of devices (e.g., emphatic stress, repetition, sound effects, and comments such as "lo and behold").

In a later study (Diehl, Bennetto, & Young, 2006) that examined narrative and story-recall abilities of children with HFASD in comparison with children with TYP (mean CA = 8 years), for the most part the findings resembled those of Capps et al. (2000). In Diehl et al. (2006), children listened to an audiotaped story while looking at a wordless picture book, and they were asked to retell the story with the expectation that they would refer to the story's causal connections and general gist. No differences emerged between the two groups on narrative length or syntax complexity, but the children with HFASD identified fewer causal connections, and, although they recalled the story's gist, they did not use it to aid their narratives, as did the children with TYP. The children with HFASD related to the concrete here-and-now facts of the story rather than to the more complex overall context; therefore, their narratives were less coherent and sounded more like a listing of events.

Even when compared with children with specific language impairment, children with HFASD showed poorer narrative skills, especially in relaying the story's content and the character's goals and actions (Manolitsi & Botting, 2011). Craig and Baron-Cohen (2000) examined adolescents' ability to tell imaginative stories spontaneously and found that adolescents (mean CA = 12.9 years) with ASD were impaired in their ability to introduce imaginary elements into a spontaneous narrative. Limited narratives may be part of a wider deficit in ToM or information processing; yet, whichever underlying mechanism offers an adequate explanation, it is clear that limited narrative abilities hold implications for the academic functioning of children with ASD.

ACADEMIC ABILITIES

Patterns of academic achievement in children with HFASD have not yet been clearly demarcated. A wide range of academic achievement outcomes, from significantly above expected levels to far below expected levels, has been reported for this population (Estes et al., 2011; Griswold, Barnhill,

Myles, Hagiwara, & Simpson, 2002). The relations between IQ level and academic achievement found in the normal population do not appear as clear-cut within ASD, especially in reading and mathematics (as elaborated later in this section). In one study examining the IQ, reading, and arithmetic abilities of 100 adolescents with HFASD, significant "peaks" and "dips" emerged that were unrelated to the adolescents' IQ profiles (Jones et al., 2009). Similar findings appeared in a later study of children with HFASD (CA = 6–9 years; nonverbal IQ > 70), who demonstrated significant discrepancies (in both directions) between their actual academic achievement and the achievement levels predicted from their overall intellectual ability (Estes et al., 2011).

Whitby and Mancil's (2009) review of studies related to the academic abilities of students with HFASD concluded on the one hand that basic reading, encoding, and rote skills were intact for the most part and on the other hand that the main deficits were in the areas of comprehension, written expression, graphomotor skills, processing of complex materials in all academic domains, and problem solving (Barnhill, Hagiwara, Smith Myles, & Simpson, 2000; Griswold et al., 2002; Mayes & Calhoun, 2003a, 2003b). Furthermore, in many cases, deficits arose when academic requisites shifted from rote tasks to abstract tasks that demanded conceptual understanding.

Some children along the spectrum are said to have special skills, or what have been called "savant skills," such as an exceptional mastery of mathematics and calculation or an impressive expertise in music or art, along with enhanced visual-spatial skills. Vital, Ronald, Wallace, and Happé (2009) examined the relations between these special skills and autistic traits among 6,426 children (CA = 8 years) reported by parents as having such special abilities. They found that those children with special skills showed more ASD traits, especially repetitive and restricted interests and activities. According to the authors, special interests and insistence on sameness may underscore the obsessive factor leading to the special abilities, because children may practice obsessively until reaching perfection. However, these children's focus on details may also suggest that their special skills may result from a detail-focused, localizing cognitive style (Vital et al., 2009).

Mayes and Calhoun (2006) examined the frequency of reading, math, and writing disabilities in 949 children with clinical disorders, of whom 124 were diagnosed with ASD. They found that 30% of the ASD group had various levels of mental retardation (IQ < 80) and that 67% had learning disabilities, showing a severe discrepancy between academic achievement and intellectual ability. The highest percentage of learning disability was in written expression (60%), then in math (23%), spelling (9%), and reading (6%). The following sections highlight these children's strengths and weaknesses in the three major academic domains: reading, writing, and mathematics.

Reading

Reading is a cognitive process in which the reader understands that what can be said via speech can be written and then read again and understood by the writer or by someone else. In order to become a proficient reader, one must acquire an understanding of print, the skills to decipher the printed message into sounds, and the ability to comprehend its meaning (Nation, Clarke, Wright, & Williams, 2006; Whalon, Al Otaiba, & Delano, 2009). In the United States, the No Child Left Behind Act of 2001 and the Individuals with Disabilities Education Improvement Act of 2004 mandated that all children, including those with ASD, be taught to read in ways that are consistent with reading research, targeting the five components of evidence-based reading instruction: phonemic awareness, phonics, reading fluency, vocabulary, and comprehension strategies (Whalon et al., 2009). This book does not discuss the process of becoming a proficient reader in detail, yet it is important to emphasize that beginning readers learn to associate letters with sounds in order to access the written information represented by the written word and to comprehend the written message. Comprehension of the text is the goal of reading, and readers at all levels are expected to utilize their own knowledge and life experience in order to comprehend what is read.

Underlying cognitive deficits typical of ASD—weak central coherence, ToM, and executive function—may also delay acquisition of reading skills. Due to central coherence weakness, children with ASD may tend to focus on single words rather than global meaning (Randi et al., 2010). Deficits in readers' ability to understand others' perspectives (ToM) may hinder comprehension of even simplistic, mundane texts. Executive functioning components such as planning, inhibition, cognitive shifting, and working memory have also been linked with reading (decoding) and reading comprehension (Swanson, 1999). Moreover, children with ASD often reveal difficulties in processing and integrating sensory information (irregular sensory profiles), which may affect their ability to learn (Brown & Dunn, 2010). Additionally, specific reading instruction activities that are effective for some students may be ineffective for others, depending on students' individual characteristics (Connor et al., 2011).

In this section, we discuss the strengths and weaknesses of children with ASD throughout the various stages of reading, from literacy skills to proficiency. Literacy covers a wide range of skills, from exposure to print material to formal reading instruction. Visual literacy is the ability to establish meaning that is relayed by images and includes the use of photos, pictorial and simple graphic symbols and signs, and film. In the context of reading abilities, picture reading and logo reading are considered to be basic literacy skills (Alberto, Frederick, Hughes, McIntosh, & Cihak, 2007).

Students with ASD may fail to acquire literacy and reading skills for a number of reasons. For example, they may lack sufficient understanding of the instructional reading and writing tasks that they are asked to perform, which may reduce comprehension or interest (Basil & Reyes, 2003). Teaching literacy enables students with disabilities to develop a range of abilities based on their individual skills (Kluth & Darmody-Latham, 2003). When teaching literacy skills, it is important to involve the children in the learning experiences in a manner that is relevant and makes sense to them (Basil & Reyes, 2003). For example, in a study on preschoolers with LFA, Koppenhaver and Erickson (2003) found that the provision of a rich literacy environment increased children's understanding and use of print materials and tools. When natural opportunities for engagement with printed materials and writing tools were increasingly supplied, the children's emergent literacy skills improved.

We next elaborate on several areas of strength and deficiency that have been identified in the literacy skills of students with ASD regarding sight word, decoding, phonological awareness, and reading comprehension skills, as well as the unique characteristic phenomenon of hyperlexia. It is important to stress that the vast heterogeneity in reading ability across the spectrum requires utmost caution when interpreting test scores for this student population (Nation et al., 2006).

Sight-Word Skills

Sight-word instruction is the teaching of the whole word in a global manner, by memorization or by understanding it through its context instead of sounding it out through decoding strategies. Spector's (2011) review of evidence and expert opinions on sight-word instruction for children with ASD identified several potential benefits, especially its usefulness in teaching the communicative intent of print and in providing motivation for learning to read (Broun, 2004). According to Spector's overview, the sight-word approach may be considered a better starting point for students with ASD than the typical phonics-based approach, because the latter relies on abstract, auditory-based concepts that are more difficult for children with ASD. After children acquire a sufficient inventory of known sight words, this inventory may serve as a foundation on which teachers can instruct the abstract alphabetic concepts and principles of phonetics and reading (for further strategies, see Chapter 8).

Decoding Skills

Many children with HFASD have strengths in visual learning and decoding skills, which are the more concrete aspects of reading, whereas they are weaker in auditory learning, language, and comprehension, the more abstract aspects (Heumer & Mann, 2010; Nation et al., 2006; Whalon et al., 2009). Heumer and Mann (2010) examined the decoding and comprehension abilities of 384 children with HFASD (mean CA = 10.08 years) in comparison with 100 children with dyslexia (mean CA = 11.2 years) and found, as predicted, that the participants with HFASD achieved lower scores on all comprehension measures, whereas the participants with dyslexia showed lower scores on all decoding measures. Interestingly, the HFASD group showed relatively high achievement in isolated word reading, which in the general population is considered to be an important predictor of successful reading and reading comprehension but which is not a good predictor in HFASD.

Although decoding skills are considered to be a strong academic point in HFASD, some children are unable to perceive letters as the "building blocks" of words and hence are unable to combine letters into meaningful units (Broun, 2004). Although they may recognize various letters individually, some children have difficulty in combining the letters coherently into a comprehensive unit that builds a meaningful word. In these instances, the decoding abilities are lacking, and words are sometimes read as a combination of separate sound units (Broun, 2004).

Phonological Awareness Skills

This metalinguistic ability refers to the awareness of syllables and phonemes within spoken words and to the ability to manipulate the word at the levels of both the syllable and the individual phonemes. Phonological awareness is critical in learning to read and write in any alphabetic system, both in decoding and spelling unfamiliar words and in the expansion of known sight-word vocabulary. Gabig (2010) examined phonological awareness and single-word recognition in children with HFASD in comparison with an age-matched group with TYP at the early stages of reading acquisition. The children with HFASD scored below the children with TYP on the phonological awareness tasks, as predicted. Interestingly, this study also reported no significant correlations between measures of phonological awareness and measures of word recognition for either real-word identification or nonword reading for the children with HFASD, whereas high correlations emerged for the children with TYP. As for the groups' word recognition and decoding abilities, no statistical intergroup difference emerged on the word recognition task, but the children with HFASD showed more difficulties when reading nonwords than real words, suggesting problematic decoding abilities when trying to read an unfamiliar word. According to Gabig (2010), word recognition involves reading words by visual memory or sight. Children with HFASD may thus be assumed to possess rote memory for visual forms of words and can thus recall from memory the spelling patterns and pronunciations of the sight words shown. In sum, this study demonstrated that complete word analysis skills, including phonological awareness, were less developed for the children with HFASD than for the children with TYP.

Reading Comprehension Skills

During the third grade, reading comprehension demands usually become more intense, as reading instruction in the general classroom shifts from decoding skills to comprehension skills. At this point the child is expected to understand the main idea, make inferences, and grasp the cause-and-effect relations within the text (Whitby & Mancil, 2009; Whitby, Travers, & Harnik, 2009). There are many reports that children with HFASD experience reading comprehension difficulties (Heumer & Mann, 2010; Mayes & Calhoun, 2003a, 2003b; Nation et al., 2006; Randi et al., 2010; Wahlberg & Magliano, 2004). However, in many cases reading comprehension is only impaired and not entirely lacking (O'Connor & Klein, 2004). To read for understanding, readers apply a wide array of cognitive abilities, such as inference and attention, motivational strategies, knowledge of vocabulary, and prior knowledge of the topic (Randi et al., 2010). Comprehension difficulties in HFASD may stem from problems in integrating information with a coherent context (Frith & Snowling, 1983; Randi et al., 2010); difficulty comprehending linguistic units beyond the word level (O'Connor & Klein, 2004); general language impairment; deficits in ToM (Mason et al., 2008; see also Chapter 1, this volume); and, when reading longer texts, memory dysfunction (Randi et al., 2010). Executive dysfunctions such as poor cognitive flexibility may hinder readers' ability to shift flexibly between phonological and semantic processing on the one hand and decoding and comprehension strategies on the other (Randi et al., 2010; see also Chapter 1, this volume). According to Heumer and Mann (2010), reading comprehension difficulties in children with HFASD apparently stem from difficulties that are not related solely to phonological or decoding abilities.

In a study analyzing reading skills and abilities (word decoding in and out of context, answering factual and inferential questions following aloud and silent reading) among children and adolescents with Asperger syndrome (mean CA = 9.4 years), both silent reading level and independent reading level (defined by the authors as the reading-aloud level at which one reads comfortably, with 95% word recognition and 75% or more comprehension) were lower than those of the TYP control group (Smith-Myles et al., 2002). Although reading comprehension improved on the factual-questions measure in the Asperger syndrome group when they read the text out loud, they continued to give erroneous responses on two-thirds of the inferential questions, exhibiting a difference between their factual understanding and their high-order inferential comprehension of texts. Inasmuch as the majority of academic demands require silent reading and inferential comprehension, the authors asserted that youngsters with Asperger syndrome need appropriate study and testing accommodations and structure in order to succeed academically (see Chapter 8 regarding intervention strategies).

Saldana and Frith (2007) examined the ability of adolescents with HFASD to make inferences from their own world knowledge in comparison with adolescents with TYP who were matched on word reading accuracy, CA, and vocabulary, but not on text comprehension (on which the HFASD group scored lower). The authors constructed two-line vignettes with either physical content that necessitated inferences (i.e., cowboys and Indians, books and boxes), followed by a general question that was either primed by the inference (e.g., "The Indians pushed the rocks off the cliff onto the cowboys. The cowboys were badly injured. Can rocks be large?") or not primed by the inference (e.g., "The Indians pushed the cowboys off the cliff onto the rocks. The cowboys were badly injured. Can rocks be large?") or social content (i.e., "Maria had never won a race before. The tears streamed down Maria's face. Can people cry because they are happy?"). Response accuracy was not scored; only reading speed and response time were measured. When the question was not primed, reading and response speeds were expected to be slightly longer than for primed questions. No differences emerged between the HFASD and TYP groups; both groups read and answered the primed questions more quickly than unprimed questions, regardless of the physical or social world knowledge context. These findings contrast with previous outcomes that pinpointed a difficulty making inferences among individuals with HFASD (Nation et al., 2006; Smith-Myles et al., 2002). Saldana and Frith (2007) suggested that one possible explanation for this discrepancy was intact automatic processing at the sentence level. Nevertheless, when presented with longer passages, many students with HFASD have shown a better ability to answer literal comprehension questions than inferential questions (Carnahan, Williamson, & Haydon, 2009).

In addition to text length, text genre also influences comprehension. Narrative texts appear to be more complex for readers with HFASD than informative and expository texts (Carnahan et al., 2009; Gately, 2008). A prerequisite to understanding narrative texts is the understanding of the various social cues given by the author through which the reader must understand the author's intent, as well as the characters' social situations, motivations, experiences, and more (Gately, 2008).

Hyperlexia

The phenomenon of superior word reading skills that extend far above the individual's reading comprehension ability is termed "hyperlexia." This concurrence of very high decoding skills on the one hand but low comprehension skills on the other may therefore be referred to as a comprehension disorder (Cardoso-Martins & da Silva, 2010; Grigorenko, Volkmar, & Klin, 2003; Newman et al., 2007). There appears to be a higher frequency of hyperlexia among children with ASD in comparison with children with TYP or with other clinical disabilities, and between 5 and 10% of children on the spectrum exhibit hyperlexia (Grigorenko et al., 2003). Many children with hyperlexia are described as having an unusual passion for and interest in the printed word.

Newman et al. (2007) compared the decoding and reading comprehension abilities of three different groups: children with HFASD and hyperlexia (mean CA = 10.4 years), children with HFASD without hyperlexia (mean CA = 12.3 years), and children with TYP (mean CA = 9.9 years). The single-word recognition skills of the HFASD hyperlexic group were higher than those of the HFASD nonhyperlexic group but were matched to those of the TYP group. Furthermore, children as young as 3 years of age in the HFASD hyperlexic group had single-word recognition skills that enabled decoding abilities. On the reading comprehension measure, the two HFASD groups performed similarly, both scoring lower than the TYP group. The authors concluded that word recognition at a young age is an isolated skill that is typical of children with hyperlexia, who may develop this particular skill as a result of deliberate and often obsessive practice (Newman et al., 2007).

Cardoso-Martins and da Silva (2010) conducted two studies to investigate the correlation between hyperlexia and LFA, one in school-age children with LFA and with TYP and one in preschoolers. The results of both studies suggested that children with hyperlexia learn to read by processing and recognizing letter–sound relations in words. The authors concluded that the phonological abilities of the children with LFA, along with their restricted interests and obsessiveness, enhance their precocious and outstanding single-word reading. In addition, the authors underscored the hyperlexic readers' disregard of meaning as a key to their early development of word decoding ability, explaining that the children regard reading solely as a decoding process without emphasis on comprehension.

Writing Abilities

Reading and writing are interrelated skills within the larger competency domain of literacy. One cannot relate to one skill without the other, and writing instruction should occur in the context of reading instruction. Writing—the ability to form letters and words—is used to express oneself and communicate. In school, writing is a necessary activity, without which one cannot participate as a pupil. As in reading, writing involves two main stages. The first stage is motor-graphic and cognitive (including planning, language, and orthographic abilities), in which the child learns how to form letters and spell words. In the second stage, writing itself becomes an automatic process, and the cognitive demands become of higher order, leading to composition (Kushki, Chau, & Anagnostou, 2011). Therefore, writing correlates with academic achievement.

Kushki et al. (2011) reviewed the existing literature to identify those factors that may potentially contribute to handwriting (the first stage of writing) in children with ASD. Most of the potential factors that lead to handwriting ability were those found to be impaired in ASD, including fine motor skills, motor control, visual-motor integration, and, in some cases, kinesthesia. Their research review uncovered only seven articles related to handwriting abilities in ASD, and all of these studies showed lower legibility, specifically poorer letter formation and handwriting quality, in ASD.

With regard to the higher-order stage of writing, Brown and Klein (2011) compared the written composition ability of adults with HFASD (mean CA = 25.75 years) and adults with TYP (mean CA = 26.56 years). After watching a video showing a problematic interpersonal situation, participants were asked to complete two writing tasks in different genres. In the expository task, they wrote an essay on the topic of problems between people, and in the narrative task they wrote a personal story about a problem that they had encountered with someone. The most important finding was that the quality of writing in both genres was significantly lower in the HFASD group than in the control group. In the expository texts, adults with HFASD had difficulty keeping focused on the main idea and transitioning from idea to idea. In the narrative texts, they had difficulty organizing the texts and supplying readers with sufficient background information, and the texts themselves were simplistic. Furthermore, the narrative texts written by the HFASD group were significantly shorter than those of the TYP group. As to the mechanics of text writing (i.e., spelling scores, grammar, clauses per measured unit), Brown and Klein (2011) found a nonsignificant trend toward lower abilities in the HFASD group.

Academic demands on children are not limited to reading and writing skills, and in the course of their academic learning, they are also expected to develop mathematical abilities.

Mathematics

Research concerning the mathematical ability of individuals with ASD is sparse. Chiang and Lin's (2007) review of cumulative empirical evidence on overall mathematical abilities and disabilities of individuals with HFASD demonstrated that the majority of these students showed average mathematical ability compared with their peers with TYP. In 8 of the 18 studies presented in their review, standardized tests were administered, thus enabling the authors to examine the relative strengths or weaknesses of these students in mathematics in comparison with their IQs. They found that the arithmetic scores were significantly lower than the mean of the WISC scaled scores (Wechsler, 1991), showing that their mathematical ability was relatively lower than their intellectual ability, although the clinical significance of the difference was small. Furthermore, their findings also suggested that some individuals with HFASD have mathematical giftedness. For example, James (2003, 2010), a professor of geometry at Oxford University who studied autism and mathematical talent, referred to the small but unique percentage of individuals with HFASD who possess outstanding mathematical abilities.

Considering the risk of underachievement in mathematics for this population, it is important to recognize the various areas of instruction regarding mathematics. According to Whitby and Mancil (2009), computational skills seem to be intact in the majority of students with HFASD, whereas difficulties emerge in solving complex mathematical problems. Cihak and Foust (2008) reported that when these students are taught mathematical skills, they can acquire functional activities such as counting, managing time, and money skills. Also, once competent in basic computational math, they can learn to manage banking, purchasing, and budgeting.

Among the difficulties that students with ASD may display when solving mathematical problems is the inability to randomly state a number that fits given parameters (e.g., stating a number that is larger than X but smaller than Y). Williams, Moss, Bradshaw, and Rinehart (2002) examined this ability among adolescents and adults with ASD (mean CA = 23.2 years; mean MA = 5.98 years) compared with a TYP group (mean CA = 25.7 years) and compared with an MA-matched intellectual disability group (mean CA = 23.9 years; mean MA = 5.99 years). When asked to generate random numbers, those in the ASD group committed more repetitions than in the other two groups.

SUMMARY AND CONCLUSIONS

As seen in all the academic domains and also in the cognitive characteristics reviewed, the achievements and abilities of children with HFASD may vary from very low to very high and even gifted (Foley-Nicpon, Assouline, & Stinson, 2012). Yet two major themes characterize the empirical literature on cognitive-academic functioning. First, when tasks are more complex, more impairment appears in HFASD relative to TYP. This finding emerges, among others, in the areas of memory, information processing, language, concept formation, reading, and mathematics. Second, children with HFASD show more impairment in abstract learning than in concrete tasks. This phenomenon appears in their information-processing, imitation, general language, and narrative abilities and in sight-word instruction, decoding skills, and reading comprehension.

Throughout this chapter, we discussed the complex cognitive and academic abilities of students with HFASD and how they compare with those of students with TYP. The prominence of reading, writing, and mathematical skills at school underscores the importance of further research alongside investigation of appropriate instructional strategies for these students with HFASD. For some, specific academic tasks may seem to be insurmountable; yet understanding the nature of the specific learning disabilities and difficulties that students with HFASD exhibit may assist educators in developing more individualized and effective interventions. Chapter 8 illustrates examples of appropriate learning interventions specific to students with HFASD.

Chapter 6

Associated Comorbid Conditions

Comorbidity is defined as the co-occurrence of two (or more) independent clinical diagnoses in the same person (Matson & Nebel-Schwalm, 2007). Comorbidity in ASD means that, in addition to meeting the full criteria for autism disorder, the child receives a diagnosis of another disorder, such as a mood disorder, ADHD, or OCD. The identification of comorbidity in ASD has important clinical–therapeutic implications. If a child does have another disorder, that comorbid disorder should receive specific treatment in addition to the interventions and educational strategies that the child receives based on the autism diagnosis. For example, individuals with HFASD who have comorbid psychiatric conditions may demonstrate a more complex neurodevelopmental disorder than those with HFASD alone (Matson & Nebel-Schwalm, 2007). Some research indicates that comorbidity may occur at higher frequencies among individuals with HFASD than among lower-functioning individuals on the spectrum (e.g., see Mayes, Calhoun, Murray, Ahuja, & Smith, 2011, for comorbid depression and anxiety disorders). Thus the existence of a comorbid disorder may significantly impact the design of educational and treatment plans to address the social-emotional and cognitive-academic functioning of children with HFASD.

Although ASD does co-occur with different psychiatric disorders such as ADHD, mood disorder, anxiety disorder, OCD, and others, the exact rates of co-occurrence are somewhat unclear because of several complications. The first complication is methodological. The vast majority of individuals who participated in empirical studies were recruited through clinical referral rather than from the wider community, suggesting that those who came to a clinic for diagnosis most likely exhibited more severe symptomology than those who did not. This selection bias may have resulted in elevated rates of psychiatric comorbidities reported for ASD. Second, differential diagnosis is challenging because many symptoms overlap between ASD and other psychiatric disorders. For example, inattention is a feature of both ASD and ADHD; social withdrawal characterizes both ASD and depression; obsessions and rituals appear both in ASD and in OCD; and so on. Adding to this complexity is the difficulty involved in establishing valid, specialized screening and evaluation measures and psychiatric diagnostic tools to account for the complex possible overlaps between ASD and other psychiatric disorders (e.g., Stewart, Barnard, Pearson, Hasan, & O'Brien, 2006).

In this chapter, I describe the major related conditions that have been empirically explored as comorbid with HFASD: ADHD, mood disorders, anxiety disorders, and OCD. For each of these comorbid conditions, this chapter (1) provides its clinical description, (2) discusses its symptom overlap with HFASD, (3) furnishes guidelines for making differential diagnosis, and (4) describes its frequency of comorbidity with ASD. Finally, I describe the instruments commonly utilized to evaluate comorbidity in HFASD. This review mainly covers findings related to HFASD or to the contribution of IQ to comorbid conditions in ASD.

MAJOR COMORBID DIAGNOSES

HFASD with Comorbid ADHD

Definition of ADHD

The estimated prevalence of ADHD in school-age children ranges between 3 and 7%, indicating a very common childhood neurodevelopmental disorder. Children with ADHD may have one of several presentation specifiers, including an inattentive presentation (e.g., failing to attend to details, losing things, getting distracted, being disorganized), a hyperactive–impulsive presentation (e.g., moving or speaking excessively, fidgeting, intruding into others' activities, having difficulty staying seated), or a combined inattentive and hyperactive–impulsive presentation (e.g., Tannock, 2013).

Some ADHD symptoms overlap with some HFASD symptoms, thus hindering differential diagnosis. More specifically, HFASD and the predominantly inattentive type of ADHD seem to share symptoms such as difficulties in following instructions, problems in listening when spoken to directly, and executive functioning difficulties such as poor planning and organizational skills (Mayes, Calhoun, Mayes, & Molitoris, 2012). Overlap between HFASD and the predominantly hyperactive–impulsive type of ADHD may exist regarding symptoms such as excessive talking, problems awaiting one's turn, or interrupting others (e.g., Reiersen & Todd, 2011).

Differential Diagnosis

A closer look at symptom quality and underlying mechanisms may help in determining a differential diagnosis between ADHD and HFASD. For one, the source of distraction to attention is usually external in ADHD (e.g., noises, others' activity), whereas it is usually internal in HFASD (e.g., a strong preference for one's own idiosyncratic interests, such as spending hours reading a book). Inattention in HFASD takes the form of overfocusing on particular stimuli of interest and underfocusing on other aspects of the situation (most likely social aspects of stimuli such as facial expression, intonation, or body gesture). Yet such inattentiveness alone would not lead to a consideration of comorbid ADHD (Murray, 2010). In addition, symptoms of hyperactivity are not considered to be defining characteristics of HFASD. Hyperactivity in ASD may be seen in highly repetitive motor stereotypies or as a result of anxiety or agitation during highly demanding social or sensory environments, but these would not be considered indicators of the hyperactive–impulsive ADHD type among individuals with HFASD (Murray, 2010).

Prevalence of ADHD in HFASD

The DSM-IV-TR (APA, 2000) disallowed the co-existence of ADHD and ASD in the same person, but empirical studies have demonstrated evidence of a high prevalence of ADHD in individuals with HFASD, whether community-based studies (e.g., Mattila et al., 2010; Reiersen, Constantino, Volk, & Todd, 2007; Ronald, Simonoff, Kuntsi, Asherson, & Plomin, 2008; Simonoff et al., 2008) or clinic-based research (e.g., de Bruin, Ferdinand, Meester, de Nijs, & Verheij, 2007; Gadow, DeVincent, & Pomeroy, 2006; Lee & Ousley, 2006; Leyfer et al., 2006; Mattila et al., 2010; Sturm, Fernell, & Gillberg, 2004; Yoshida & Uchiyama, 2004). For example, Yoshida and Uchiyama (2004) found that 69% of school-age children with HFASD in their clinic-based sample (CA = 7–15 years) met diagnostic criteria for ADHD: 38% with inattentive type, 8% with hyperactive–impulsive type, and 23% with combined type. Similar results emerged from Sturm et al.'s (2004) study of the medical and psychiatric records of school-age Swedish children with HFASD (CA = 5–12 years), where 75% met criteria for ADHD, of whom the majority (95%) showed attention problems and about half (56%) demonstrated hyperactive–impulsive problems. Similar findings emerged in Lee and Ousley (2006) for smaller clinical samples defined as HFASD; 7 of the 12 children and adolescents with Asperger syndrome (58%) met criteria for ADHD, and 10 of the 13 children and adolescents with PDD-NOS (77%) met ADHD criteria. In their study, as in the former findings, the inattentive type of ADHD was the most common type in Asperger syndrome (42%) and in PDD-NOS (46%).

Likewise, de Bruin et al. (2007) reported that 45% of school-age children with PDD-NOS (CA = 1.5–12.11 years, mean = 8.5 years; Full Scale IQ = 55–120, mean = 91.22 IQ; with diagnosis verified by ADOS; Lord et al., 2000) met the criteria for ADHD: 15% inattentive type; 8.5% hyperactive–impulsive type; 21.3% combined. Yet, as their IQ range indicates, not all of these participants were high functioning, even though their mean IQ exceeded retardation level. Similar percentages (53%) of ADHD comorbidity were reported by Gadow et al. (2006) for a clinical sample of children with ASD (CA = 3–12 years; 35% autism; 22% Asperger syndrome; and 43% PDD- NOS), although no specific percentages were reported for the more cognitively able children in the sample. In a like manner, Leyfer et al. (2006) also found that 31% of their ASD sample (CA = 5.1–17.0; mean = 9.2 years) met the criteria for comorbid ADHD; however, this percentage referred to the whole sample, whereas only 67.7% of the sample met criteria for HFASD (IQ > 70).

Population-based studies, unsurprisingly, show lower frequencies of comorbidity. Providing a somewhat different point of view to the co-occurrence of ADHD and HFASD, Reiersen et al.'s (2007) twin study (N = 495) demonstrated elevated autistic traits in children with ADHD from the general population, as measured by the Social Responsiveness Scale (SRS; Constantino & Gruber, 2005). Although it is difficult to determine whether these children with autistic traits would have met the full criteria for ASD, this finding is interesting and supports the link between the two disorders. Another study derived from a population-based twin sample in the United Kingdom reported 41% ADHD comorbidity in individuals with Asperger syndrome (Ronald et al., 2008). Mattila et al. (2010) found that 38% of their Finnish participants with Asperger syndrome or HFASD in a combined community- and clinic-based sample (n = 50, CA = 9–16 years) met criteria for ADHD, with 68% showing ADHD combined type and 32% showing inattentive type (and none meeting criteria for hyperactive–impulsive type). A similar picture emerged for each sample separately: In the community-based sample (n = 18, CA = 12–13 years), 33% met criteria for ADHD, comprising 83% combined type and 17% inattentive type. In the clinic-based sample (n = 32, CA = 9–16 years), 40% met criteria for ADHD, comprising 62.3% combined type and 37.5% inattentive type. Simonoff et al. (2008) found lower rates of ADHD (28.2%, with 84% combined type) in their large population study of children with ASD (N = 112, CA = 10–14 years), but many of these participants were not high functioning (IQ = 19–124; mean = 72.7). Interestingly, no associations emerged between IQ and ADHD in their study.

In sum, clinic-based studies specific to HFASD have indicated rates of comorbidity with ADHD that range from 40 to 75%, whereas studies that were not HFASD-specific yielded somewhat lower rates (31–53%), resembling the rates obtained for community-based HFASD-specific samples (33%). Thus, even if it is difficult to precisely estimate the prevalence of

ADHD in individuals with HFASD, it is clear that a significant percentage of children with HFASD do meet a diagnosis for ADHD. This clear outcome justifies the modified perception suggested in DSM-5 (APA, 2013) to allow the co-occurrence of these two diagnoses.

Moreover, when these two disorders co-occur, they may affect children's social and adaptive functioning, as well as their executive control, leading to a more severe clinical profile and possibly to poorer outcomes, especially socially. For example, children's autism-linked insistence on playing games with peers that are oriented toward their own peculiarities may be exacerbated by their ADHD-linked tendency to move quickly between peer activities (Murray, 2010). Thus children with HFASD who demonstrate comorbid ADHD features may require specialized intervention efforts for both disorders, indicating that treatments should be tailor-made (Murray, 2010; Reiersen & Todd, 2011).

HFASD with Comorbid Mood Disorders

Higher IQs have been linked with greater levels of depression in individuals with ASD (see review in Szatmari & McConnell, 2011). For example, in a study of adults with ASD (CA = 18–44 years), Sterling, Dawson, Estes, and Greenson (2008) found that individuals with less social impairment, higher cognitive ability, and higher rates of other psychiatric symptoms were more likely to report depressive symptoms. Indeed, researchers have suggested that individuals with HFASD are at higher risk of developing comorbid mood disorders than their less cognitively able counterparts, due to their more developed awareness of their social deficit and isolation (e.g., Hedley & Young, 2006). Barnhill and Smith-Myles (2001) found that adolescents with Asperger syndrome who felt responsible for their social failure at school experienced heightened levels of depression. This subsection describes the most common mood disorders: major depressive disorder and dysthymic disorder.

Definition of Mood Disorders

Most studies on the comorbidity of mood disorders with HFASD have reported co-occurence with major depressive disorders (MDD), involving depressed affect and/or diminished interest or pleasure in almost all life activities. MDD causes clinically significant impairment in important domains such as social or occupational functioning. HFASD can also co-occur with dysthymic disorder, which involves milder but consistently depressed mood most of every day for a minimum of 2 years. Both disorders involve symptoms such as sleep or eating disturbances, feelings of unimportance and low self-esteem, concentration difficulties, and a sense of hopelessness (APA, 2013).

The diagnostic criteria for depression are similar in children and adults; however, symptom profile may differ with age. Children and adolescents may manifest agitation, irritability, and bad temper, whereas adults may exhibit sadness or depressed mood. In addition, somatic complaints and social withdrawal are more frequent in children than in adults (APA, 2000). A recent nation-based survey by the National Comorbidity Survey—Adolescent Supplement showed a prevalence of 11.2% for major depression among adolescents (CA = 13–18 years) in the United States (Merikangas et al., 2010). In children, clinical depression affects girls and boys at about the same rate, but over the lifespan major depression is twice as common in females as in males, with overall population rates of 8–12% (e.g., Kessler et al., 2003, 2005).

Differential Diagnosis

Social withdrawal is a common symptom of both HFASD and depression. In addition, individuals with HFASD are characterized by atypical and restricted means of emotional expression, such as inadequate, flat, or mechanical intonation; atypical range and clarity of facial expression; and difficulties in expressing and communicating emotions (e.g., Begeer et al., 2008; Hubbard & Trauner, 2007; see also Chapter 2, this volume, on social cognition and emotions). On the one hand, these atypical emotional expressions may mask depressive symptoms at times, but on the other hand, they may mislead significant others to conclude that the individual with HFASD has depression even when that is not the case (e.g., Ghaziuddin, Ghaziuddin, & Greden, 2002; Matson & Nebel-Schwalm, 2007). Other symptoms, such as sleep and appetite disturbances, may also characterize both disorders (Stewart et al., 2006).

Change in symptoms' severity or profile is a key guide for differential diagnosis between HFASD and depression. Symptoms may indeed overlap between the two disorders, but they are chronic in HFASD and not episodic, as in most cases of depression (Mayes et al., 2011). The most common symptoms found to signify depression in HFASD according to Stewart et al.'s (2006) review of studies up to 2003 were depressed mood (reflected in sad facial expression and an increase in crying and irritability); loss of interest in activities; and deterioration in adaptive functioning, especially in self-care behaviors and personal hygiene. Interestingly, symptoms such as worthlessness, guilt, diminished ability to concentrate, and suicidal thoughts—which are frequent in individuals with depression—were not frequent in HFASD (Stewart et al., 2006). Along with fatigue and hypoactivity (slowing down or even stopping one's usual activities), individuals with HFASD may also become more active. They may show an increase in the intensity and severity of such symptoms as obsessive–compulsive behaviors (e.g., Ghaziuddin, Weidmer-Mikhail, & Ghaziuddin,

1998) or aggression, irritability, and oppositional behaviors (e.g., Kim, Szatmari, Bryson, Streiner, & Wilson, 2000; Lainhart, 1999; Matson & Nebel-Schwalm, 2007). Kim et al. (2000) found that children with HFASD and comorbid depression (CA = 9–14 years) demonstrated higher levels of aggressive behavior that had an influence on parental participation in social activities, as well as on the child's relationships with teachers, peers, and family members.

Prevalence of Mood Disorders in HFASD

Mood disorders are a prevalent comorbid condition in children, adolescents, and adults with HFASD (e.g., Ghaziuddin et al., 1998; Kim et al., 2000; Leyfer et al., 2006; Mayes et al., 2011; Mazefsky, Conner, & Oswald, 2010; McPheeter, Davis, Navarre, & Scott, 2011; Sterling et al., 2008; Wing, 1981), and they are more likely to appear in families with a history of depression (Ghaziuddin & Greden, 1998). Furthermore, among children with HFASD (mean CA = 11 years, mean IQ = 75.3) depression was linked with a higher frequency of negative life events (e.g., bereavement, parental marital discord) in the 12 months before onset of depression (Ghaziuddin, Alessi, & Greden, 1995). Measuring depression, Kim et al. (2000) reported that 16.9% of children with Asperger syndrome and HFASD (CA = 9–14 years, IQ > 70) scored at least two standard deviations above the mean of a random community sample (N = 1,751). Several other studies demonstrated even higher depression rates in HFASD at similar ages. For example, Mayes et al. (2011) collected maternal reports on children's depressed mood, yielding rates of 54% for children with HFASD compared with 42% for children with LFA and only 19% for children with TYP (n = 233; CA = 6–16 years, mean = 8.3 years; mean IQ = 103).

In order to understand the rates of depression in HFASD, it is important to make a distinction between a syndromal profile of depression, which meets the full DSM-5 criteria (APA, 2013) for MDD, and a subsyndromal profile, which falls short of meeting the DSM criteria (Leyfer et al., 2006). Syndromal rates of depression were somewhat lower (10%) than subsyndromal rates (24%) in Leyfer et al.'s study (CA = 5–17 years, mean = 9.2 years), but only two-thirds of that sample were high functioning (Full Scale IQ > 70). Based on a sample including only youngsters with HFASD (CA = 10–17 years, mean = 11.90 years; Verbal IQ = 71–147, mean IQ = 106.35; Full Scale IQ = 71–144, mean = 104.84), Mazefsky et al. (2010) reported that 32% met criteria for syndromal or subsyndromal diagnosis under the "any depression" category (including dysthymia and depression not otherwise specified), whereas only 19% met criteria for a full MDD syndromal diagnosis. Also, 40% of Green, Gilchrist, Burton, and Cox's (2000) sample of adolescents with Asperger syndrome had chronic unhappiness, but only an additional 5% met criteria for MDD. Thus it seems that children with

HFASD more often tend to show depressed mood or a subsyndromal profile of depression rather than full-blown MDD. Alternatively, current methodologies may not be reliably capturing the symptoms of MDD in HFASD, due to the lack of specific depression measurements adapted to HFASD.

Among adults with HFASD, percentages of depression are somewhat higher than those of children or adolescents. In Sterling et al.'s (2008) sample, based mostly on adults with HFASD (CA = 18.33–44.75, mean = 26.82 years), 43% exhibited a significant level of depressive symptoms. These authors found that individuals who qualified for a mood disorder diagnosis were older, more cognitively able (had higher Verbal and Full Scale IQs), and scored higher on the ADOS social domain (Lord et al., 2000) than individuals who did not meet the diagnostic criteria. Wing (1981) reported that depression was the most common comorbid psychiatric diagnosis among adults with Asperger syndrome, occurring in 30% of her sample (N = 34). Ghaziuddin et al. (1998) reported similar rates of depression (37%) for a sample including individuals between the ages of 8 and 51 years (mean = 15.1 years; mean Verbal IQ = 105.9; mean Full Scale IQ = 102.7), where 23% met criteria for MDD, 11.4% met criteria for dysthymic disorder, and 2.8% (n = 1) met criteria for bipolar disorder.

Most of the reported rates of depression were derived from clinic-based samples; however, a more recent study (McPheeter et al., 2011) estimated the prevalence of depression among children ages 4–17 years with ASD using a national U.S. sample of 125,000 parents during the years 2003–2004. Of these parents, 40% reported having been told by a health care provider that their child had depression or anxiety in addition to autism, although the frequency of such reports was low in early childhood (5.6%, ages 4–6; 48.4%, ages 7–10; 46.0%, ages 11–17; see similar reports in Ghaziuddin et al.'s [2002] review.) However, these outcomes should be taken with caution because (1) information is lacking on how diagnoses were obtained, (2) percentages referred to the whole ASD spectrum, without differentiating HFASD, and (3) these data mixed depression and anxiety diagnoses. Indeed, anxiety is another frequent comorbid disorder in individuals with HFASD, as described next.

HFASD with Comorbid Anxiety Disorders

Among the various anxiety disorders, the following have been considered to co-occur more frequently with HFASD (APA, 2000): a specific phobia (i.e., significant fear of a distinct, well-defined object/situation) or a social phobia (i.e., significant fear of a potentially embarrassing performance/social situation); a generalized anxiety disorder (i.e., disproportionate anxiety or worry about multiple incidents or activities that is hard to control and continues for a minimum of 6 months on more days than not); and OCD (i.e., repeated unwelcome compulsions such as hand washing or obsessions such as intrusive thoughts that require a significant investment of time or lead to discernible distress or impairment). Thus, in this section, I focus on these anxiety disorders.

Definition of Anxiety Disorders

All people experience anxious feelings from time to time, but fear or tension are considered pathological when they are intense, excessive, irrational, and uncontrollable and when they affect people's ability to manage daily tasks and relate to others. Anxiety may be accompanied by a range of physical and affective symptoms such as increased heart rate, tensed muscles, rapid breathing, and intensive fear without a noticeable reason. Such anxiety may lead to a change in the person's behaviors (e.g., avoidance) and cognitions (e.g., compulsive thoughts).

Anxiety disorders are common within the general population. In the United States 18% of adults show an anxiety disorder at some point in their lives, and 4.1% of them present with severe disorder (Kessler et al., 2005). A full quarter (25.1%) of adolescents in the general population (CA = 13–18 years) exhibit an anxiety disorder, of which 5.9% are severe (Merikangas et al., 2010). Among these adolescents, percentages for the different anxiety disorders range from 2.2% for generalized anxiety disorder to 19.3% for specific phobia. The earliest onset is defined as young as 6 years, with elevating risk toward older adolescence and among adolescents whose parents were divorced or separated (Merikangas et al., 2010). As in the case of mood disorders, anxiety disorders are more common in females than males across the lifespan (e.g., Kessler et al. 2005; Merikangas et al., 2010).

Differential Diagnosis

Avoidance of social interaction is a characteristic of individuals with ASD, yet is not necessarily a sign of social phobia. Crowded situations involving many people are overwhelming and fearful for many children on the autism spectrum, as are noises that may provoke distress (e.g., school bell, vacuum cleaner). Thus social and specific phobias are not easy to differentiate from HFASD. Even more difficult is the challenge of differentiating between OCD and HFASD, because both disorders share the existence of obsessive and compulsive behaviors as a defining criterion.

DIFFERENTIAL DIAGNOSIS BETWEEN HFASD AND OCD

The key to differential diagnosis between HFASD and OCD lies in both emotional reactions and contents. First, in OCD but usually not in HFASD, the obsessive–compulsive preoccupation is painful, and performing the compulsion results in anxiety reduction or prevention, whereas in ASD it may provide some gratification and pleasure. Thus children's emotional reaction to the perseverative thoughts may be a criterion for differential diagnosis (Spiker, Lin, Van Dyke, & Wood, 2012; Wood & Gadow, 2010). However, for some children on the spectrum, repetitive behaviors can increase in frequency and intensity during stressful situations, as a reaction to change, or during transitional periods, which only adds to the complexity of differential diagnosis based on emotional reaction (Wood & Gadow, 2010). As a result, children's emotional reaction cannot be the only criterion for differential diagnosis, and the contents of the obsessions should also be considered.

Contents of obsessions and compulsions may differ between OCD and HFASD. Taylor and Hollander's (2011) recent review of work in the field provided a helpful summary of repetitive behaviors that may be comparable or dissimilar in OCD and ASD. Their classification of repetitive stereotypical behaviors in ASD into high order (cognitively mediated) versus low order (primitive brain processes) may specifically help in differential diagnosis of the two disorders. High-order repetitive behaviors include complex behaviors such as circumscribed interest and preoccupation, a need for sameness, adherence to rituals and routines, and repetitive language, whereas low-order behaviors include repetitive sensory and motor behavior such as stereotypical movements (e.g., body rocking, finger flicking, hand flapping) and repetitive use of objects (Taylor & Hollander, 2011).

Taylor and Hollander's (2011) review reported that low-order repetitive sensory and motor behaviors such as touching, rubbing, stereotypical body movements, repetitive use of objects, unusual sensory interests, and self-injuring behaviors were linked only to ASD. High-order behaviors in the category of sameness (e.g., resistance to change) were also linked to ASD. However, high-order cleaning behaviors and fear of contamination, as well as forbidden thoughts, such as thoughts about aggression, sex, religion, and somatic symptoms, were identified as unique to OCD. Nevertheless, both high- and low-order subtypes of repetitive behaviors can be identified in OCD; for example, intrusive repetitive thoughts may be considered high-order behaviors (e.g., of harm—"Did I hurt him?"—or of doubt—"Did I close the oven?"), whereas engagement in repetitive actions (e.g., hand washing) may be considered low-order repetitive behaviors, thus impeding differential diagnosis. Several symptoms that were found to overlap between OCD and ASD included hoarding and higher-order symmetry such as repeating, counting, or checking.

DIFFERENTIAL DIAGNOSIS BETWEEN SPECIFIC
AND SOCIAL PHOBIA AND HFASD

Not many studies have explored the types of fears that characterize children with ASD. Parental reports (Evans, Canavera, Kleinpeter, Maccubbin,

& Taga, 2005) highlighted that children with ASD exhibited a distinct profile of fear and anxiety compared with children with Down syndrome and to children with TYP matched for CA and MA (mean CA = 9.20 years; mean MA = 5.53 years; mean IQ = 59). This ASD profile included more situational fears, such as fears of crowded transportation and medical situations (e.g., shots, blood tests, physician's exam), but fewer fears of harm or injury (e.g., fears of one's own or a parent's death, fear of fire). In addition, externalizing problem behaviors such as conduct, impulsive, and hyperactive symptoms were associated with these fears only in ASD. Likewise, Matson and Love (1990) also identified a fear profile for ASD (CA = 2.5–17.0 years) that differed qualitatively from the fear profile of CA-matched children with TYP. Children with ASD feared thunderstorms, dark places, large crowds, dark rooms or closets, going to bed in the dark, and closed places; whereas children with TYP feared failure or criticism (social anxiety), harm and injury, small animals, and punishment.

These two studies are helpful in starting to delineate a fear profile in ASD, but their participants were not high functioning. Specific examination of fear profiles for more cognitively able children is important because they may differ (e.g., including higher rates of social anxiety; see, e.g., Gillott, Furniss, & Walter, 2001) based on their higher social awareness and understanding.

Symptoms of social phobia and those of ASD may be differentiated based on the phobia's content. If the anxiety has social attributions (negative evaluation from peers or worry about "looking stupid"), it is more likely a social phobia, whereas in ASD such anxiety, as described in the aforementioned profiles, usually relates to nonsocial aspects of the situation, such as unfamiliar people, noise, or changes in routine (e.g., Szatmari & McConnell, 2011).

In sum, differential diagnosis of ASD from the various anxiety disorders (mainly specific and social phobia or OCD) relies heavily on clinical judgment of the anxiety's content and functionality. Hence, careful attention should be given to the identification of genuine versus apparent comorbidity of anxiety disorders (specifically of OCD) with HFASD.

Prevalence of Anxiety Disorders in HFASD

Although exact prevalence rates of anxiety disorders in HFASD may be unclear due to overlapping symptoms, Wood and Gadow's (2010) research review concluded that prototypical manifestations of clinical anxiety may be identified in children and adolescents with HFASD. These authors also emphasized this anxiety's significant impact on life quality regardless of the severity of the ASD symptoms, thereby underscoring the need for serious consideration of comorbidity. Several empirical studies have reported a higher prevalence of anxiety disorders in HFASD compared with TYP (e.g., Gillott et al., 2001; Kim et al., 2000; Kuusikko et al., 2008; Mattila et al., 2010; Mayes et al., 2011; Mazefsky et al., 2010; Russell & Sofronoff, 2005) and a higher prevalence in HFASD compared with LFA (e.g., Mayes et al., 2011; Sukhodolsky et al., 2008).

For example, Kuusikko et al. (2008) examined differences in self-reported social anxiety and parent-reported internalizing difficulties between Finnish children (CA = 8–12 years) and adolescents (CA = 12–15 years) with HFASD (*n* = 21 with HFA and *n* = 35 with Asperger syndrome) and their agemates from a large community-based TYP sample (*n* = 353). The self-report findings pinpointed a higher risk for social anxiety in the sample of adolescents with HFASD, with over half (57.1%) exceeding the clinical cutoff scores for social anxiety versus only 17% of the TYP sample. This difference did not emerge for the younger children in the study. Differently, according to parent reports using the Child Behavior Checklist (CBCL; Achenbach & Rescorla, 2001), both younger and older participants with HFASD were rated higher than the TYP group on internalizing symptoms that exceeded the U.S.-defined clinical borderline status. Between one-half and three-fourths of the HFASD group were rated with clinically elevated internalizing symptoms on the CBCL's total Internalizing scale and on its subscales (e.g., Withdrawn, Somatic, Anxious/Depressed subscales). Thus the adolescent age group with HFASD appears to be at specific risk for developing social anxiety, whereas internalizing difficulties (including both depression and anxiety) should be a concern in HFASD across development. Interestingly, to exclude possibly overlapping symptoms between HFASD and social anxiety, Kuusikko et al. (2008) analyzed their measures twice, once with the original scales and a second time using a revised scale that accounted for symptom overlap. Both analyses yielded comparable outcomes.

Similarly, significant percentages of children and adolescents with HFASD (CA = 9–14 years) extracted from a large random community sample (*N* = 1,751) scored at least two standard deviations above the population mean for anxiety disorders based on parental report: 13.6% for generalized anxiety disorder and 8.5% for separation anxiety (Kim et al., 2000). Two other studies reported anxiety disorders among about 40% of HFASD samples, as follows: Mattila et al. (2010) reported anxiety disorders in 42% of a combined community and clinic sample of HFASD in Finland (CA = 12–13 years in the community-based study and 9–16 years in the clinic-based study). Specific phobias were the most common anxiety disorder, found in 28% of the participants (e.g., fears of animals, darkness, heights, confined spaces, bridges, needles, injections), and OCD was present in 22% of the participants. Interestingly, 14% of the participants revealed two to three different concurrent anxiety disorders. According to maternal reports in Mazefsky et al. (2010), 39% of clinic-based adolescents with HFASD (CA = 10-17 years) met the criteria for lifetime history of an anxiety disorder (e.g., syndromal and subsyndromal generalized anxiety disorder, social phobia, or specific phobia).

Somewhat higher percentages of anxiety symptoms (79%) were reported in Mayes et al. (2011) based on maternal reports for children with HFASD and for children with anxiety disorder (CA = 6–16 years). Interestingly, in this study, the frequency of mother-reported anxiety symptoms was similar for children in the two groups, attesting to the high prevalence of anxiety in HFASD. In addition, as found for depression rates, Mayes et al. (2011) reported that more children with HFASD had symptoms of anxiety than did children with LFA. Differences in anxiety were also reported between participants with LFA (IQ < 70, n = 106) and HFASD (IQ > 70, n = 48) in Sukhodolsky et al.'s (2008) large sample of parental reports for children and adolescents with ASD (N = 171; CA = 5–17 years). Altogether, 43% of the participants met the cutoff criteria for at least one anxiety disorder, with the HFASD group showing a significantly higher prevalence of generalized anxiety disorder (25%) and of overall anxiety disorders (58%) compared with the LFA group (4% and 39%, respectively).

Higher IQs have been linked with greater anxiety in ASD (see review in Szatmari & McConnell, 2011). Indeed, researchers have conjectured that individuals with HFASD may be at higher risk for developing comorbid anxiety than their less cognitively able peers as a result of their greater awareness of their social deficit and isolation (e.g., Hedley & Young, 2006). Gadow, DeVincent, and Schneider (2008) found that higher IQ was associated with more severe anxiety in children with PDD-NOS, and Sukhodolsky et al. (2008) underlined an association between higher levels of anxiety in children with HFASD and greater impairment in social responsiveness and more frequent stereotypical behaviors. Similarly, Bellini (2004) found that greater anxiety symptoms were related to social skill deficits.

Taken altogether, rates of any anxiety disorders (syndromal or subsyndromal) in HFASD differ somewhat between studies, due to difficulties in differential diagnosis related to overlapping symptoms and variability in the methods used to determine comorbid status along the different studies. However, a common parameter in all studies is that anxiety frequently co-occurs with HFASD and that the child with both comorbid conditions is at greater risk for maladjusted social functioning. Thus comorbid anxiety disorders may increase the social impairment of children with HFASD and impede their actual social involvement with peers in natural social situations (White, Oswald, Ollendick, & Scahill, 2009). Adolescents with HFASD seem to be at greater risk for such influences (Kuusikko et al., 2008).

The picture is even more dramatic when looking at the higher rates of overall mood and anxiety disorders in HFASD, which place the child and especially the adolescent—even the adult—with HFASD, as well as their families, at greater risk for negative short- and long-term outcomes. Regarding childhood, this comorbidity is associated with higher levels of withdrawal, noncompliance, and aggression and with increasing stress and conflict for the family (Matson & Nebel-Schwalm, 2007). These outcomes coincide with recent efforts to develop effective treatment endeavors that target reductions in anxiety and depression and increases in social competence in order to enhance these individuals' social participation (see more in Chapter 7 on social intervention).

MEASURES TO ASSESS COMORBIDITY IN HFASD

As mentioned earlier, the development of instrumentation to tap comorbid conditions in HFASD remains inadequate in terms of ruling out the possible overlapping criteria between HFASD and other psychiatric disorders while implementing a dual diagnosis. However, several instruments have been used for ASD (not for HFASD specifically), and some preliminary efforts were made to validate these diagnostic tools for the ASD population and to pinpoint cutoff scores that would identify potential risk for comorbid conditions. Importantly, higher scores on such screening instruments would still need to be clinically verified. The next section provides a short review of such instruments, divided into general and specific measures for assessing psychopathology.

General Measures of Psychopathology

Child Behavior Checklist

The 113-item Child Behavior Checklist (CBCL; Achenbach & Rescorla, 2001) is frequently used to evaluate various emotional and behavioral disorders across the lifespan. It can be implemented as a questionnaire or as an interview, and it includes forms for self-report or for reports by significant adults (e.g., caregivers, teachers, other professionals) who are familiar with the child. Two versions are available: the preschool checklist version (termed the CBCL—1.5–5 years or CBCL—Preschool) and the school-age checklist version (termed the CBCL—6–18 years or CBCL—Youth). Each version contains two empirically derived overall broadband syndrome scales—Internalizing and Externalizing—and eight norm-referenced narrowband syndrome scales that were derived through factor analysis of data from the general pediatric population. Three subdomains (withdrawal, somatic complaints, and anxiety/depression) form the broadband internalizing syndrome, which evaluates emotional problems. Two subdomains (delinquency and aggressiveness) form the broadband externalizing syndrome, which evaluates behavior problems. The remaining three other mixed syndrome subdomains (social difficulties, thought problems, and attention problems) do not belong to either broadband scale because they had sizeable factor loadings on both broad domains in Achenbach and Rescorla's (2001) factor analyses. A Total Problems scale, quantifying overall impairment, is also obtained.

Despite the fact that its psychometric properties have not been extensively evaluated in ASD, the CBCL has been used in autism research to evaluate comorbid psychiatric conditions—for example, in Kuusikko et al. (2008) to assess the internalizing syndrome and its three subdomains, or in Schroeder, Weiss, and Bebko (2011) to assess psychiatric comorbidities in individuals with Asperger syndrome. Previous studies showed that the caregiver form of the CBCL—Youth checklist could differentiate between youngsters with ASD and those with other psychiatric conditions (e.g., Duarte, Bordin, de Oliveira, & Bird, 2003; Mazefsky, Anderson, Conner, & Minshew, 2011; Petersen, Bilenberg, Hoerder, & Gillberg, 2006). Also, two recent studies that evaluated the psychometric qualities of the preschool and school-age checklist versions among children with a confirmed diagnosis of ASD supported both versions' factorial validity for the broadband and subdomain syndromes (Pandolfi, Magyar, & Dill, 2009, 2012, respectively). The CBCL—Youth checklist's diagnostic accuracy was sensitive but low on specificity in differentiating ASD symptoms from other emotional behavioral symptoms. That is, only general scale elevation was noted, which may be taken as evidence of a significant emotional and/or behavioral problem; however, the general low specificity found for usage of the CBCL—Youth with the ASD population underscores the need for further diagnostic assessment using measures specific to ASD and to particular emotional and behavioral disorders. Only further assessment can complement the CBCL to differentiate between ASD symptoms and the presence of co-occurring emotional and behavioral disorders (ADHD, depression, anxiety) that may require specific treatment.

Schedule for Affective Disorders and Schizophrenia for School-Age Children (6–18)—Present and Lifetime Version and Autism Comorbidity Interview—Present and Lifetime Version

The Schedule for Affective Disorders and Schizophrenia for School-Age Children (6–18)—Present and Lifetime Version (K-SADS-PL) is a semistructured "gold standard" diagnostic interview (Kaufman et al., 1997; Lauth et al., 2010) designed to assess current and past psychiatric disorders, including affective disorders (e.g., MDD, dysthymia), psychotic disorders, anxiety disorders (e.g., generalized anxiety disorder, OCD, social phobia), behavioral disorders (e.g., ADHD), substance abuse disorders, eating disorders, tic disorders, and ASD (PDD-NOS and Asperger syndrome). The K-SADS-PL is administered by interviewing the parent(s) and then the child and compiling summary ratings that include all information sources (parent, child, school, and other). The K-SADS-PL has also been used in

ASD studies to evaluate comorbid psychiatric disorders (e.g., Joshi et al., 2010; Mattila et al., 2010).

In light of the paucity of "gold standard" measures for validly and reliably assessing present and lifetime psychopathology in ASD, Leyfer et al. (2006) recently suggested the Autism Comorbidity Interview—Present and Lifetime Version (ACI-PL) as a modification to the K-SADS-PL. The ACI-PL is a parent interview adapted in several ways for specific use with ASD:

1. This scale considers the unique way in which psychiatric symptoms may be manifested in ASD, such as MDD expressed through increased agitation, self-injury, and temper outbursts, rather than simply by showing depressed mood.

2. The scale regards children's described behaviors or emotional reactions as psychiatric symptoms only if they differ qualitatively and quantitatively from the children's baseline behaviors or emotions; that is, symptom manifestation is measured as change from baseline. For example, coding for social phobia in the ACI-PL requires that children's fear and/or avoidance relate to situations' social aspects (e.g., fear of "looking stupid") rather than its nonsocial aspects (e.g., noise). Thus the ACI-PL distinguishes impairment due to comorbid psychiatric disorders from impairment due to core features of ASD.

3. The scale acknowledges that ASD makes some questions irrelevant for some children (due to limited language or self-reflection capabilities); therefore, symptoms are probed only if a child is capable of demonstrating them (e.g., increased guilty feelings are not an applicable symptom of depression in a child who does not understand guilt). Moreover, criteria for subsyndromal disorders are applied (i.e., when significant psychiatric impairment falls just short of meeting full DSM criteria; APA, 2000). Utilization of subsyndromal criteria enables identification of treatment needs that may be overlooked by relying solely on DSM criteria.

Altogether, the ACI-PL modification includes the addition of an introductory section that explores children's behavior and emotion at baseline, as well as supplementary questions at the beginning of each disorder section assessing further observable features and applicability of symptoms to the child. Leyfer et al. (2006) examined the instrument's psychometric qualities for 109 fairly high-functioning children (67% had Full Scale IQ > 70, CA = 5–17 years) with a diagnosis of autistic disorder based on the ADI-R (Lord et al., 1994), ADOS (Lord et al., 2000), and DSM-IV-TR (APA, 2000) criteria. The ACI-PL demonstrated good interrater reliability, test–retest reliability, and criterion and concurrent validities for the diagnosrs of MDD, OCD, and ADHD. Recently, using the ACI-PL, Mazefsky et al. (2010) was able to identify high percentages of depression and anxiety in youth with HFASD (CA = 10–17 years). Further validity and reliability testing are needed for DSM disorders across the age, IQ, and verbal ability spectra found in autism and for subsyndromal disorders.

Behavior Assessment System for Children—Second Edition

The Behavior Assessment System for Children—Second Edition (BASC-2; Reynolds & Kamphaus, 2004) is a standardized multidimensional rating system using children's self-reports, teacher ratings, and/or parent ratings to assess a broad range of children's skills, adaptive behaviors, and problem behaviors at home and in the community. It is available for three age ranges: preschool (2–5 years), child (6–11 years), and adolescent (12–21 years). The BASC-2 provides information on nine clinical scales—aggression, Anxiety, Attention Problems, Atypicality, Conduct Problems, Depression, Hyperactivity, Somatization, and Withdrawal—and five adaptive scales: Activities of Daily Living, Adaptability, Functional Communication, Leadership, and Social Skills. Together, the nine clinical and five adaptive scales are used to generate four composites: Externalizing Problems, Internalizing Problems, Behavioral Symptoms Index, and Adaptive Skills. To supplement interpretation of the core scales, additional scales were added: six new clinical scales (Anger Control, Bullying, Developmental Social Disorders, Emotional Self-Control, Executive Functioning, and Negative Emotionality), one adaptive scale (Resiliency), and seven new content scales. Of these, the Developmental Social Disorders content scale is of particular relevance to HFASD because it captures such aspects of ASD as deficits in social skills, interests, activities, and communication.

BASC-2 items are oriented toward DSM-IV-TR (APA, 2000) symptomology and can be used in screening and as part of a comprehensive assessment procedure. This measure has been shown as reliable and valid for persons ages 2–24 years of age; children with ASD were included in the general and clinical norm samples, as well as in the reliability and validity studies (Reynolds & Kamphaus, 2004). Solomon, Miller, Taylor, Hinshaw, and Carter (2012) used the BASC-2 to assess the depression, anxiety, and internalizing problems (a composite of anxiety, depression, and somatization items) among boys and girls with HFASD (CA = 8–18 years). They found a specific risk for affective disorders in the teen years for girls with HFASD. Adolescent girls with HFASD had higher internalizing symptoms compared with boys with HFASD and with girls with TYP and higher symptoms of depression than girls with TYP. Volker et al. (2010) explored the prototypical profile on the BASC-2 of students with HFASD (*n* = 124; CA = 6–16 years, mean IQ = 105) and found significant differences between HFASD and TYP groups on all BASC-2 parent version scores except for the Somatization, Conduct Problems, and Aggression scales. Mean HFASD scores were in the clinically significant range on the Behavioral Symptoms Index, Atypicality, Withdrawal, and Developmental Social Disorders scales. Screening indices suggested that the developmental social disorders scale was highly effective in reliably differentiating between HFASD and TYP. Even so, the task remains to explore the instrument's ability to discriminate between HFASD and other childhood disorders. Thus the sensitivity and specificity data obtained by Volker et al. (2010) would not necessarily apply to screening for other potential comorbid clinical conditions.

Diagnostic Interview Schedule for Children–IV

The Diagnostic Interview Schedule for Children–IV (DISC-IV; Shaffer, Fisher, Lucas, Dulcan, & Schwab-Stone, 2000) is a highly structured respondent-based interview for the assessment of more than 30 childhood and adolescent psychiatric disorders (e.g., anxiety, mood disorders, schizophrenia, disruptive behavior disorders) derived from the DSM-IV (APA, 1994) and the ICD-10 (World Health Organization, 1992). The DISC-IV includes two versions: the Parent version (DISC-IV-P) for parents of children ages 6–17 and the Child version (DISC-IV-C) to be administered to children ages 9–17. The DISC-IV showed moderate to good reliability (Shaffer et al., 2000). Using a Dutch version of the DISC-IV-C to assess anxiety disorders, mood disorders, schizophrenia, and disruptive behavior disorders in a sample of children ages 6–12 with ASD, a high prevalence of at least one comorbid psychiatric condition (80.9%) was found (de Bruin et al., 2007). However, despite the sample's mean Full Scale IQ score in the high-functioning range (91.22), not all participants were high functioning (Full Scale IQ ranged from 55 to 120), and the psychometric qualities of the Dutch DISC version have yet to be explored.

Child Symptom Inventory–4

The Child Symptom Inventory–4 (CSI-4; Gadow & Sprafkin, 2002) offers a teacher and a parent version of a behavior rating scale that assesses the behavioral symptoms of a broad range of childhood psychiatric disorders (e.g., ADHD, oppositional defiant disorder, conduct disorder, generalized anxiety disorder, and MDD) based on DSM-IV-TR classifications and symptoms (APA, 2000), providing indication of diagnosis and severity for each disorder. The findings of numerous studies indicate that the CSI-4 (targeting children ages 5–12) demonstrates satisfactory psychometric properties in community-based normative, clinic-referred non-ASD and ASD samples (see literature review in Gadow & Sprafkin, 2009). This scale was extensively used with children with ASD, but with mixed IQ capabilities, not specific to HFASD. These studies showed the scale's construct validity for ADHD, oppositional defiant disorder, separation anxiety, and tics (see summary in Gadow, DeVincent, Olvet, Pisarevskaya, & Hatchwell, 2010). Confirmatory factor analysis supported the internal validity of the DSM-IV model of behavioral syndromes in a large sample of children with diagnosed ASD (*n* = 730; Lecavalier, Gadow, DeVincent, & Edwards, 2009). Parent and teacher ratings have shown modest convergence. A revised version—the CSI-4R—was recently suggested to combine the CSI-4 with its sister symptom inventory for adolescents (the ASI-4, targeting ages 12–18 years) in a single measure spanning ages 5–18 years (the Child and Adolescent Symptom Inventory–4R [CASI-4R]; Gadow & Sprafkin, 2012). Another version of the symptom inventory is also available for children as young as 3–5 years (the Early Childhood Inventory–4; Sprafkin, Volpe, Gadow, Nolan, & Keely, 2002).

Measures to Assess Specific Psychopathologies

Several measures have been used in the study of HFASD to evaluate specific psychiatric disorders, including the following:

1. The *Children's Depression Inventory* (Kovacs, 1992) is a self-report assessing depression level in children ages 7–17, which also provides evaluation of areas relevant to depression (negative mood, interpersonal problems, ineffectiveness, anhedonia, and negative self-esteem). Kovacs (1992) reported a Cronbach's alpha of .86 for this inventory in a normative sample, and Hedley and Young (2006) presented similar results for children with Asperger syndrome (see also Solomon et al., 2012).

2. The *Conners 3rd Edition* (Conners, 2008) consists of observer ratings (parents, teachers, caregivers) and adolescents' self-reported ratings to assess ADHD and to evaluate problem behaviors in children and adolescents. Ronald et al. (2008) utilized the parents' version of this scale to identify ADHD traits and suspected cases in individuals with Asperger syndrome, and the scale showed good internal consistency (Cronbach's alpha = .92).

3. The *Children's Yale–Brown Obsessive Compulsive Scale* (Scahill et al., 1997) is a semistructured parent and child interview assessing a range of possible OCD symptoms for obsessions (e.g., contamination, aggression, hoarding/saving, magical thoughts/superstitions, and possible obsessive thoughts—somatic, religious, sexual) and for compulsions (e.g., cleaning/washing, checking, repeating, counting, ordering/arranging). This scale has shown good internal consistency (Cronbach's alpha = .90) and a significant correlation with other measures of OCD in the general population. In Zandt et al. (2009), children with HFASD (CA = 7–16; mean Verbal IQ = 96.45) scored lower on both the obsession and compulsion scales compared with children with OCD. Recently, a modified scale for

ASD was developed, the *Children's Yale–Brown Obsessive Compulsive Scale–PDD* (Scahill et al., 2006). This modified scale's symptom checklist was expanded to include repetitive behaviors associated with autism, such as spinning objects, staring, twirling, and repeating words and phrases, which can help ascertain differential observation between repetitive behaviors associated with ASD or with OCD. Scahill et al. (2006) reported that the modified version was found to be reliable, distinct from other measures of repetitive behavior, and sensitive to change, but these outcomes were not yet specifically tested for HFASD.

To sum up, this section presented a list of psychiatric measures to assess comorbidity in HFASD that is not all-inclusive but does delineate some of the major general and specific self-report and other-report (parents, teachers) instruments that have been most commonly implemented in the study of individuals with HFASD. As seen, there is a great need for researchers in the field to establish "gold standard," reliable, valid diagnostic tools to assess comorbid conditions associated with ASD. Such assessment measures should take into account the possible overlaps in symptoms between HFASD and comorbid disorders, as well as the unique manifestations of psychiatric symptoms in the HFASD population.

SUMMARY AND CONCLUSIONS

Overall, the co-occurrence of psychiatric conditions such as ADHD, mood disorders, and anxiety disorders with HFASD is high, probably higher than in LFA. Moreover, at least for depression and anxiety, risk seems to increase with age in HFASD. Reasons for the high rates of such comorbidities with one or more psychiatric disorders in HFASD are still speculative. The contribution of potential genetic, cognitive, and environmental risk factors should be studied further, as should potential underlying neurobiological mechanisms involved in psychiatric disorders in HFASD. Despite some recent efforts, most of the instruments to evaluate comorbidity in HFASD were not specifically designed for ASD and definitely not for HFASD. Thus the need exists to develop such assessment systems that are valid and reliable in children along the spectrum and that take into consideration the possibly unique form, content, and function of symptoms in the high-functioning population in order to enhance differential diagnoses between ASD and other psychiatric disorders.

Currently, diagnosis of comorbidity relies heavily upon clinicians' judgment, based on changes over time in symptom manifestations, deterioration in functioning, demonstration of behaviors that are outside the spectrum, and lack of responsiveness to treatments targeting children with ASD. The self–other and observation scales that are available make it hard to achieve objective diagnoses of comorbidity in HFASD. Yet, having said all this, it is impossible to ignore the significant percentages of children with HFASD who exhibit significant comorbid syndromal or subsyndromal psychiatric conditions. Furthermore, those characterized by such conditions clearly appear to be at greater risk for more severe impairment and for both social-emotional and cognitive-academic maladjustment. Consequently, specific intervention models should be developed to target these complex comorbidities. Specifically, instructional methods should be oriented toward helping children and adolescents overcome both their difficulties based on their ASD and those based on their comorbid conditions. For example, cognitive-behavioral models to reduce anxiety and depression are a recent important experimental trend, as described in Part II of this book, "Intervention Models," and in Chapter 7, "Interventions to Facilitate Social Functioning."

INTERVENTION MODELS

Interventions to Facilitate Social Functioning

MAJOR CHALLENGES AND COMPONENTS OF SOCIAL INTERVENTION

Social intervention for school-age children with HFASD is challenging and essential. Many children with HFASD are "loners," and social isolation increases toward adolescence (Bauminger & Kasari, 2000; Lasgaard et al., 2010). Moreover, as described in the previous chapter, affective disorders such as anxiety and depression characterize the majority of adolescents with HFASD—65%, according to Attwood (2004), and even higher (up to 84%) according to a more recent review by White and Roberson-Nay (2009). In addition, high percentages of adults with Asperger syndrome suffer from "gelotophobia," the fear of being laughed at (45% vs. 6% in adults with TYP). Gelotophobia is highly connected to traumatic experiences of being laughed at or being ridiculed in past social experiences (e.g., Samson, Huber, & Ruch, 2011). Such research indicates that high-functioning adults may have a long history of experiencing ridicule, mainly due to their social peculiarities, thus highlighting the deep need for professionals to implement interventions as early as possible and over the years of development in an attempt to avert the multiple interpersonal and affective by-products of chronic social dysfunction.

A major challenge facing interventionists is to design treatments based on what these youngsters actually do and what they know, rather than on what youngsters do not do or know. Many children with HFASD are already involved in peer interactions (even if of poor quality) and do have some social and emotional knowledge; therefore, interventions should focus on "fine tuning" of participants' social-emotional functioning and communication. Treatment aims include helping participants correct distorted perceptions, deepen their partial understanding of social and emotional constructs, and learn to perform "good enough" synchronized joint interactions with peers that may even evolve into friendships. In this chapter, I touch on these challenges and present intervention models and techniques that have been implemented in the field to meet these challenges. Throughout, I also illustrate how to translate these intervention principles into actual practice by describing specific examples derived from my own individual and group multimodal cognitive-behavioral-ecological (CBE) interventions (Bauminger, 2002, 2007a, 2007b).

CONCEPTUAL BASIS OF SOCIAL INTERVENTION

Generally speaking, recent developments in social skills training (SST) interventions have shown a shift from focusing on the enhancement of specific social behaviors—such as listening, eye contact, conversational skills, or gestures—to a multidimensional perception of social functioning. This multidimensional perception encompasses the child's capacity to integrate behavioral skills (e.g., social interaction), cognitive skills (e.g., accurate processing of information, perspective taking, social understanding), and affective skills (e.g., emotional regulation, knowledge, and recognition) in order to adapt flexibly to diverse social contexts and demands (Bierman & Welsh, 2000; Spence, 2003). This shift stems not only from a growing understanding that "social competence" is a multidimensional construct with interlinks between social-cognitive and social-behavioral capabilities but also from increasing knowledge about the multilevel social-emotional difficulties of children with HFASD. In line with this general multidimensional direction, social interventions for children with HFASD are also shifting from skills-oriented SST programs based mainly on social behaviors to more comprehensive, holistic interventions based on modifications of classic cognitive-behavioral treatment (CBT) models.

Indeed, many valuable empirical evaluations of SST-oriented interventions have shown improvements in specific behaviors such as social interaction and conversation among children with ASD; however, several methodological issues limit the extent to which these important interventions may be specifically relevant to the multidimensional profile of social deficits characterizing youngsters with HFASD in particular:

1. The majority of SST studies targeted specific vital social behaviors such as children's social interaction, play, social conversation, and collaboration (e.g., Charlop-Christy & Kelso, 2003; Chin & Bernard-Opitz, 2000; Ganz, Kaylor, Bourgeois, & Hadden, 2008; Kamps et al., 2002; LeGoff, 2004; Licciardello, Harchik, & Luiseli, 2008; Owen-DeSchryver, Carr, Cale, & Blakeley-Smith, 2008;

Terpstra, Higgins, & Pierce, 2002), but mostly without emphasis on the integration of social-cognitive aspects.

2. For the most part, SST evaluations investigated a single participant or a small sample (e.g., Charlop-Christy & Kelso, 2003; Chin & Bernard-Opitz, 2000; Kamps et al., 1992; Loftin, Odom, & Lantz, 2008; Owen-DeSchryver et al., 2008).

3. Most SST research studies included a mixed sample with regard to cognitive functioning (high and low), and in many cases children's level of functioning was not systematically assessed, thus precluding distinctive conclusions about HFASD (e.g., Kamps et al., 2002; LeGoff, 2004; Morrison, Kamps, Garcia, & Parker, 2001; Thiemann & Goldstein, 2004).

4. Few SST interventions directly focused on school-age children and adolescents with HFASD (e.g., Barry et al., 2003; Charlop-Christy & Kelso, 2003; Chin & Bernard-Opitz, 2000; Ganz et al., 2008; Loftin et al., 2008; Owens, Granader, Humphrey, & Baron-Cohen, 2008). Therefore, efforts in treatment models should be directed toward a comprehensive, multidimensional perception of social competence to explicitly help the more cognitively able school-age youngsters with HFASD to integrate both social-cognitive and social-interactive skills (see review in Klinger & Williams, 2009).

As mentioned earlier, the contemporary shift to more comprehensive, holistic social interventions for HFASD derives from modifications of classic CBT models. Historically, CBT grew out of classical behavioral therapy. Cognitive variables (beliefs, cognitions, attributions, expectancies, images) and emotions are considered to be fundamental concerns of CBT intervention, with an emphasis on cognitive-mediation processes in the acquisition and regulation of social behavior (Dobson & Dobson, 2009; Hart & Morgan, 1993). The CBT orientation assumes reciprocity between the ways in which an individual thinks, feels, and behaves in social situations (Hart & Morgan, 1993). Also, CBT presumes that social perception processes can be taught cognitively and can influence behavior (Hart & Morgan, 1993). The child is perceived as an active "cognitive constructor" of his or her social world; hence CBT focuses on correcting distorted perceptions of the social world and teaching more efficient ways to perceive and respond to the vast variety of verbal and nonverbal stimuli existing in that social world (Dobson & Dobson, 2009; Spence, 2003). Children, through CBT, become "scientists" who observe and study their own behavior, learn to identify its components, test their own belief systems, seek effective techniques to achieve change, and combine skill learning with hands-on experiencing of each skill.

Accordingly, CBT offers a multimodal social intervention (e.g., Ronen,

1998; Spence, 2003; Spence & Donovan, 1998) that emphasizes learning and experience. As seen in Figure A1 in Appendix A, CBT-based social interventions include cognitive techniques such as cognitive reconstruction, interpersonal problem solving, and affective education. CBT-based social interventions also include behavioral techniques through which children can practice social interactive skills in a safe environment, such as modeling, behavioral rehearsal through role play in dyads and in small groups, and feedback and reinforcement to increase appropriate response strategies and to learn from mistakes. Table A1 in Appendix A presents the definitions and aims of these various techniques, along with examples from general studies, as well as from studies implementing them specifically for HFASD (particularly from my CBE interventions, as elaborated later). Overall, growing evidence supports the effectiveness of multimodal SST that combines behavioral and social-cognitive techniques over monomodal SST that focuses on only one technique—either social-cognitive or social-behavioral (Beelmann, Pfingsten, & Lösel, 1994; Bierman & Welsh, 2000; Spence, 2003; Spence & Donovan, 1998). As seen in Figure A1 in Appendix A, CBT social-skills-based intervention can be applied by incorporating three main change agents or their combinations: adult–child mediation, dyadic peer mediation, and small social groups (Barry et al., 2003; Paul, 2003; Rogers, 2000). Adult mediators may be teachers, parents, clinicians, counselors, or other professionals. See Table A2 in Appendix A for expansion on the main change agents of each intervention.

Working through cognitions to influence behaviors and emotions, as suggested by the CBT conceptual principle, seems to be advantageous for children with HFASD, who can use their relative cognitive strengths to help them make sense of their social world (e.g., Hermelin & O'Connor, 1985; Kasari et al., 2001). One anecdote clearly exemplifies this advantage: When asked to share an example of a time when he felt embarrassed, a child in our intervention program said: "I do not know what the meaning of embarrassment is, but I can look at the dictionary." As detailed in Chapter 1, cognitive compensation strategies can be used by these children to promote their social-emotional understanding, and CBT's emphasis on systematic analysis of thoughts, feelings, and behaviors can help this cognitive compensatory mechanism operate more efficiently. A dictionary definition cannot help children identify and recognize embarrassment in real situations, in themselves or others. However, a systematic, pragmatic definition of embarrassment, accompanied by exposure to practice of situations in which embarrassment is experienced, as well as explanations of how people look when experiencing embarrassment, may be well suited to the cognitive strengths of children with HFASD. Despite the general acceptance of the potential utility of integrating CBT components into SST programs for HFASD, it is only recently that more studies are being published that have empirically tested the effectiveness of such multimodal SST programs. The next section reviews such studies.

CBT-BASED STUDIES IN HFASD: LITERATURE REVIEW

Empirical studies emphasizing cognitive-mediational processes in the acquisition and regulation of social behavior for children with HFASD have focused on the enhancement of four main areas of functioning—ToM capabilities, executive function–problem solving, emotion recognition, and social-emotional understanding—either with or without direct training in social-behavior skills such as collaborative and conversational skills.

Cognitive-Oriented Training

A first group of studies in HFASD focused mainly on cognitive training while enhancing key social-cognitive capabilities, such as ToM (e.g., Gevers, Clifford, Mager, & Boer, 2006; Begeer et al., 2011), emotion recognition (e.g., Ryan & Charragáin, 2010), or ToM and executive function (e.g., Fisher & Happé, 2005). For example, in Gevers et al., children with HFASD who had average verbal functioning (CA = 8–11 years) studied ToM skills in small groups in a clinical setting during 21 weekly 60-minute meetings. In addition, their parents received psychoeducational training focusing on understanding autism, ToM development, and how to promote ToM capabilities at home through game playing and storytelling. Main findings showed an improvement in some ToM areas, such as describing first-order beliefs (i.e., what people think about real events) and understanding pretense and humor, but no improvement emerged on second-order beliefs (i.e., describing what people think about other people's thoughts and emotions) or on emotion recognition. Parents did report improvement in children's socialization capabilities concerning interpersonal relationships, play, and social skills, but, considering parents' deep involvement in the treatment, their reports should be regarded carefully. Parental inclusion in the treatment appears important but possibly not sufficient alone to obtain comprehensive change in children's ToM capabilities or to enable transfer from one taught area (ToM) to another (emotion recognition). Similar results were presented by this group of researchers (Begeer et al., 2011) using the same ToM intervention for children with HFASD (CA = 8.5–13.7 years, mean = 10.3 years), but this time using a randomized controlled design (experimental versus wait-listed groups). Overall, the experimental group did better than the control group on conceptual ToM capabilities, but their self-reported empathetic skills or parent-reported social behavior did not improve, furnishing little support for the soundness of ToM instruction as an effective means for actually improving children's overall social competence.

To examine children's ability to transfer social-cognitive skills from one area to another, Fisher and Happé (2005) used a short individual training (5–10 days, 25 minutes/day) for two groups of children with ASD, one focusing on ToM (mean CA = 10.50 years) and the other focusing on executive function (mean CA = 10.68 years). Both groups significantly improved on ToM tasks, whereas a control no-treatment group revealed no progress. However, none of the groups demonstrated improvement on executive function. Of specific interest were the participants trained on executive functioning, who were able to transfer learned skills to the domain of ToM but could not improve their executive function capabilities. Note that this sample of children was not an HFASD sample; their verbal abilities were below age norms (verbal MA = 7.23 years for the group that received ToM treatment and 6.57 years for the group that received executive function treatment).

The third study that focused mainly on cognitive training in HFASD (Ryan & Charragáin, 2010) was a short group intervention (1 hour per week for 4 weeks) targeting emotional recognition in children with average IQ levels (CA = 6.75–14.25 years). To help them learn to identify differently expressed emotions, children were taught various verbal and nonverbal components of expressions via affective education, and they received role-play techniques, workbooks for home use, and recordings of emotional expression at home. Assessment included only an emotional recognition measure, which showed improvement immediately after treatment and a trend toward improvement at follow-up 3 months later. Generalization of treatment gains to other settings (such as home) or to other social-cognitive capabilities was not measured.

To sum up, specific cognitive training seems to be efficient to some degree in improving the learned skill; however, generalization to various settings, as well as to other untrained social-cognitive capabilities, has yet to be discovered.

Multimodal Intervention

ToM and SST

In a different line of studies, cognitive training was combined with behavioral skill-oriented training that focused on the enhancement of social interaction behaviors such as play, collaboration, and social conversation. The effectiveness of this combination of ToM and SST was examined in several studies (e.g., Crooke, Hendrix, & Rachman, 2008; Feng, Lo, Tsai, & Cartledge, 2008; Mackay, Knott, & Dunlop, 2007; Ozonoff & Miller, 1995). Among the first to conduct such an intervention study for adolescents with HFASD (mean CA = 13.8 years), Ozonoff and Miller (1995) taught perspective taking at different levels, as well as social interaction and conversation skills, using role play and organized social activities (parties). Although the children worked both on social-cognitive and social interaction skills, only ToM capabilities improved.

Feng et al. (2008) presented different results for a single-case study of a sixth-grade boy with HFASD, who improved both his ToM and his social interaction capabilities. He was able to show increases in social interaction behaviors in terms of frequency (rising from 5.7% to 18.4% in a 40-minute observation period), appropriateness (rising from 29% appropriate behaviors at pretest to 73% at posttest), complexity (increasing his inclusion of empathetic statements, help seeking, pretend play), and transfer to settings that were not part of the treatment (i.e., recess and lunchtime). This treatment included systematic teaching of ToM through animated presentation of ToM scripts (i.e., a birthday party) via computer software for viewing multimedia and through a teacher's verbal explanation of the script, followed by modeling of the appropriate response, practicing in role play, and receiving feedback on performance. The training was implemented by the teacher in one-on-one child–adult mediation settings, accompanied by small-group intervention to facilitate generalization. Treatment took place in four 40-minute sessions per week, resulting in 32 one-on-one sessions and 29 small-group sessions. Although generalization from a case study is difficult, several factors may have contributed to this treatment's successful results. First, treatment components were sequenced so that the child initially learned new skills in the one-on-one setting and then practiced them experientially in the group, but only after gaining an 80% success rate, thereby practicing each learned skill in two settings. Second and most importantly, the teacher was the therapist, which enabled the inclusion of many "real-life" situations into the intervention content.

A school-based group intervention aiming to enhance a large number of participants' ($N = 46$) social-emotional perspective taking, together with conversational and friendship skills (SST), included cooperative games, group discussion, role play, home practice with parents, and outings into the community (Mackay et al., 2007). The intervention yielded improvement on parent-reported and self-reported social competence questionnaires, but no control group was included, nor any objective observational outcome to examine children's real-life improvement in social interactions or friendships.

Social Cognition and Social Interaction

Several studies have suggested that multimodal interventions combining social interaction training with the enhancement of various social-cognitive capabilities may foster more holistic social functioning in children with HFASD. Multilevel, hidden, as well as exposed, social and emotional behaviors and cognitions have been at the focus of these intervention studies. For example, some such interventions targeted emotional understanding and regulation, as well as social understanding, social problem solving, and social perception skills (Bauminger, 2002, 2007a, 2007b; Beaumont & Sofronoff, 2008); others targeted ToM, emotion recognition, and executive function (Solomon, Goodlin-Jones, & Anders, 2004; Stichter et al., 2010). Many similarities can be found between Solomon et al. (2004) and

Stichter et al. (2010) for preadolescents (CA = 8–12 years) and adolescents (CA = 11–14 years) with HFASD. Both interventions aimed to enhance youngsters' emotional recognition, executive function, and ToM using a group treatment delivered by therapists in a clinical setting, as well as parent training. Intervention comprised 20 sessions in both studies: twice weekly for 10 weeks in Stichter et al.'s (2010) study and once weekly for 20 weeks in the study by Solomon et al. (2004). Both implemented various CBT-driven techniques and principles, such as metacognitive strategies for problem solving (i.e., the ability to react to stress appropriately, identify problem situations, and determine appropriate means to respond to problem situations, as well as analyze perspectives of others within collaborative situations); self-monitoring; affective education (i.e., recognition of facial expressions and emotions in self and other, the ability to identify and interpret the contextual variables for emotional recognition across perspectives of emotional range and variance); and structured learning (i.e., each concept that was learned in a previous unit was incorporated into a later unit). In an example of structured learning of conversational turn-taking skills (Stichter et al. 2010), the curriculum included discussion not only on the importance of reciprocal exchanges but also on the importance of interpreting facial expressions (understanding whether another person is bored or interested in the conversation, which was taught in a prior unit), as well as on the importance of sharing ideas in order to develop a conversation. Thus, through structured learning, competencies were built gradually and were scaffolded through in vivo interactions with the staff and other group members and through role play. In both studies, curriculum combined social-cognitive capabilities (ToM) and social-interaction behaviors such as social conversation.

Results of the two studies were somewhat similar. Both showed improvement in facial recognition and executive function measures. Results for ToM capabilities were mixed: Children in Solomon et al.'s (2004) treatment group improved to a similar extent as did a no-treatment control group, and in Stichter et al. (2010) the difference between pretest and posttest for ToM measures was marginal. Children in Stichter et al.'s study were also reported by their parents as demonstrating improvement on all subscales of the Social Responsiveness Scale (Constantino & Gruber, 2005): social awareness, social cognition, social communication, social motivation, and autistic mannerisms. This finding may suggest some generalization of treatment gains to the home environment; however, generalization of treatment gains to the school environment remains unknown based on these studies. Likewise, both sets of researchers recommended replication in the child's natural social environments, such as at school.

Expanding on issues of generalization, careful attention was given to this issue in Beaumont and Sofronoff 's (2008) study that targeted emotional recognition and regulation, as well as conversational skills, in children with HFASD (CA = 7.5–11 years). Their study implemented a parent–child computer game ("Junior Detective") on recognizing and regulating emotions, followed by small-group training that enforced generalization of treatment gains through problem solving and role play. In addition, teachers received handouts of treatment content, and children were asked to record various emotional expressions in the home environment. Study results demonstrated improvement on parent-reported social skills and emotional management strategies (coping with anxiety and bullying at school), both immediately after intervention and at follow-up 5 months later. However, no significant improvement was noted in the experimental group compared with a wait-listed control group regarding recognition of facial expressions and body postures. This outcome may relate to the difficulty in transferring skills from a computer game to real-life expressions. Also, despite the fact that teachers were involved through handouts, their role in supporting the process of treatment in the children remains unclear.

CBE INTERVENTION: TAKING CBT FROM THEORY TO PRACTICE

In line with the literature available on social-emotional interventions for children with HFASD, I developed a multimodal CBT-based ecological dyadic and group intervention to be operated in the school setting by trained teachers over an entire academic year. It is now well over a decade since I began implementing the CBE intervention across Israel, in regular education schools that include children with HFASD.

Overview of the CBE Intervention Rationale

Based on the multifaceted social-emotional deficit characterizing children with HFASD—encompassing social-emotional perception and understanding, emotional difficulties such as anxiety and regulation, and difficulties in peer interaction and friendship (see Chapters 2 and 3 for elaboration)—the CBE social intervention was designed as a multidimensional, comprehensive intervention aiming to simultaneously enhance both school-age children's understanding and their actual behavior (e.g., Dobson & Dobson, 2009). The CBE intervention thus adopts a holistic perspective, providing treatment concurrently in three integral areas of social functioning, namely social cognition (with an emphasis on social understanding), emotions (with an emphasis on emotional knowledge and recognition), and social behavior (with an emphasis on dyadic and group interactions and on collaborative and social conversational skills). This multimodal CBE intervention blends a developmentally oriented cognitive-behavioral (CB) treatment orientation that matches components and techniques to children's heterogeneity of social-emotional functioning, together with an ecological (E) perspective that serves as the model's conceptual guide (e.g., Bronfenbrenner,

1979, 1992; Sontag, 1996; Dobson & Dobson, 2009). That is, teaching takes place in the child's natural ecology—in the school and the home social environments—and involves the child's main social partners: the peers, teachers, and parents. Thus the CBE intervention encompasses adult mediation (by teachers and parents) and peer mediation (through dyadic work and through small-group work), which enables the integration of children's learning, practice, and experiencing of new skills and also squarely addresses issues of generalization and maintenance. Figure B1 in Appendix B illustrates this multimodal intervention model.

Intervention Design

Over the years, our multimodal CBE intervention for children and adolescents with HFASD has developed in two main directions: (1) empirical evidence-based trials and (2) widespread field applications. Initially, three empirical studies were conducted to carefully examine the pretest–posttest effectiveness of the two main training modes in the CBE intervention: the dyadic treatment mode (Bauminger, 2002, 2007b) and the group treatment mode (Bauminger, 2007a). Both modes are mediated by trained, supervised facilitators, and both incorporate peers with TYP. To assess the two treatment modes' effectiveness, each mode was initially implemented by trained teachers and was tested separately in inclusive educational settings.

In terms of field applications, following the promising initial findings yielded by the separate empirical evaluations of the two treatment modes, which highlighted their effectiveness (Bauminger, 2002, 2007a, 2007b; see detailed description following), we began implementing an integrated CBE social curriculum for youngsters with HFASD that combines both the dyadic and the group modes into one holistic developmental model, applying this model into an ever-widening circle of schools in the Israeli regular education system. Over many years, Bar-Ilan University faculty, in collaboration with the Israeli Ministry of Education, have been providing instruction, support, and supervision (see subsequent elaboration) to develop a cadre of CBE facilitators (mainly teachers but also other professionals such as speech therapists, occupational therapists, and psychologists) who implement the holistic CBE intervention into regular elementary, junior high, and high schools that include youth with HFASD.

Since those initial empirical studies, additional research projects have been initiated in my Behavioral Research Laboratory to continue critical assessment of the integrated CBE intervention model. Ongoing research includes studies examining the effectiveness of a modified CBE intervention for young preschool children, investigating the efficacy of a CBE intervention adapted to nonverbal adolescents, and conducting a controlled study comparing participants' progress with that of a wait-listed control group. Thus empirical evidence, as well as vast clinical experience, has been gathered through the implementation of CBE. Based on this experience, in this section, I describe the CBE intervention's structure, contents, procedures, and techniques, followed by reports on empirical results indicating treatment efficacy.

Dual Treatment Modes

The holistic CBE intervention model combines two modes of treatment for children with HFASD, initially assessed separately for empirical purposes: the dyadic treatment (tested in Bauminger, 2002, 2007b) and the group treatment (tested in Bauminger, 2007a). As clarified before, field applications since these initial studies combine the two modes into one holistic intervention.

DYADIC TREATMENT

The major aim of the dyadic treatment mode is to develop social interaction capabilities, as well as basic social-emotional processing and understanding, in a one-on-one dyadic peer setting. As initially assessed empirically, this manualized CBE intervention comprised three teacher–child lessons per week (totaling 3 hours) for 7 months and two meetings per week with a peer. The manualized three-topic curriculum (see summary and examples of topics in Appendix B, Table B1) began with two preliminary consecutive stages, implemented through teacher–adult lessons (concept clarification and affective education) as described in Appendix A, Table A1:

1. The social-understanding stage consisted of concept clarification of important social constructs such as *What is social listening?* and *Why are friends important?*
2. The emotional understanding and recognition stage was taught through affective education, focusing mainly on basic emotions.
3. The lessons then focused on the third intervention topic, teaching social initiations essential for peer interaction, such as initiating a conversation with a friend and sharing experiences, thoughts, and feelings with a friend through self-instruction and problem solving, role play, and practicing with the peer as a change agent. In this third stage, each of the defined social-interpersonal goals was first taught individually by the child's teacher through social problem-solving vignettes (see examples in Appendix A, Table A1, and see the social topics for problem solving in the bottom row of Table B1). Second, each skill was practiced in role play with the teacher. Third, the new skill was practiced with an assigned peer at home and at school, in dyadic peer mediation that was supported by an adult (by the teacher at school, by the child's parents at home). Each child with HFASD met with an assigned peer with TYP twice weekly, once at home and once during a school break, to practice

learned social skills. The adult (teacher at school, parent at home) provided scaffolding for the dyad's social activities and furnished support to the peer with TYP during the peer mediation (Paul, 2003).

The manualized small-group intervention mode aims to foster complex social and emotional understanding and recognition skills, as well as peer-group interactions. As initially assessed empirically, the CBE group intervention comprised teacher–child lessons that focused on understanding social-emotional group behavior and small-group sessions at school for practicing such behavior The small group, mediated by the child's teacher, met twice weekly for an hour each time. Each group included three to five peers, comprising one to three children with HFASD and two children with TYP (preferably classmates of the child with HFASD) matched for age and preferably for sex. In addition, the child with HFASD met separately once weekly for an hour with the teacher only to pretrain the child individually on the skills to be learned next by the group and to enforce areas that the group had previously learned. The intervention covered six main topics, as presented in Appendix B, Table B2. Each group lesson included both a teaching process and practice. The teaching process aimed to provide a "definition" and a set of "rules" to help the children understand the social context of each learned social construct or skill through concept clarification, problem solving, and affective education (see Appendix A, Table A1). Practicing enabled rehearsal of each learned skill within the small-group setting. Group interaction was taught through participation in cooperative social group activities and through role play with the child's agemates.

Intervention Procedures: Integration of Construct Learning and Skill Experiencing

The CBE approach asserts that interplay between learning about social and emotional constructs and actually experiencing and practicing such constructs is essential to the development of adaptive social functioning in children with HFASD. The CBE intervention combines learning and experiencing of each social construct or skill through multiple cognitive and behavioral techniques, as well as through dyadic and group social games and activities (see Figure B2, Appendix B, for an example of such interlinks between learning and experiencing of the skills for social conversation).

The multitude of social-emotional and social-cognitive processes that determine the actual behavior of children in social situations necessitates direct learning of social concepts and constructs as fundamental to any social intervention (Spence, 2003). This need for direct teaching of social constructs may seem self-evident; yet, in the CBE intervention, emphasis is placed on avoiding any assumptions about children's prior knowledge and on systematically teaching each and every construct and skill, however basic. The rationale for this approach stems from the often distorted or partial understanding that children with HFASD exhibit (see Chapter 2 for elaboration).

For example, in our cross-cultural friendship studies (Bauminger, Solomon, Aviezer, Heung, Brown, et al., 2008; Bauminger, Solomon, Aviezer, Heung, Gazit, et al., 2008) we asked children to play a construction game in which they built a model together, and we specifically asked them to collaborate with their peer-friend. After a while, when we saw that each child tended to focus on his or her own part of the model, we again prompted them to work together, and they affirmed: "We *are* working together." Thus they seemed to consider working in close proximity and doing the same activity as collaboration. What they actually missed was the "joint engagement" or "coregulation" aspect of collaboration. Thus cognitive reconstruction through concept clarification of social concepts and constructs is an essential ingredient in the CBE intervention.

Another related issue concerning the learning aspects of the CBE is to help children figure out the "why" beyond each of the social constructs: Why is it is important to listen to a friend? Why is it important to collaborate? Why should I negotiate at times and compromise at others? The "why?" and the "what?" are two main components that children need to acquire through the systematic learning process of the CBE intervention. However, mere learning of the meaning and importance of social constructs such as social conversation, collaboration, and social listening is insufficient without actually practicing them. It will leave the child with only a theoretical level of understanding of the social constructs, which will not automatically be translated into real social behavior in authentic social interactions. In line with Krasny, Williams, Provencal, and Ozonoff's (2003) recommendation to make the abstract concrete when teaching social competence to children with HFASD, the CBE incorporates experiential activities as an integral part of its structure to help children work on translating their theoretical knowledge into more pragmatically useful social behavior in actual peer interactions. These social experiences include role play with an adult mediator and then actual practice of newly learned skills in dyadic and small-group environments.

It is important to note that the CBE intervention contains no specifically dedicated lessons aiming to teach or experience either ToM or executive function capacities, inasmuch as the CBE approach considers both of these to be core, cross-topic capabilities that must be enhanced throughout each and every topic studied in the intervention. For example, reciprocity is enforced throughout the intervention as a means of practicing ToM capabilities. In a like manner, while working on problem solving, children develop planning skills, as well as capabilities for solving problems, which strengthen executive function skills.

Intervention Emphases: Children's Developmental Stages and Heterogeneity

The CBE social curriculum design is developmentally oriented in order to help children with HFASD meet the social and emotional challenges characterizing each developmental period. In TYP, social and emotional functioning increases in complexity over the years (see Chapters 2 and 4). For younger children such as preschoolers with TYP, the link between behavior and its stimulus is often fairly direct and automatic ("I'm happy because I got something I like"), whereas for older children, especially from middle childhood and up, much of their social and emotional behavior in peer interaction is concealed, and they invest considerable effort in learning the rules for displaying emotions to peers in order to avoid embarrassment (Harris, 1989). Thus the challenge of making sense of such behaviors is much harder for older youngsters with HFASD.

Furthermore, the CBE intervention model takes into account the fact that within the population of children with HFASD, levels of social-emotional and social-cognitive capabilities range along a large continuum that extends even beyond CA, IQ, and verbal capabilities (see Chapters 2 and 3). Some children may possess better capabilities than others and can begin working in small social-skill groups, whereas others may still need help in the basic building blocks of dyadic interaction. Some may possess good knowledge of only basic emotions (happiness, sadness, fear, anger), whereas others may have some higher-level emotional understanding about complex emotions (e.g., see review in Begeer et al., 2008; Hobson, 2005) or even about hidden emotions and sarcasm (e.g., Barbaro & Dissanayake, 2007).

Thus the CBE developmentally oriented social curriculum incorporates a continuum of social functioning levels, ranging from the more basic social capabilities such as understanding basic emotions and experiencing one-on-one interactions to the more complex social capabilities such as understanding complex, hidden, or mixed emotions and experiencing small-group peer interactions or the development of friendship. This continuum—both with regard to increasingly difficult constructs and with regard to gradually more challenging settings for social engagement—aims to enhance the social intervention's usefulness for children located at different levels of functioning in terms of their peer-interaction skills. For example, with regard to emotional understanding and recognition, the CBE intervention starts with basic emotions in individual, adult-mediated treatment and in one-on-one interaction with a same-age or older peer with TYP, followed by facilitation of complex emotions and higher-order emotional understanding processes such as hidden emotions, cynicism, and irony in a small group of children with HFASD and TYP.

Another important yet often overlooked aspect of heterogeneity in social functioning in children with HFASD that has emerged from the

CBE multimodal social intervention is the consideration of uneven functioning within the individual. For example, one child who participated in our social-group intervention revealed high sensitivity to others' emotional states and could recognize a fairly wide range of emotions in others and in himself; however, that same child, at other times, was sure that the music he was mentally listening to in his head was also playing in his friend's head. Thus, according to the CBE intervention approach, particular attention must be paid to each child's unique developmental stage and performance profile when systematically teaching the various concepts through the diverse treatment activities and lessons.

However, despite efforts to provide a systematic, developmentally oriented model that considers between-child and within-child heterogeneity, the CBE school-based curriculum is not inclusive. Other important areas still need to be included in fuller future interventional curricula, especially areas that hold specific significance for older adolescents and young adults with HFASD beyond the school years. Specific lessons have not yet been developed on understanding and experiencing issues of self-disclosure and intimacy, the development of friendship and romantic relationships, and emotional regulation. Such studies are reviewed in a later section of this chapter.

Ecological Basis for the Intervention

The majority of children's social life transpires in school settings or in school-related activities such as group homework projects. Based on the noted difficulties in spontaneous transfer between settings among children with HFASD (from home to school, from small in-class group to school recess, etc.), the ecological perspective (Bronfenbrenner, 1979, 1992; Sontag, 1996) serves as a conceptual guide for the CBE intervention. Namely, treatments are delivered in environments that resemble the children's natural social settings as closely as possible, meaning at school, and with teachers and peers. It is not enough to operate an intervention in a school setting, because if the interventionist is a research assistant who is unrelated to the child's actual social life, then the intervention in school may look very much like an intervention in a clinical setting. Thus the mediating adult should be the child's own teacher or a familiar professional such as the child's own speech therapist or psychologist. Moreover, inasmuch as skills for peer interaction are best learned and acquired during actual interactions with other children, obviously peers should be a key component of every social intervention (e.g., Rogers, 2000). However, it is now abundantly clear that mere proximity between children with HFASD and children with TYP (i.e., inclusion in the same classroom or on the same playground) results only in very limited improvement, if at all, in the social interaction skills of children with HFASD (see review in Bass & Mulick, 2007; see also Paul, 2003). Thus the participating peers with TYP should be guided, instructed, and supported by an adult in their efforts to enhance social interactions in children with HFASD. Hence, the combination of adult (teacher, parents, other familiar professional) support and mediation, together with peer training and participation (classmates), seems to be an important aspect of the ecological perspective of treatment for teaching and practicing social interaction in HFASD. This section examines these major CBE change agents in more detail.

ADULT FACILITATORS

According to the holistic CBE model, the child's teacher (or a familiar professional) mediates both the dyadic and the group treatment modes under supervision by the research team. In the dyadic intervention, teachers teach the social-problem module and the affective-education module for 3 hours per week, support and guide the peers with TYP who are assigned to each child with HFASD participating in the training, inform the child's parents about homework for each learned skill, and obtain feedback from parents and the peers about the child's performance of homework in the home environment. During the group treatment, teachers mainly lead the group sessions. Teachers also help children with HFASD to transfer activities from the small-group social intervention to the classroom. For example, when children develop a game to practice collaboration in the small group, the teacher supports them in playing the game with the whole class at a later stage. In both treatment modes, teachers are instructed to create links between real-life school social events and the social tasks that are taught through the intervention. Adult mediation, as provided by teachers in the CBE, may be considered an effective method for the stage of construct acquisition and for learning the various social skill capabilities. Utilization of teachers as adult mediators maximizes the learning process and the facilitation of transfer from what was learned in the training to spontaneous real-life social situations. Teachers can also observe whether the child indeed uses and applies the learned skills in various social situations (Paul, 2003).

Training and Supervision. Throughout the years of field applications for the holistic CBE intervention in regular schools, we developed a model of inservice training and supervision for facilitators (mostly teachers), provided by the School of Education at Bar-Ilan University in collaboration with the Israeli Ministry of Education. Trained faculty who are experts in CBE teach and supervise teachers' administration of the holistic CBE intervention (combining both dyadic and group modes) for children with HFASD in an elementary, junior high, or high school setting throughout an entire academic year. The teacher-training curriculum integrates both treatment modes, thus helping teachers adapt social topics and structure (dyad or group) to individual children's needs. The year-long training is conducted at the School of Education for 3 hours once a week, plus monthly onsite supervision sessions in the schools.

Each university training session comprises theory and practice. For the first half of every weekly meeting, teachers receive theoretical instruction on issues related to the social characteristics of children with HFASD and with TYP (e.g., emotional development, social cognition and information processing, major characteristics of social interaction, development of play), as well as explanations of the main CBT techniques—both cognitive and behavioral. For the second half of every weekly meeting, using the CBE manuals, teachers practice CBT techniques and the various social curriculum topics to be implemented in the coming week. During these practice hours, teachers also present case studies from their dyadic or group work and receive feedback from their peer teachers and from the instructor. In addition, teachers share supplementary materials with each other that they had developed during their work. Thus the practice hours offer a forum for brainstorming and for support in solving problems that arise during ongoing work in the schools.

In collaboration with the Ministry of Education in Israel, teachers also receive onsite supervision of their work in the schools by a trained CBE staff member through monthly school visits during the implementation of the holisitic CBE intervention. Immediate feedback is provided to the teachers on completion of the observed intervention sessions.

PEERS

Children with TYP play an essential part in the CBE intervention model. Peers are considered to be very powerful mediators in fostering children's ability to participate in social interactions in natural settings (e.g., see reviews in Rogers, 2000, and in Kasari, Rotheram-Fuller, Locke, and Gulsrud 2012). In Kasari et al. (2012), mainstreamed children with ASD (CA = 6–11 years, grades 1–5, IQ > 65) who had undergone social intervention using peer mediation in regular schools were shown to obtain better results than children who underwent social intervention using adult mediation. The peer-mediated children were more salient in their classroom social network, had more friends, were evaluated by their teachers as having better social skills in class, and, most importantly, were less isolated on the playground compared with adult-mediated children.

Several formats for mediation of children with HFASD by peers with TYP have been presented in the literature, ranging from a more structured cotherapist role to the role of merely remaining in close proximity to children with HFASD to enhance their spontaneous social interaction and play (see review in Bass & Mulick, 2007; see also Paul, 2003; Rogers, 2000; Rubin & Lennon, 2004). In our CBE dyadic treatment mode, the child with TYP meets with the child with HFASD twice a week, once during a school recess (20 minutes) and once during home visits (duration was relative to the social task). Dyadic peer meetings offer structured opportunities to experience social activities during school time and after school, consistently with the same peer, and to practice learned social skills. During these two dyadic meetings, under adult supervision, the peer with TYP initiates social activities with the child with HFASD; these activities are related to the social topic being learned, with the teacher using problem-solving stages. Thus, for example, if the topic to be learned is collaboration, the peer with TYP is instructed by the teacher to initiate and be involved in collaborative activities with the child with HFASD (e.g., playing cards during recess and making pizza at home). The peer with TYP and the teacher meet once weekly (for 45 minutes). In this meeting, the teacher informs the peer with TYP about the social tasks for the coming week, instructs the peer on the task's implementation, listens to the peer's feedback about the performance of the former social task learned in the week before, and provides support for any difficulty that emerged during the enactment of the prior social task. In the group intervention mode, two children with TYP, usually of the same age and from the same class as the target child, are equal members of the group, along with the target children with HFASD. The peers with TYP serve as role models of adaptive social interactional behavior, fully participating in all group social activities and role playing. Criteria for selecting these peers—who act as mediators, aides, cotherapists, or change agents—are described in Appendix B, Table B3, for both CBE modes.

Peer involvement in both CBE treatment modes permits strong emphasis on reciprocity and perspective taking (in line with ToM capacities). Children in both modes are guided by the teacher or parent to select social activities that are pleasant both for children with HFASD and their peers with TYP. Thus peers' interests and preferences are taken into consideration throughout all intervention activities. The fact that practice always occurs in dyads or peer groups allows activities to remain other-focused, as suggested by Krasny et al. (2003), to foster cooperation and partnership.

The involvement of peers in the CBE intervention also enables the creation of a safe environment for the children with HFASD in which they can practice the learned skills and gain a sense of success. Inasmuch as the peers with TYP are "enforced collaborators" who volunteer to meet repeatedly and consistently with the child with HFASD, this reduces the anxiety generally elicited by experiencing social tasks with an unfamiliar child. Thus emphasis is placed on building up relationships with the peers with TYP within the group or dyadic treatment environment, as well as on forging a sense of social efficacy in the children with HFASD—the belief that they are able to start a conversation, join a group activity, and so on. To foster this safe environment, special attention is given to creating group rules, such as respecting each other and keeping what children share in the dyad or group confidential (loyalty and discretion). Furthermore, the well-being and sense of enjoyment of the peers with TYP are carefully considered throughout the work. Based on our experience, a key factor to the success and stability of participation among peers with TYP within the groups or dyads throughout the school year is the allotment of specific time in the program to teacher-support sessions for the peers with TYP regarding any difficulty that emerges (e.g., lack of cooperation of the child with HFASD despite the peer's efforts). On the whole, we learned that it is indeed important to choose an appropriate peer aide with TYP, but it is even more important to support that peer's social experience throughout the intervention and to ensure the peer's enjoyment no less than the completion of the intervention goals.

PARENTS

In the CBE intervention model, parents are more involved in the dyadic mode, due to technical complexities in including parents in the group treatment. However, parental involvement is highly significant for any type of intervention aiming to increase generalization of treatment effects into the home environment and to provide the child with another social setting in which to practice learned social competencies. Parents in both intervention modes receive an explanation about the intervention curriculum and procedure before the school year. During the school year, parents of children in the dyadic treatment receive weekly instructions from the teacher on that week's learned tasks, using a "contact notebook" passed back and forth from teacher to parents via the child. These parents' role is to motivate and support their child in the process of practicing those tasks with the assigned peer in the weekly dyadic session at home, as well as practicing the new skills directly with their children and encouraging the child's siblings to do so, too, if possible. Parents help their child implement each social goal at home with the assigned peer by suggesting ideas for social activities, by physically bringing the assigned peer to their home, by helping their child to find conversational subjects for a telephone call, and so on. Parents may consult the teacher freely for guidance.

Issues of Generalization and Maintenance

Spontaneous transfer between settings and persons is difficult for children with HFASD (e.g., Rogers, 2000). Social intervention, then, should include mediation in different social settings within school (e.g., to foster transfer from the small group to school recess) and also in settings outside school, such as after-school activities at home, in order to increase the likelihood of generalization to children's spontaneous social-interaction capabilities (e.g., Attwood, 2003; Paul, 2003; see also Spence, 2003, who expounded on increasing generalization of treatment to settings and persons but not specifically to HFASD). Indeed, generalization of treatment gains is the most difficult issue related to treatment efficacy.

Although individual differences in response to treatment have not yet been systematically explored for holistic CBE interventions, clinical observations of the numerous children with HFASD who have participated thus far (in over 100 classes) demonstrated these children's fairly rapid progress in social-cognition capabilities. They are rather quick to show understanding of a variety of emotions and to use the problem-solving technique in various social settings. However, actual change in their social interaction behaviors usually lags behind this relatively fast improvement in the social-cognitive domain. We have also observed that different children exhibit very different rates of improvement in targeted treatment domains, in demonstrating a real change in behavior, and in maintaining that change after treatment termination, even if these children show similar verbal and nonverbal capabilities. Our clinical impression is that these improvement rates are influenced by an accumulation of social-emotional competencies (e.g., motivation, self-esteem, self-awareness, sensory issues, support at home) and social-cognitive competencies (e.g., learning profile, memory capabilities, attention span, executive function, and baseline ToM skills).

Further empirical studies are crucial to help delineate the factors related to these individual differences in response to treatment, as well as to follow up on treatment gains. However, based on current knowledge, the CBE design incorporates the three aspects currently assumed to increase generalization of treatment gains: ecological treatments that encompass various social change agents in the child's life (teachers, peers, parents); implementation in diverse natural social settings (school, home); and use of different techniques and activities to practice each social task (Duncan & Klinger, 2010; Krasny et al., 2003; Paul, 2003). On the other hand, although this mixture of people, settings, and treatment modalities and techniques through multimodal treatment models may indeed contribute to generalization, it simultaneously poses a challenge to researchers trying to determine the relative contributions of each separate treatment component. This remains an important challenge for future studies. For example, based on clinical impressions indicating that problem-solving techniques are very helpful to children on the spectrum—perhaps because these tools bring order and structure into these children's "chaotic" social world—such techniques have been used frequently in several CBT-based interventions for children on the spectrum, as reviewed in the preceding section; however, their unique contribution has not yet been systematically examined.

Another issue related to generalization concerns the possible conflict between the need to create a safe environment in the treatment, as discussed earlier, and the need to move beyond sheltered treatment environments out into more natural, spontaneous environments in order to promote generalization, which therefore exposes these children to potentially more threatening social situations. Thus, clinically, one of the most challenging decisions in CBE intervention is to decide when the child is strong enough to cope with social demands outside the peer-dyad or small-group treatment milieu involving children who are not part of the treatment setting. For example, when is the right time to add homework tasks such as inviting peers who are not part of the intervention or joining peer play on the playground? Transitions from the "safe" environments into real-life social situations should be planned very carefully. For example, it is very important for the teacher to work with the target child on mapping classmates into potential collaborators and noncollaborators by helping them identify classmates' personal characteristics (e.g., funny, gives help, makes fun of other children, aggressive, patient). Transition from the small-group and dyadic social activities to "real-world" social interactions are based on the teacher's clinical judgments throughout the intervention but contribute tremendously to the child's ability to generalize and transfer learning from the safe treatment environment into a more natural social environment.

In sum, in line with other recent multimodal social interventions in the field for children with HFASD, as reviewed earlier, the CBE is a comprehensive and multilevel intervention (integrating social cognition, emotions, and social behavior) that incorporates learning and experiencing of each social or emotional construct, considers developmental issues and between- and within-individual differences, and plans for generalization and maintenance of social gains, within an ecological orientation. The three initial empirical examinations of the dyadic and group CBE treatment modes are presented next.

Empirical Studies Testing the Effectiveness of Implementation of the CBE Multimodal Social Intervention

Three pretest–posttest studies examined the efficacy of the school-based CBE intervention: (1) a pilot study of a dyadic intervention (Bauminger, 2002); (2) a replication of the pilot study (Bauminger, 2007b); and (3) a study of the group intervention (Bauminger, 2007a). The first empirical study evaluated the effectiveness of a 7-month dyadic CBE intervention targeting a pilot sample of 15 youngsters with HFASD (CA = 8–17 years) implemented by trained, supervised teachers in regular schools. Preintervention and postintervention measures included observations of social interaction during school break, social-cognition measures of problem solving and emotional understanding, and teacher ratings of children's social skills. Results demonstrated progress in all three areas of intervention. After treatment, children were more likely to initiate positive social interaction with peers unrelated to the treatment; in particular, they improved eye contact and their ability to share experiences with peers and to show interest in peers. When solving social problems after treatment, children provided more relevant solutions and fewer nonsocial solutions to different social situations. In emotional knowledge after treatment, children provided more examples of complex emotions, were able to supply more specific than general examples, and included an audience more often for the different emotions. Children also obtained higher teacher-rated social skills scores in assertion and cooperation after treatment.

The 2007b study replicated the 2002 intervention model (7-month dyadic intervention mediated by trained, supervised teachers in regular schools) for 26 preadolescents with HFASD (CA = 7.7–11.6 years) and yielded even better improvement rates both in social cognition and in social interactions. The 2007b study also provided strong support for the intervention's impact on generalization of learned social interaction skills, because teachers who were unrelated to the intervention reported improvements in the children's social behavior. Interestingly, in the 2007b study, children's interaction skills were better 4 months after treatment than immediately after treatment.

However, both the 2002 and 2007b studies provided one-on-one mediation by the teacher and practice in a dyad with an older peer with TYP, thus furnishing little data about progress in children's conversational or cooperative skills in peer groups. As a result, the 2007a study extended the CBE model beyond dyadic interactions to target peer-group interactions in groups comprising two peers with TYP and between one and three children with HFASD and also to target more complex social-emotional capabilities. This 7-month small-group intervention, mediated by trained, supervised teachers in regular schools, targeted two groups of preadolescents with HFASD. The first group consisted of preadolescents with HFASD who had participated in the first-year CBE dyadic treatment and then continued into the group treatment (n = 11, mean CA = 8.78 years). The second group comprised new recruits with HFASD (n = 15, mean CA = 9.23 years). Groups were matched according to CA, Full Scale IQ, and the three ADI-R subscales of Social, Communication, and Behavior (Rutter et al., 2003). We examined the group treatment's direct effects (e.g., social problem solving) and indirect effects (ToM, executive function) on social-cognitive capabilities, as well as on children's abilities to maintain group interactions not only within the group treatment setting but also during school break with peers unrelated to the treatment. Study results demonstrated direct and indirect treatment effects on social cognition for both groups. In terms of direct treatment effects, after the intervention, children showed a more advanced ability to define and recognize emotions, social situations, and constructs (such as what a friend is and how to solve social problems by relating to social solutions more often), and they revealed a better understanding of others (by better justifying a person's activities along different social scenarios) and an improved awareness of others' presence (by more frequently including an audience for complex emotions). Thus treatment appeared to be efficient in promoting socioemotional perceptions and problem-solving capabilities, which comprise essential components of social cognition.

In terms of indirect effects, children's enhanced ability after treatment to provide higher levels of justification to explain another person's motivation to tell a lie suggests that these children improved in their ToM capabilities and in their facility in relating to and considering social norms (such as telling a lie to avoid hurting parents' feelings). Regarding executive functions, after treatment, children showed a tendency to better sort card sets and clearly demonstrated a better capacity to conceptualize sorting strategies and to recognize the examiner's strategies. Perhaps their ability for concept formation improved through treatment. Inasmuch as the sorting measure did not include social stimuli but rather objective verbal and nonverbal stimuli, it examined more conceptual cognitive capabilities—to solve problems and to flexibly restructure concepts by shape, by size, by verbal content, and so forth.

Outcomes of the group intervention regarding children's social interaction capabilities were mixed. Although children's cooperative capabilities within the intervention group itself improved, dyadic and group social interactions during school recess did not. When companionship capabilities were examined within a structured situation such as working together on a shared design, children demonstrated an overall improvement in their ability to collaborate with peers and specifically in their abilities for mutual planning, cooperative work with peers, and sharing. Working together and mutual planning may have resulted directly from the treatment's focus because during the CBE intervention children practiced different activities that required them to plan together and work cooperatively. However, their improved sharing capability is of great interest. Perhaps friendships evolved between the children within the group, and thus they felt more secure in sharing. In addition, their lack of generalization into spontaneous dyadic or group interactions with peers who were not associated with the treatment is especially interesting in light of the generalizations demonstrated by the aforementioned research (Bauminger, 2002, 2007b). Perhaps the fact that children's social agents outside the intervention group (such as parents and peers) were not actively involved in the group treatment (Bauminger, 2007a) may have reduced children's capacity to transfer what they learned in the small group to their day-to-day interactions with peers during recesses. Thus generalization merits further investigation.

In summary, we identified several issues that deserved consideration: First, multimodal CBE dyadic and/or group intervention seems to offer promising possibilities in facilitating social-cognition processes in HFASD. Second, the enhancement of spontaneous peer interaction appears to require careful consideration of setting and person generalization within the CBE intervention. Differences between the 2002 and 2007a studies in children's spontaneous interactions may be attributable to meetings with the assigned older peer during school recess and the more active involvement of the child's parents in the first study (Bauminger, 2002). Thus the learned behaviors underwent practice in different social settings (class, school recesses, and home), possibly fostering generalization of social behaviors to school recesses. During the group (2007a) study, children met with their peers in the small group during treatment, but group activities did not require playing together during school recesses. Indeed, in the holistic CBE approach, we directly include mediation to different social settings within school (e.g., school recess) and maybe even outside school (e.g., home), in order to increase the likelihood of children's spontaneous generalization of social interaction capabilities.

Third, a noticeable pitfall of CBE research efforts must be considered: the lack of control groups across studies. In order for us to obtain approval to implement these studies in schools, many stakeholders in the educational system and community had to give consent, such as school principals, children's educational inspectors in the Ministry of Education and local municipalities, children's teachers, parents both of children with HFASD and children with TYP, and the children themselves. It was hard to obtain their consent to run all evaluation procedures with a group of children who would not receive treatment. In addition, due to the fact that treatments took place throughout an entire school year, it was impossible to include a wait-listed group. This lack of control groups thus far has precluded the possibility of concluding that the CBE treatment's efficacy goes beyond the effects of children's natural maturation processes. This is indeed an important shortcoming, and currently we are conducting research with a wait-listed comparison group to better develop evidence-based methodologies for CBE.

Finally, one other issue emerging from these studies is that, despite the CBE curriculum's breadth, it does not yet cover several important topics with specific relevance to older adolescents with HFASD, such as understanding social rules for self-disclosure, understanding intimacy, forming same-sex and opposite-sex relationships, and coping with anxiety. These are all future possible expansions for CBE. The secondary gains in social functioning elicited by recent treatments that have focused on reduction of anxiety are discussed next.

SOCIAL IMPLICATIONS FOR CBT-BASED TREATMENT OF COMORBID ANXIETY DISORDERS

> In one of our group sessions, we worked on a problem-solving scenario that included group entry into a conversation. The vignette was very simple: "John went outside during recess and saw his friends gathering and talking together. He really wanted to join them but did not know how. What can he do?" In the group discussion, we asked the group members to identify the task, and they did, but when we asked "How do you think John feels?," suddenly one girl with Asperger syndrome replied, "For me, when I need to join a group conversation, I feel so afraid that I imagine that the earth is opening its mouth and swallowing me up! At that moment, I cannot think of anything to do because I feel paralyzed!"

Clearly, this example demonstrates how a very bright, high-functioning girl with Asperger syndrome withdraws from joining social conversation due to her anxiety. Indeed, as detailed in Chapter 6, anxiety has frequently been identified as a comorbid condition for children with HFASD (e.g., White et al., 2009), which may create a real obstacle to most social intervention efforts. Recently, studies have been published describing attempts to reduce affective disorders, mainly anxiety disorders, in children with HFASD (e.g., Chalfant, Rapee, & Carroll, 2007; Drahota, Wood, Sze, & Van Dyke, 2011; Moree & Davis, 2010; Reaven, Blakeley-Smith, Culhane-Shelburne, & Hepburn, 2012; Sofronoff, Attwood, & Hinton, 2005; Sze & Wood, 2007; White et al., 2010; Wood, Drahota, Sze, Har et al., 2009). Fewer HFASD interventions have implemented CBT-based models to treat OCD—another frequent comorbid disorder in HFASD (e.g., Lehmkuhl, Storch, Bodfish, & Geffken, 2008; Reaven & Hepburn, 2003). For the purpose of the current discussion of social and emotional functioning in HFASD, two main questions should be posed regarding the utility of CBT in treating these children's anxiety: Do such CBT-based interventions effectively diminish anxiety? Do they lead to enhanced social functioning in these children? It seems that the answer to the first question is easier than the answer to the second question, despite the diversity of methodologies that have been implemented, such as case studies (as in Sze & Wood, 2007) or experimental group studies using wait-listed control groups (as in Chalfant et al., 2007; Reaven et al., 2009; Sofronoff et al., 2005; Wood, Drahota, Sze, Har, et al., 2009).

Do CBT-Based Interventions Effectively Diminish Anxiety in Children with HFASD?

Overall, study results thus far have presented consistent success in reducing anxiety among children and preadolescents with HFASD through the use of CBT-based models modified for children with HFASD, in that high percentages of children who met criteria for anxiety disorders before treatment no longer did so after treatment. For example, in Chalfant et al. (2007), 71.4% of the CBT-treatment group did not meet anxiety disorder criteria after treatment, whereas 100% of the wait-listed children showed no change. Likewise, in Wood, Drahota, Sze, Har, et al. (2009), 92.9% responded positively to the CBT intervention in the experimental group, with 80% no longer meeting the diagnostic criteria, versus spontaneous improvement shown in only 9.1% of the wait-listed group. Children's self-reports also revealed reduced anxiety as a result of treatment; for instance, in Sofronoff et al. (2005), children reported a higher number of strategies for coping with anxiety compared with the wait-listed group, and in Chalfant et al. (2007) children reported lower anxiety level after treatment, whereas the wait-listed control group showed no change in anxiety level. Significant reduction in anxiety after CBT treatment was also reported using parental reports and interviews (e.g., Chalfant et al., 2007; Reaven et al., 2012; Sofronoff et al., 2005; Wood, Drahota, Sze, Van Dyke, et al., 2009) and teacher reports (e.g., Chalfant et al., 2007). Thus CBT-based models to treat anxiety in children with HFASD have shown good efficacy in reducing anxiety.

In a recent review of CBT-based studies, Moree and Davis (2010) suggested that CBT interventions targeting anxiety should undergo four main modifications to suit children with HFASD. The first recommended modification involves taking disorder-specific hierarchies into consideration, meaning that interventionists should relate to the child with HFASD as a whole and thus consider treating other areas in addition to anxiety (which may be equal in importance or even of higher importance for the child's well-being), such as children's lack of adaptive social skills. For example, Wood, Drahota, Sze, Har, et al. (2009) developed an integrative curriculum that included not only a modification of a traditional CBT protocol utilizing cognitive reconstructing and in vivo exposure to feared situations but also components aiming to treat children's poor social skills (i.e., emotion recognition and friendship skills), increase self-help skills, and reduce stereotypical behaviors. Recently, White et al. (2010) also proposed an integrative multimodal treatment targeting both anxiety and social skills, although this intervention has not yet been experimentally scrutinized. In White et al.'s (2010) suggested curriculum, the social-skills-building modules included lessons on how to initiate with peers, conversational skills, recognizing others' cues, and handling rejection. Their group curriculum included issues such as emotional regulation and group entry (e.g., White et al., 2009).

The second recommended HFASD modification for CBT-based anxiety interventions involves an increased emphasis on concrete, visual, and affect-related cognitive and behavioral techniques for teaching social-emotional skills. Moree and Davis (2010) highlighted the need to concretize concepts, use visual tactics such as the "emotion toolbox" or the "emotion thermometer," and extensively utilize emotional statements, pictures, drawings, visual worksheets, narratives, social stories, and role play (see Appendix A, Table A1). Most of the studies described in this section have utilized some of these adaptations. For example, a "tool box" to "fix" feelings was implemented in Sofronoff et al. (2005); and visual aids and structured worksheets were used in Chalfant et al. (2007).

The third recommended modification is to ensure that treatment includes parental involvement. Although parents are frequently involved in CBT-based anxiety treatments, their involvement has not been consistent, and their roles in treatment have differed. Sofronoff et al. (2005) specifically examined the differential contributions of individual treatment and parent–child treatment and demonstrated better results on some of the measures for the mode in which parents were involved. Only some interventions (e.g., Chalfant et al., 2007) provided parents with psychoeducational training (e.g., lessons on topics relating to the child's intervention) and with a parental support network, as well as with parental management training. Reaven et al. (2012) implemented multifamily group sessions, which included large-group activities (children and parents together) and small-group activities (children together, parents together), and dyadic work (parent–child pair), and this study presented a significant reduction in anxiety symptoms that were maintained at the 3- and 8-month follow-ups.

The fourth and last modification recommended by Moree and Davis (2010) involves the need for treatment to account for the child's specific areas of interest, either as a starting point for increasing motivation or else by addressing the need to reduce overly extensive interest in a narrow topic in order to increase more adaptive functioning (as in Wood, Drahota, Sze, Har, et al., 2009). Altogether, Moree and Davis (2010) seem to offer a helpful framework to be considered in the various CBT treatments that focus on anxiety in HFASD.

Do CBT-Based Interventions Targeting Anxiety Lead to Enhanced Social Functioning in Children with HFASD?

Even if CBT-based anxiety interventions have concurrently targeted additional child competencies (e.g., friendship, self-help ability), empirical research has not yet systematically measured or addressed children's progress in such skills. Therefore, succinct information is not yet available about the effects of anxiety treatments on general improvement in social functioning among children with HFASD. For example, Sofronoff et al. (2005) stated that parents gave qualitative reports about their children's progress in some areas, such as friendship development and increases in confidence in day-to-day interactions; however, these authors did not furnish data from systematic examination of these competencies. Likewise, Chalfant et al. (2007) administered both the parent and teacher versions of the Strengths and Difficulties Questionnaire (Goodman, 1997), which includes a Peer Problems scale and a Prosocial scale to measure conduct disorders and emotional problems; however, results were reported only regarding more general internalizing and externalizing outcomes. Wood and his colleagues demonstrated several preliminary findings showing a positive trend toward improvement in social interaction (Wood, 2012), in general adaptive skills of personal and daily living (Drahota et al., 2011), and in autism symptoms (Wood, Drahota, Sze, Van Dyke, et al., 2009). Thus, even if a positive trend emerged in these studies, children's improvement beyond anxiety reduction still needs to be explored more systematically.

As described thoroughly in Chapter 3, one of the major social challenges for children with HFASD is the development of friendship with peers. I now review studies that were specifically aimed at helping children with HFASD to develop such relationships.

INTERVENTIONS TO IMPROVE SOCIAL RELATIONSHIPS IN HFASD

Recently, interventionists have increased their focus on enhancing social-emotional and social relationship capabilities such as peer friendship (e.g., the UCLA the Program for the Evaluation and Enrichment of Relational Skills [PEERS]; Laugeson & Frankel, 2010) and on issues such as mutual regulation and coregulation, which comprise the foundation for developing relationships (e.g., the Social Communication Emotion Regulation Training System model [SCERTS]; Prizant, Wetherby, Rubin, Laurent, & Rydell, 2006; Rubin & Laurent, 2004). Laugeson and Frankel's (2010) recently published curriculum, the PEERS friendship curriculum, specifically aimed to enhance the ability to make friends throughout development from elementary school age up to young adulthood in individuals with HFASD. The PEERS treatment included 12 group meetings for the children and their parents, emphasizing issues such as the characterization of "good friendship"(i.e., sharing common interests, self-disclosure of private thoughts and feelings, mutual understanding and conflict resolution, equalities, affection and care, and loyalty and trust), as well as how to choose appropriate friends; how to "get together" with friends; ways to cope with teasing, bullying, and a "bad reputation"; and training on trading information, as in social conversation with friends. During this program, children were asked to initiate relationships with other children outside the treatment milieu, with the support of their parents in the process.

Several recent studies have demonstrated the promising efficacy of the PEERS with different age groups. Children at the 2nd to 5th grade level (mean CA = 8.6; Frankel et al., 2010) and adolescents with HFASD ages 12–17 years (mean CA = 14.6; Laugeson, Frankel, Gantman, Dillon, & Mogil, 2012) reported decreased levels of loneliness, improved perceptions of popularity, higher quality of friendship relationships, and higher levels of social understanding after treatment. Their parents also reported hosting an increased number of playmates and their children's decrease in disengaged behaviors. Follow-up effects should be explored more systematically. In Frankel et al. (2010), children had returned to more solitary behavior on play dates 3 months after treatment, and in Laugeson et al. (2012) improvement was noticed at the 14-week follow-up, but this was mainly according to reports by parents, who were active participants in the treatment.

Recently Gantman, Kapp, Orenski, and Laugeson (2012) presented similar results for the PEERS based on parent reports and self-reports for young adults (CA = 18–23 years), but no follow-up outcomes have been reported. Thus the PEERS looks to be very helpful in unblocking children's initial social exclusion and in providing necessary guidance tools for parents and children to help the latter develop friendships; however, children probably need longer support and further training to enable them to maintain the developed relationships, as well as to transfer their capabilities to new social settings, such as school. One other future direction may be to assess the actual quality of the peer friendships that children form as a result of participation in the PEERS by directly observing the friends' interactions at pretest and posttest to assess friendship characteristics such as sharing of thoughts and feelings to denote intimacy or mutual interests and mutual affection to denote closeness (see Chapter 3).

Emotional regulation may be an important mechanism underlying the development and maintenance of social relationships. Emotional regulation and mutual coregulation are critical mechanisms for developing social engagement (Rubin & Laurent, 2004). Difficulties in these capacities characterize many children with HFASD (Laurent & Rubin, 2004) and may be partially responsible for their problems in developing durable friendships. The SCERTS model (a comprehensive educational approach for children with ASD; Prizant et al., 2006) included a specific aim of enhancing children's coregulation, as well as self-regulation. Self-regulatory skills refer to children's ability to use different behavioral, linguistic, and metacognitive strategies to regulate their level of arousal during various familiar and unfamiliar activities; for instance, to use self-talk or self-monitoring to guide behavior, to rank emotional intensity, or to remove themselves from overstimulating activity. Mutual regulation refers to children's ability to regulate their behaviors, emotions, and thoughts by attuning to their partner's behaviors, emotions, and thoughts, resulting in joint engagement. CBT efforts have also shown efficacy in increasing emotional regulation skills, especially reducing impulsivity and increasing anger management (Scarpa & Reyes, 2011) and in Sofronoff, Attwood, Hinton, and Levin (2007).

Despite their importance for facilitating peers' joint engagement, self-regulation and coregulation have not received sufficient attention in peer-relations interventions, whereas more attention has been given to adult–child interactions (e.g., Gulsrud, Jahromi, & Kasari, 2010). Helping children with HFASD to develop more coordinated relationships with peers is indeed a challenging aim for future treatment endeavors.

SUMMARY AND FUTURE DIRECTIONS

This chapter presented a broad perspective on the recent social intervention models targeting social-cognitive and social-behavioral functioning for the more cognitively able children on the spectrum. Overall, this field has come a long way in its efforts to help these children assimilate more adaptively to their peer groups by pursuing more comprehensive and multidimensional intervention models treating social-cognitive, social interaction, and social-emotional capabilities, up to the development of social relationships such as peer friendship.

However, several questions remain unanswered. First, related to the content of intervention: What should a social curriculum include? This chapter presented the clear advantages of designing a multidimensional, developmentally and ecologically oriented curriculum that interlinks social cognition, emotions, and social behavior (interaction capabilities) to obtain integrative social functioning in HFASD. However, content selection related to which direct and indirect capabilities should be learned remains more ambiguous. For example, should ToM be a specific topic or a core overall intervention theme? Can progress in executive functioning result from teaching problem-solving techniques? To what extent does instruction in one social-cognitive capability (e.g., recognizing various emotions) promote the development of other social-cognitive capabilities (e.g., emotional regulation)?

Another important issue for future consideration is the need to explore the quality of the interactions that develop between children as an outcome of intervention efforts helping them to develop coregulated interactions. Chains of interaction may comprise a good unit of analysis for understanding what transpires in the developing social interaction. Researchers also need to move on from coregulation interventions in the peer–adult system to a coregulated interaction in the peer system. Hence more studies focusing on friendship facilitation are needed. Developing methods that increase social motivation and social involvement in school-age children and adolescents will be helpful. Identification of play-related goals and collaborative capabilities for the older children is currently missing in the literature. In particular, understanding of individual differences in treatment outcomes should be explored further, relating both to children's biological characteristics (e.g., sensory profile, temperament, speed of processing, learning capacity) and environmental characteristics (e.g., parents, teachers, school).

Another issue involves treatment techniques. This chapter showed the merit of combining a mixture of cognitive and behavioral techniques; however, the differential contribution of each technique is not yet clear-cut. For example, social stories and social problem solving are two techniques employed frequently to teach social understanding and coping strategies; nonetheless, data are currently unavailable as to which situations or social tasks are more appropriate for each technique (e.g., Should group entry be taught using a social story or a problem-solving technique?), nor regarding the optimal target population (e.g., Which situation or task is more suited to younger vs. older children?). Social stories provide a structured narrative for the child, with instructions about how to behave in a social situation, but how effective is such training if the child confronts a slightly different or even very different situation in everyday life? On the other hand, problem solving provides a social scheme for the perception of social situations, but this technique does not supply social alternatives and suggestions, necessitating their development by the child through mediation. A major issue for interventionists is helping the child to transfer theoretical knowledge of social constructs into pragmatic, more spontaneous social experiences. What helps this transfer is only partially known. For example, the use of visual support in the form of written and pictorial representations of expected activities and behaviors, worksheets, rules, comic strips, and so on are all frequently recommended and utilized learning tools; however, research has not yet demonstrated which of these tools actually leads to effective coping with real-life social experiences.

An additional important issue is, Where should social intervention take place and by whom? This chapter discussed the advantages of using more naturalistic social environments in intervention, such as the school, and the advantages of using the child's close social agents within these environments—namely, peers, teachers, and parents—to attain better generalization of treatment gains into various other social settings. However, despite acknowledgement of its importance (Lord et al., 2005), school-based intervention is not yet a common intervention model; therefore, researchers in the field are only beginning to explore how such interventions should be optimally implemented. Many questions remain open: Should social curriculum be integrated into the child's overall curriculum? Considering time and budgetary constraints, should this curriculum come at the expense of other lessons, and if so, which? Also, if teachers operate the intervention, who should support and guide their implementation? How frequent and lasting does such support need to be? Considering that social intervention for children with HFASD requires small settings, such as small social groups or even dyadic work, what are the best ways to connect between the social activities and gains in the treatment group and the child's regular class? Should peer mediators or aides be assigned for the child both in the treatment setting and during school recess? What adaptations and modifications are required in the child's social environment to better fit the child's special needs? How should teachers mentor and guide parent participation in the treatment, if at all? These are only some of the queries to be explored empirically regarding the implementation of social intervention in the school setting. Indeed, the presentation of the holistic CBE model provided some insight into the implementation of school programs; however, a deeper understanding of such models and processes is greatly needed, especially in light of the wide-ranging calls for implementing such models (e.g., Lord et al., 2005; National Research Council, 2001). It is also important to consider the need to extend such interventions to young adults and adults with HFASD, who, after high school exit, are surprisingly underresourced, as are their families (see Chapter 4). On the whole, social interventions are essential for the more cognitively able school-age youngsters on the spectrum, to reduce their loneliness and increase their social involvement and friendships with peers. The field has come a long way in developing more comprehensive multidimensional treatment models that link social cognition and social interaction to better fit the complexities in social functioning that are experienced by these children. Moving from more traditional social-skills-oriented training toward global multidimensional treatment models that concurrently enhance several social-cognitive capabilities and social behaviors also enables a focus on affective difficulties, such as anxiety, and on treatments to promote the development of ongoing friendships. It seems that children with HFASD show good progress in social-cognitive capabilities through such multidimensional interventions and also some progress in social interaction skills; however, a core dilemma remains regarding finding ways to help these children transfer new abilities and develop more efficient, responsive, durable interactions with various peers in different, unfamiliar social situations.

Chapter 8

Interventions to Facilitate Cognitive and Academic Functioning

with Yael Kimhi

Considering the high cognitive functioning level of the population with HFASD and their common inclusion in regular education settings, this chapter reviews effective strategies for helping students with HFASD to meet academic needs. Constant new lines of research are providing empirical evidence that can be implemented into daily practice in educational settings for learners with ASD (Odom, Collet-Klingenberg, Rogers, & Hatton, 2010). Pennington (2009) emphasized, in his article concerning writing instruction for students with ASD, that teachers should plan learning interventions according to relevant existing data, rather than "proceeding blindly" or using instructional products that have no research support. However, it is important to note that empirical studies concerning academic interventions for school-age children with HFASD are scarce; therefore, this chapter describes empirically validated teaching strategies found effective for facilitating learning along the wider spectrum of ASD and also covers all age groups (preschool to adult).

The majority of students with ASD require specialized services in school (National Research Council, 2001), whether they attend general or special education settings. To enable specialized professional services, school staff should possess sufficient knowledge regarding various teaching and training strategies that have been empirically proven as successful when applied to learners with ASD. The review in this chapter describes two main strategy domains: those that aim to improve academic skills in general for students with ASD and those that aim to develop various specific cognitive and academic domains such as memory, language (e.g., ability to use questions), reading, writing, and mathematics. At the end of this chapter, we include a glossary explaining the various academic professional terms used throughout the chapter (see Table 8.1 on pages 211–214).

FREQUENTLY USED STRATEGIES TO FACILITATE GENERAL ACADEMIC SKILLS IN ASD

Among the interventions that are frequently employed for learners with ASD, the following interventions derive from two major fields: structured teaching that involves organizing the environment in order to assist children in understanding what is expected of them and behavior analysis interventions (such as pivotal response training and multiple examplar training) that aim to teach children appropriate behaviors.

STRUCTURED TEACHING

The use of structured teaching for children with HFASD (called the Treatment and Education of Autistic and related Communication-Handicapped Children, or TEACCH) derived from Schopler's work in the 1970s (e.g., Schopler & Reichler, 1971). This teaching strategy modifies the class setting and instruction via emphasis on visual information and organizational support. The major components of structured teaching include the classroom's organization, visual schedules and information concerning school activities, visual work systems that refer to students' tasks, and visual task organization. All of these aim to assist students in completing required tasks and in increasing independence while working (Mesibov, Shea, & Schopler, 2005). Many children with HFASD are visual learners; therefore, visually based interventions are, for the most part, recommended to enhance and enable learning (Bryan & Gast, 2000; Ganz, 2007). The visual organizers (i.e., separate or individual work areas; visual work schedules; visual instructions for class work tasks, such as graphic maps, written instructions, color-coded organizers, pictorial cues, etc.) should assist in promoting children's attention to the task at hand. Hume and Odom (2007) executed a single-subject study for structured teaching with replication across three preschoolers with ASD, one scanning documents in the library and the other two completing individual play and work activities in their preschool. Findings showed that the use of individual work systems fostered all three participants' levels of on-task behavior, task participation, and task completion.

Behavioral Interventions

Pivotal Response Training

Behavioral intervention has shown effectiveness in producing large gains in IQ, especially in young children with ASD (Reichow, 2012; Reichow & Wolery, 2009). Pivotal response training (PRT) is a variant of behavioral intervention and aims to increase children's motivation to learn, monitoring of their own behavior, and initiation of communication with others. Furthermore, it is intended to assist the child in responding to multiple cues and stimuli, which is an essential skill necessary for learning (Koegel, Koegel, Harrower, & Carter, 1999). PRT is based on the assumption that learning depends on "pivotal" skills (specific skills targeted for learning, such as the ability to ask specific "wh" questions or the ability to read a sight word in a specific context) and collateral skills (skills that develop due to the intervention that were not targeted specifically). The development of the specific, targeted pivotal skills usually results in improvement in or expansion to various collateral, general skills. For example, the teacher could target the ability to ask appropriate "wh" questions as a targeted pivotal skill to be directly taught, and the child may develop the collateral skill of learning to answer the questions during the learning intervention (although asking, not answering, was the skill taught specifically). In other words, PRT has been found to be effective in developing certain behaviors (called pivotal responses), together with additional, nontargeted behaviors that also begin to emerge due to the intervention (Koegel, Shirotova, & Koegel, 2009).

PRT takes place in the child's natural environment (e.g., in the classroom) in order to promote collateral changes in generalized areas of functioning, such as learning and communication (Koegel, Koegel, & Carter, 1999). In a study that examined the efficacy of PRT, Koegel, Koegel, Green-Hopkins, and Barnes (2010) explored the ability of three young preschool children with ASD to ask "where" by aid of PRT and found that all three children exhibited an increase in correct use of the language structures corresponding to the questions they had asked (the pivotal skills), along with generalization that occurred at home (collateral skills).

Multiple-Exemplar Training/Instruction

The use of multiple exemplars (or examples)—different examples of the same stimulus—is important when teaching children with ASD. The use of multiple-exemplar training/instruction (MET/MEI) can assist acquisition and can facilitate generalization. For instance, when teaching a word visually (see the upcoming section, "Visual Learning Strategies"), presentation of the same word in different sizes and fonts should enable full acquisition of the word. Various studies show that MET/MEI is an efficient strategy for children with LFA, leading to increases in the ability to name objects. The recommended setting for MET/MEI is within a learning unit that includes teacher–pupil interaction in the following steps: (1) teacher presents target, (2) pupil responds, and (3) teacher responds (consequence) to the pupil's response (Hawkins, Kingsdorf, Charnock, Szabo, & Gautreaux, 2009). A recent study (Persicke, Tarbox, Ranick, & St. Clair, 2012) found that utilization of MET/MEI facilitated the understanding of metaphors in a group of young children with HFASD (see the upcoming subsection on figurative language in texts).

In addition to the interventions deriving from structured teaching and behavior analysis described previously, a number of general strategies that facilitate learning for all students (both with TYP and with impairments) have also been found to be relevant in promoting learning for pupils with ASD and HFASD. Three general strategies that have been examined empirically for ASD are detailed next.

General Strategies

Scaffolding Strategies

Scaffolding refers to the idea that when introducing a new academic subject, it is important to supply specialized instructional supports, such as modeling the task, providing prompts and cues, supplying partial solutions, sequencing the various stages of the task, and more, in order to facilitate learning. While scaffolding, the adult uses the various techniques in order to create an interesting and motivating learning environment and to develop a feeling of competence. Scaffolding often includes the adults' participation and joint engagement in the specific activity (Basil & Reyes, 2003). Bellon, Ogletree, and Harn (2000) examined the efficacy of a single-subject scaffolding intervention that included prompts, cues, and supply of partial solutions, along with a repeated storybook-reading technique (in which the same story was read repeatedly to the child; see the section on language below for elaboration), with one young preschooler with ASD (CA = 3.10 years). This scaffolding technique aimed to increase the child's use of spontaneous speech, and it included the following prompts, cues, and partial solutions: (1) *cloze,* in which the adult pauses to indicate that the child should fill the gap with relevant information; (2) *binary possibilities,* in which the adult offers the child two options and the child chooses the appropriate one; (3) *"wh" questions,* in which the adult elicits explicit information; and (4) *expansions,* in which the adult elaborates on the child's utterances. Bellon et al. found that the repeated storybook reading, along with the scaffolding techniques, facilitated and enhanced the child's ability to use speech spontaneously in general settings.

Cueing Strategies

Cueing comprises a general strategy that may relate to any given situation, whether social or pedagogical, and that is supplied by the adult to facilitate the child's understanding of the situation at hand. For the most part, cues are verbal (such as semantic cues, which supply words' context and meaning), pictorial (which supply meaning by aid of pictures or graphic symbols such as arrows, icons, and so on), and/or textual (such as underlining specific words or sections in a given text). The clues are intended to help children understand instructions, texts, and language. The efficacy of cueing as a strategy in ASD and HFASD is described throughout this chapter (see the upcoming sections on memory, question asking, and reading comprehension).

Embedded Instruction

This general strategy promotes the child's engagement in learning activities by identifying times and activities that can be used to implement learning tasks in the context of ongoing academic activities. The teacher identifies appropriate and relevant times to apply chosen instructional procedures (e.g., teaching odd and even numbers when children line up in pairs to go out of the class). Embedded instruction is believed to maximize children's motivation because teachers take children's preferences into consideration. Studies have supported the notion that embedded instruction could be efficient for children with disabilities (Horn, Lieber, Li, Sandall, & Schwartz, 2000; McDonnell, Johnson, Polychronis, & Riesen, 2002) and specifically for children with ASD (Hundert & van Delft, 2009). (See the sections on language and mathematics later in this chapter for a full review.)

Up to now, we have described strategies that were aimed at increasing academic skills in general. The following sections describe the main empirical strategies found to enhance specific cognitive and academic skills in HFASD and ASD.

STRATEGIES TARGETING MEMORY SKILLS

The ability to remember information is essential for academic achievement. Several studies show that learning and memory performance of individuals with ASD diverges from that of comparison participants with TYP (for elaboration, see Chapter 5). Various strategies have been found to be effective in learners with TYP for improving memory performance, whether internal—such as rehearsal, mental imagery, and word grouping—or external—such as visual aids and cueing. The effectiveness of each of these strategies was examined for learners with ASD as well.

Rehearsal is considered to be one of the most important memory strategies, and children with TYP use it spontaneously and effectively by the age of 6 years. This language-based strategy involves verbal repetition (Bebko & Ricciuti, 2000). Bebko and Ricciuti (2000) examined the spontaneous use of a rehearsal strategy in three groups: preadolescents with HFASD (mean CA = 9.7 years, mean verbal MA = 9.6 years), preadolescents with LFA (mean CA = 11.8, mean verbal MA = 6.7), and younger children with TYP (mean CA = 6.0). Overall, findings showed that children who had rehearsed recalled significantly more information than children who had not rehearsed. Spontaneous use of the rehearsal strategy revealed differing outcomes according to level of functioning: Of the two ASD groups, the high-functioning group outperformed the low-functioning group (63% vs. 9% spontaneously used rehearsal), and the TYP group significantly outperformed them both (73%), thus enhancing memory performance. To evaluate the efficacy of supportive conditions, participants were then asked to recall the words in a modified supportive condition, in which they could look at the stimuli (six pictures) for any amount of time (as opposed to the first condition, in which each picture was shown once for only 3 seconds) and as many times as they wanted (Bebko & Ricciuti, 2000). This unlimited support led to a slight increase in strategy use in the HFASD group (from 63% in the first study to 82% in the second study)—slight only because the majority of participants had already implemented the rehearsal strategy in the first condition. However, a significant increase in strategy use was seen in the LFA group (from 9% in the first study to 64% in the second study), showing that a change in task constraints can have an important impact on strategy use in children with ASD. Furthermore, recall rate was higher in all groups when using a rehearsal strategy. From this the authors drew two main educational implications for memory recall tasks: Learning conditions should be optimized by external aids (visual aids and cues) and by sufficient learning time, and explicit instruction of the relevant rehearsal strategy is necessary to facilitate children's generation of the appropriate strategy.

Another study with implications for academic learning investigated the effectiveness of appropriate strategy learning for the recall of three different lists of words—unrelated words, phonologically related words, and semantically related words—for adults with HFASD and adults with TYP matched for age, Verbal IQ, and Full Scale IQ (Smith et al., 2007). During the learning stage and prior to the recall task, participants received instruction in specific rehearsal strategies: repetition aloud of the words for the list of unrelated words, a semantic clustering strategy (word grouping) according to categories for the semantically related list, and a rhyming strategy (clustering the words according to their final syllable) for the phonologically related list. Furthermore, participants were taught and then advised to make use of mental imagery (i.e., forming an abstract mental image of the word, thus visualizing it) as a mnemonic device to encourage relational techniques that aid recall for the unrelated and semantically related word lists. Contrary to the authors' expectations, the strategy training implemented during the learning phase, prior to the recall testing, did not bring the HFASD group's level of recall up to that achieved by the matched controls. The authors explained these findings as further evidence of impaired organizational strategies or central coherence weakness in HFASD, which may prevent full understanding of the phonological or semantic relations between words presented in a list.

A later study examined the efficacy of external semantic cueing by which participants trying to learn a shopping list were cued by the authors to listen for categories such as fruit or animals (Phelan, Filliten, & Johnson, 2011). The participants were adolescents with HFASD (mean CA = 13.02 years, mean estimated IQ = 112.07) and a control group with TYP matched for age and estimated IQ (on the basis of the Wechsler Abbreviated Scale of Intelligence [WASI]; Wechsler, 1999). Using the California Verbal Learning Test—Children's Version (CVLT-C; Delis, Kramer, Kaplan, & Ober, 1994), participants were first presented five times with a 15-item shopping list representing three semantic categories and then were asked to repeat as many items as they could remember. Next, a distracter word list was presented once to the participant, and immediate free recall of this list was assessed. After this distraction, both free and cued recall (based on an external category cue) of the original shopping list were assessed. Twenty minutes later, free and cued recall and recognition recall of the original shopping list were assessed. Results showed that the HFASD group improved significantly from the free recall to the cued recall trial, although they also used semantic clustering during the free recall trial. The HFASD group benefited significantly from the external semantic cueing support given by the authors at the retrieval phase when they were asked to say the words aloud themselves.

The main difference between the two studies just described was the timing of the cueing strategy. In Smith et al.'s (2007) study, the strategy was implemented during the learning phase, whereas in Phelan et al.'s (2011) study the task support and strategy were implemented during the retrieval phase of the memory task. The finding that the HFASD participants showed improvement following retrieval support suggests that individuals with HFASD may have a deficit in retrieval rather than in encoding. In another study, Whitehouse et al. (2007) found no significant differences in the semantic and phonological cued recall ability between children with HFASD (mean CA = 10.11 years) and children with TYP (mean CA = 8.4 years) who were matched on verbal and nonverbal MA. These findings corroborate the conclusion that individuals with HFASD resemble children with TYP on free recall tasks when given phonological or semantic cues as retrieval support. Externally cued recall at the retrieval stage appears to provide the "missing link" that children with HFASD cannot provide for themselves, thereby triggering unimpaired recall.

In a related avenue of memory research, Bruck et al. (2007) reported that children with HFASD (CA = 5–10 years) evidenced impairments in generating autobiographical memories using two different paradigms (see Chapter 4, section concerning memory). The authors examined the children's ability to recall past events via open-ended questions and specific yes–no questions. In light of the children's sparse provision of information during free recall of events (via open-ended questions), Bruck et al. (2007) expected that the utilization of direct, leading yes–no questions would elicit more information. Yet their study's results indicated that this binary strategy only emphasized the participants' error rates (corroborating accuracy according to parents' recall), whereas no between-group differences emerged on error rates for free recall of events. Therefore, the authors recommended developing relevant open-ended questioning strategies to enhance autobiographical memory.

In summary, when facilitating memory performance, it is important to note the following:

1. External cueing can promote recall, especially if given at the retrieval stage rather than the learning–storage stage.
2. Learning conditions can be optimized by providing visual cues and sufficient learning time.
3. Autobiographical memory can be supported by appropriate open-ended questions that serve as cues for responding.

STRATEGIES TARGETING QUESTION ASKING AND ANSWERING

Question asking is an important element in social and academic growth, and children with TYP make competent use of questions by the age of 3–5 years; yet children with ASD tend to make use of only a few questions, and some children do not use questions at all (Chiang & Carter, 2008; Koegel et al., 2010). Various strategies for enhancing question-asking and question-answering abilities have been examined empirically, as elaborated in this section. Importantly, these studies relate to different age groups and different levels of cognitive abilities.

Question Asking

Several studies have found different strategies to be successful for increasing question asking in ASD and HFASD. In one study, three young preschoolers with ASD who each possessed a vocabulary of 50 words were taught to ask and answer "Where?" questions by use of PRT (see earlier discussion) and intrinsic reinforcements such as candy or small favored objects (Koegel et al., 2010). The investigator first prompted the children to ask the question (e.g., "Where is the apple?"), fading the prompt gradually. After the child asked the question correctly, the investigator prompted them to answer the question with the appropriate preposition (e.g., "The apple is *on* the box") and, in one case, with the appropriate ordinal marker. Following the intervention, participants showed a generalized use of the targeted question ("Where?") and appropriate use of the language structures (prepositions and, in one case, ordinals) corresponding to the questions they had asked.

In another study to facilitate question asking, Palmen, Didden, and Arts (2008) implemented a visual cue by aid of a flowchart for young adults with HFASD (CA = 17–25 years, IQ = 90–130). The flowchart depicted a structured diagram for asking an appropriate question during a conversation (e.g., Introduction of topic; Do you have a question for this topic? If yes—ask your question; if no—tell the coach). During the training, participants viewed cards presenting three criteria for correct questions: (1) The question should be asked within a 5-second silence interval presented by the trainer; (2) the question should be related to the topic of the conversation; (3) the question should begin with "wh-" or a verb (e.g., "Do" or "Is"). In the next stage of the intervention, participants were asked to evaluate questions as correct or incorrect when listening to a recorded conversation that had a fixed order, in which each introduced topic was followed by a question being asked and answered. The last stage was role playing, in which participants were expected to respond to a topic according to the flowchart. Results showed a significant improvement in question asking, including generalization from the therapy room with the trainer to the natural setting of tutorial conversations with their personal coach.

The skill of generating questions can also be taught with a visual cue card that is paired with a script. At first, children are shown a cue card that reminds them to ask a question, along with a full script of the expected question (e.g., "What did the child do?"). After the question-asking structure is implemented, it can be systematically faded—first to a visual cue paired with a signal word, then to a visual cue alone, and so forth, until the child is able to generate questions independently (Whalon et al., 2009).

Question Answering

The following studies describe visual and verbal strategies that were found to enhance question-answering abilities in children with ASD and HFASD. Secan, Egel, and Tilley (1989) found that children with ASD (CA = 5–9 years) with varying levels of intelligence (IQ = 40–95) could learn to answer specific "wh-" questions ("Why?" "Who?" and "What?") if pictorial cues were shown; yet without the pictorial cues the children could not answer the questions. Similarly, Jahr (2001) examined the ability of young children with ASD (CA = 4–7 years) with varying levels of intelligence (IQ = 56–70) to answer "wh-" questions ("What?" "Where?" "Who?" and "Why?")

without pictorial cues. Each "wh-" question was learned separately, and correct answers were expected to include part of the question (i.e., "What do you like to eat?" "I like to eat pizza"; "Who do you sing with?" "I sing with my mother"). The results showed that, following training, the children were able to answer novel questions with complete sentences within each "wh-" question type. They also demonstrated transfer of their skills to new settings and persons, although they had been trained in one setting with only one teacher. However, they did not transfer their acquired ability from one question type to the other (i.e., transfer from "what" to "where").

The ability to answer a question based on inferential knowledge (knowledge concerning information that is not directly stated) is considered to be a more complex skill in comparison with factual knowledge (as described earlier). In answering inferential "why" questions, a correct answer would be any plausible one based on the child's general knowledge, rather than a definite right or wrong answer (Hundert & van Delft, 2009). Hundert and van Delft (2009) examined the ability to answer three formats of inferential "why" questions among children with HFASD (CA = 7–13 years, IQ = 70–103). The first format asked "why" following a sequence of three pictures. For example, there were pictures of a bus stopped with open doors; of the bus driving away; and of children running in an indefinite direction, with the departing bus in the background. The question was "Why were the children running?" Possible correct inferential answers would be "The children were trying to catch the bus" or "The children were running to school." The second format asked "why" following verbally presented stories. For example, the story might say, "Ricky was completing work in his classroom. He raised his hand." The question would be "Why did Ricky raise his hand?" Possible correct inferential answers might be "He needed help with his work" or "He wanted to go to the bathroom." The third format asked "why" following general information questions. For example, the question might be "Why shouldn't you eat food that falls on the floor?" Possible correct inferential answers could be "Because it may be dirty" or "You might get sick."). All the questions had more than one possible answer inasmuch as the focus of the intervention was to teach inferences.

Hundert and van Delft (2009) used embedded instruction throughout the training sessions (see the previous section, "Frequently Used Strategies to Facilitate General Academic Skills in ASD"). In this study, the participant chose a preferred activity (card or table game), and during that activity the trainer paused approximately every 90 seconds to ask a question in one of the three formats. If children gave an irrelevant answer, they were first asked to describe the information that had been presented and then answer a prompt (e.g., in relation to the picture sequence about the bus, the prompt was "What would happen if the children missed the bus?"). The children first mastered one type of question format (picture sequence, verbal story, or general information) before learning the other two. Results of this study demonstrated that the children learned how to answer inferential "why" questions following training, yet they could not generalize their ability from one format to another. As expected, the lowest frequency of correct answers emerged for the verbal story format.

Summary of Question-Related Skills

When facilitating question asking and answering in ASD and HFASD, it is important to note the following:

1. External visual cueing (such as flowcharts and pictorial cues) can enhance question asking and answering.
2. External verbal prompts and cueing can support appropriate question answering.
3. Each question type (yes–no; different "wh-" types) should be taught separately.
4. Intrinsic motivation and embedded instruction were found to be supportive strategies in developing question asking and answering.

STRATEGIES TARGETING READING

Reading is a critical skill for student success in school; nevertheless, much heterogeneity exists across the autistic spectrum in reading ability (Nation et al., 2006; Whalon et al., 2009). Likewise, a range of strategies is available to teach reading, such as visually via whole words, phonologically via decoding, or both visually and phonologically. Selection of the optimal strategies must take into account the individual child's learning profile. It is beyond the scope of this chapter to discuss the various ways to teach decoding abilities; therefore, this chapter concentrates on strategies that were found to effectively facilitate whole-word recognition in ASD. To date, we have found no specific studies that examined strategies for teaching decoding along the autistic spectrum.

Visual Learning Strategies

These strategies enable teachers to help children with ASD to read, based on their visual strengths. The basis is sight-word instruction, or the "whole-word" learning approach, which encompasses visual, auditory, and kinesthetic components. Sight-word instruction is recommended as the first part of a wider literacy program that includes other components such as phonemic awareness, phonics, fluency, and comprehension.

The ability to read sight words may enable students who are unable to master the alphabetic principle to perform functional tasks such as reading environmental signs, lists, items on a menu, schedules, recipes, and so forth. The data from the nine studies that Spector (2011) reviewed showed that all the participants with ASD learned to read varied sets of words, even children who had no prior history of reading instruction or who had failed when taught with classic reading methods. Spector concluded that although sight-word instruction alone is insufficient for students to achieve high literacy standards within general education, sight word instruction may motivate participation and enhance a feeling of belonging to the class curriculum.

To motivate the child, it is usually important to choose words that are relevant and meaningful to that child (such as names of preferred persons, favorite foods, familiar TV characters, and so on). These words serve as the vocabulary base, on which the teacher adds "sentence builders" such as pronouns, verbs, and so forth (for a more comprehensive review, see Broun, 2004; Oelwein, 1995). Whalon et al. (2009) reported that once children with ASD were able to decode or had a sufficient bank of sight words, reading texts aloud was found to be a strategy that increased oral reading fluency on the one hand and reading proficiency on the other hand.

Basil and Reyes (2003) examined the advantages of reading instruction via an intervention program based on a multimedia software program (Delta Messages) and a scaffolding approach. In this approach, six students with various severe disabilities (including two with LFA) who had very low or no literary skills participated in a 10-session program during which they learned to create sentences. The program was designed to create noun–verb–noun sentences; hence, no matter what combination of words the children chose, they formed a coherent, even if somewhat absurd, sentence (e.g., "The vulture chases the carrot"; "The carrot chases the vulture"). The children received immediate positive feedback, consisting of their coherent sentence displayed immediately by comic characters on the computer screen. The intervention results showed that within a short period of 3 months, the children's reading and writing skills improved significantly. Another important result was that, although the program was based on the "whole-word approach," the children also made phonological gains.

According to the authors, the intervention was successful for several reasons:

1. Activities were meaningful to participants from the beginning of the acquisition process. The children could immediately create sentences that they understood; they also made something interesting happen on the computer screen, and the sentences' contents were not related in any way to their prior, usually unsuccessful, learning experiences.
2. The computer characters were motivational to the children because they were similar to cartoon TV characters. Furthermore, the teacher–student interaction during the learning procedure was motivational because it was based on success and shared fun. The

scaffolding enabled the child's active learning via the adult's joint engagement during the acquisition stage.

3. The intervention design differentiated between acquisition and evaluation. During acquisition, the children worked at their own individual pace and received immediate feedback via the cartoon characters, and there was no opportunity for them to err. Only during the evaluation stage were children expected to supply a correct sentence to a given cartoon, which was evaluated as right or wrong.

Basil and Reyes (2003) concluded that a major implication of their study is that the children's poor reading skills cannot be explained only by their cognitive deficits. These interventionists asserted that when reading is motivational and meaningful for students, the relevant processes necessary for reading can be activated, and the underlying cognitive abilities (i.e., phonological awareness, sight-word acquisition, and decoding skills) can be developed.

In summary, when a child with ASD has difficulty acquiring whole words and phonological reading skills, it is recommended to use:

1. Visual supports.
2. Motivational words (based on the child's interests or high attractiveness).
3. Computer-assisted or computer-based interventions.

Reading Comprehension Strategies

According to Randi et al. (2010), general reading comprehension strategies and interventions that are relevant to children with TYP are also relevant to children with ASD. These authors underscored the necessity of reading-comprehension instruction, and not just posing reading comprehension questions. Many readers with HFASD focus on the decoding aspect of reading and disregard its comprehension elements. One reason for this neglect may be their executive function deficits in cognitive shifting and flexibility; therefore, one of the basic strategies recommended by Randi et al. is implementing cognitive flexibility strategies following Cartwright's (2006) word exercises. In these exercises, the child is requested to sort a set of words twice, once based on phonological rules (i.e., beginning sound— all the words beginning with D) and once based on semantic categories (i.e., all the words that are fruit).

When teaching children with HFASD to read, it is important to emphasize the search for meaning as an instructional priority, from the first stages of sight-word and decoding acquisition (Whalon et al., 2009). Considering these children's range of strengths and weaknesses in general, and in reading in particular, a single reading comprehension intervention may not be appropriate for all (Randi et al., 2010). As seen next, reading comprehension in HFASD may require different strategies, such as visual support, cueing, and focus on texts' figurative language.

Visual Support Strategies

Students with HFASD may benefit from visual supports to enhance textual comprehension, for example, flowcharts, graphic organizers, concept maps, story maps, and so on. The use of graphics and colors may provide concrete visual information that can aid in focusing attention. An important visual support is the written word itself, and in many instances provision of written information is fruitful in ASD, such as written texts in auditory comprehension situations or written instructions delineating classroom and homework assignments (Kluth & Darmody-Latham, 2003).

The use of a story map—a visual graphic organizer that maps a story—helps children with HFASD to understand the intricate relations within a narrative text (Gately, 2008). In a study that examined the efficacy of story map usage, the authors found that children with HFASD who had learned how to use a story map succeeded in answering appropriate class-level quizzes after reading the story (Stringfield, Luscre, & Gast, 2011). Whalon and Hanline (2008) examined the effect of a reciprocal-questioning comprehension strategy in an inclusive environment with the aid of a story map for children with HFASD and children with TYP (CA = 7–8 years). In a group, one child with ASD and two peers with TYP were taught to generate and respond to questions based on a story map. All the participants increased their frequency of unprompted question asking and responding during reading; however, HFASD needed more prompting when asking and responding to inferential questions, such as identifying the problem posed in the story, than they did when stating facts (concerning the characters, setting, or events) from the story itself. The authors concluded that the reciprocal-questioning intervention has the potential to increase question generation and responding of children with HFASD in the context of storybook reading with peers.

Another type of visual graphic organizer is concept mapping, in which readers construct a visual map that displays their knowledge in relation to a specific concept or concepts. Interconnectivity between concepts is also shown by various links on the map. Roberts and Joiner (2007) examined the use of computer-based concept mapping as a learning strategy in comparison with conventional teaching methods for children with HFASD (mean CA = 12.8 years). Findings showed that participants could successfully retain and recall information following the concept-mapping intervention, whereas they exhibited difficulties following conventional teaching methods. A further significant effect emerged on children's performance on class tests following the intervention. According to the authors, this outcome indicated participants' ability to generalize their newly acquired knowledge in the mapping format to other methods of recall.

Asberg and Sandberg (2010) examined the efficacy of a classroom-based intervention to support comprehension of narratives, delivered via answering informative questions and discerning their origin, for students with HFASD (CA = 10–15 years). Teachers underwent specific training to learn the linguistic and cognitive basis for comprehension difficulties in HFASD and how to implement scaffolding strategies. Over the course of the intervention, teachers gradually passed academic responsibility over to participants after modeling the appropriate strategies both for answering the questions and for understanding the questions' origin. Teachers worked with children three times weekly for 4 weeks. The children received a booklet with 13 stories arranged hierarchically, of increasing length. After reading each story, they had to answer questions and decide whether the origin of the question and answer was: (1) directly in the text, (2) inferred by integrating different sentences in the text, or (3) inferred from the individual's world knowledge. The authors found significant improvement after training for the children with HFASD. Furthermore, the teachers who participated in the study reported that they would continue to use the same or similar comprehension instruction, thereby extending the efficacy and utility of this strategy's implementation.

Colasent and Griffith (1998) examined the efficacy of a thematic reading intervention based on a specific topic (in this case, rabbits) on the comprehension ability of students with ASD (CA = 12–15 years) who functioned (according to the authors) at the social and developmental age of 5- to 8-year-olds. The intervention design included three consecutive parts. In line with its thematic approach, first the general topic of rabbits was introduced in class. Then a story about rabbits was read aloud to the children over a 3-day period. Finally, the children retold the story, answered informative questions, and were asked to relay their favorite part using writing and drawing. The second and third parts of the intervention were repeated three times, presenting three different stories. The authors found that the children demonstrated gains in oral retelling following the thematic intervention. After the third story, the children revealed an increase in their ability to answer a wide array of questions concerning the stories they heard (such as naming the characters, stating the problem and the setting, stating the events, naming a favorite character or favorite part of the story). Drawing and writing served as facilitating strategies that enhanced the retelling. These researchers also found both a quantitative and qualitative improvement in the children's writing ability following the intervention. The children wrote longer passages and used more sophisticated vocabulary after the third story. Furthermore, the authors noted behavioral changes during the last stages of the intervention, including less stereotypical behavior while listening to the stories; fewer verbal outbursts; relevant verbalizations; and emotional expressions appropriate to the characters' feelings.

Understanding a text often depends on readers' ability to apply their own knowledge in relation to the information included in the specific text, thus creating an inner mental representation of the text. Consequently, when background knowledge is inaccurate, comprehension of the text is likewise disrupted. The more knowledge readers possess on a specific topic (e.g., rabbits), the likelier they are to connect the text with that knowledge (Gately, 2008). Therefore, interventions concerning specific topics should include topic-related teaching. One strategy that was found to be effective in two different studies for readers with HFASD was cueing individuals to draw on their individual background knowledge to facilitate text comprehension.

Cueing Strategies

As stated at the beginning of this chapter, cueing strategies are general strategies given by an adult to facilitate children's understanding of a given task. As demonstrated in the sections related to memory and to question asking and answering, the cues can be verbal or pictorial. O'Connor and Klein (2004) examined the efficacy of anaphoric cueing (see Table 8.1)—words that refer to other words, such as pronouns—among adolescents with HFASD (mean CA = 15.11 years, mean IQ = 88). Altogether, they examined the efficacy of three different reading comprehension strategies: (1) anaphoric cueing that related pronouns to antecedent nouns (i.e., the pronoun "it" referred to the noun "dog" that appeared earlier in the text); (2) the use of prereading questions to activate prior knowledge, which children with ASD have difficulty accessing; and (3) cloze tasks within the text, which left blanks for words that appeared earlier in the text (other than a pronoun). Each student read five stories: one in the anaphoric cueing condition, one in the prereading-question condition, one in the cloze condition, and two control stories (unmodified). After reading the texts, participants received a sequence of questions that included free retelling, identifying the story's main idea, generating a title for the story, detecting an incongruous sentence in a paragraph from the story, four "why" or "how" questions that required students to make inferences about information not explicitly stated in the passage, and four "who, what, where, when" questions that required students to recall factual information explicitly stated in the passage.

O'Connor and Klein's (2004) results showed that anaphoric cueing was the most efficient strategy, benefiting more than half of the participants. In this condition, participants had to reread portions of the text to look for the appropriate antecedent noun, which induced self-monitoring. This seemed to lead to better comprehension and significantly better postreading comprehension. The cloze tasks, which also induced self-monitoring when participants reread the passage in search of the appropriate word to fill in the blank, were also successfully completed by a majority of the participants (80%). Yet, interestingly, the cloze strategy did not advance participants' overall comprehension of the text or their postreading comprehension. The least efficient strategy was answering prereading questions. Although these questions activated prior knowledge, as expected, in many instances the participants brought up irrelevant and inaccurate information. One solution that the authors suggested was to use advance graphic organizers, by which readers would receive an organizer with relevant information prior to reading the text.

Readers' world knowledge is often activated by the text's title; therefore, cueing a text's title is an important strategy to enhance meaning (Wahlberg & Magliano, 2004). In many cases of ambiguous texts, activation of appropriate world knowledge is insufficient as readers must examine their interpretation of the text while trying to relate the text's meaning to their knowledge. Wahlberg and Magliano (2004) examined the ability of adults with HFASD (mean IQ = 103.25) and undergraduate students with TYP matched on IQ (mean IQ = 105) to activate their world knowledge by aid of the text's title and then to integrate that knowledge when reading an ambiguous text. The participants with HFASD showed significant impairment in dealing with the ambiguity of the text in comparison with the participants with TYP, even when provided with an informative title and an informative priming text (that contained specific background knowledge relevant to the text). Inasmuch as the HFASD group recalled a larger proportion of the text when provided with both a priming text and an informative title, the authors' educational implications stressed the necessity of providing explicit cues that include both informative titles and a priming text in order to activate relevant knowledge. It is important to note that for ambiguous texts the authors recommended supplying cues only after the readers acquire a sufficient level of proficiency such that they are able to answer questions regarding the concrete factual details of the text.

One of the major difficulties in reading comprehension is the ability to fill in information that is not stated overtly in a text, requiring inferential skills. Comprehension requires integration of meanings for words, sentences, and paragraphs and for key ideas and themes. Readers need to apply general knowledge and global processing in order to fill in the missing gaps. To understand a narrative and fill in its gaps, readers need to build an event schema that depicts the chain of events within the narrative, first as a concrete diagram and then mentally as proficiency increases.

Figurative Language in Texts

Figurative language (words or groups of words that exaggerate or alter the words' usual meanings) raises texts' complexity level. Thus strategies to facilitate the comprehension of figurative words and phrases are important. Rundblad and Annaz (2010) examined comprehension in children with HFASD of metonymies, figures of speech in which a thing or concept is not called by its own name but by the name of something intimately associated with it, and of metaphors, literary figures of speech that use an image, story, or tangible thing to represent a less tangible thing. Metonymies and metaphors are considered complex because they are ambiguous both in the lexical and the syntactic sense. A metonymy is considered to be less complex than a metaphor, as a metonymy is mapped within a single conceptual domain (e.g., car includes the concept of driver), whereas a metaphor is mapped across two conceptual domains (e.g., eyes that sparkle and jewels). The authors compared children with HFASD and children with TYP matched on CA (mean = 8.4 years). A developmental trajectory emerged for the TYP group, showing improved performance in metonymy and metaphor understanding as CA increased and development of metonymy comprehension first. In the HFASD group, children revealed significant difficulty understanding both metonymies and metaphors, yet overall they showed better understanding for metonymies than for metaphors. These findings are relevant for designing hierarchical interventions dealing with texts that incorporate figurative language, suggesting that metonymies should be taught before metaphors.

The use of MET/MEI was investigated as a strategy to enhance the understanding of metaphors within a group of young children with ASD (CA = 5–7 years) who were apparently high functioning (Persicke et al., 2012). (The authors did not report the children's IQs; yet the children's verbal abilities implied cognitive high functioning—the ability to listen and answer questions about short stories, describe everyday objects by naming three features, and discriminate between same and different.) The authors read short stories to the children that depicted simple descriptions of people or events (2–10 sentences per story) and then asked three metaphor questions. The stories described the target of the metaphor and its features. For example, one story was "One of my coworkers brought a cake to work last week. The cake had fluffy frosting, and it smelled really good, but the cake was really hard on the inside." It was followed by three questions containing metaphors:

1. If I say the cake was perfume, what do I mean? (Answer: The cake smelled really good.)
2. If I say the cake's frosting was a cloud, what do I mean? (Answer: The frosting was white and fluffy.)
3. If I say the cake was a rock, what do I mean? (Answer: The cake was hard.)

Using MET/MEI, during each of the 10 sessions the experimenter read four stories—two previously trained stories and two new stories. If the child answered incorrectly, the experimenter used leading questions to help the child realize the hierarchical relations between the target (e.g., cake) and its features, the vehicle (e.g., rock) and its features, and the relation between the one feature shared between the target and vehicle (e.g., hardness). If the child still did not succeed, the experimenter used an echoic prompt by stating the shared feature. If the children showed no progress after five trials, the experimenters added a graphic visual aid that consisted of a laminated chart divided into two columns. The children were instructed to write the target at the top of one column and the vehicle at the top of the other column. They were then told to write a list of the features of each item in the appropriate column. After writing the features, children were asked to connect a line between the matching features. The experimenter aided children via verbal prompts and gestures. The results of the study showed that children with HFASD can understand metaphorical language when taught via MET/MEI and graphic organizers.

With regard to homographs (words that have same written form but different meanings, such as "tear," which could mean "rip" or "cry"), Snowling and Frith (1986) found that when readers with ASD and HFASD read passages that incorporated homographs, they tended to read based on the most common meaning. Nonetheless, when cued to search for meaning in the context of a sentence, a major improvement in their comprehension was noted. Thus specific cueing for contextual meaning can advance the comprehension of a textual passage.

Norbury (2005) examined the ability of children with HFASD and children with TYP, who did or did not have language impairment, to comprehend lexically ambiguous texts (i.e., "dig with a spade," in which spade could mean shovel or the symbol on a playing card). A difference emerged between the two HFASD groups. Those with structural language scores in the normal range, like their peers with TYP, made use of the context in order to solve the lexical ambiguity. In contrast, those with lower scores in structural language showed an impaired ability to extract the intended meaning. These findings add a level of complexity when planning interventions to facilitate ambiguous lexical and semantic meaning, suggesting that interventionists should take the child's degree of language impairment, if any, into consideration when planning treatment.

In summary, when facilitating reading comprehension, it is important to note the following:

1. The use of visual strategies and graphic organizers can enhance reading comprehension: Story maps can assist when teaching narrative texts, and concept maps can assist when teaching informative and factual texts.
2. Thematic intervention can advance reading comprehension and writing skills in readers with ASD and HFASD.
3. Cueing is an important strategy when teaching children with ASD. Anaphoric cueing was found to be effective for dealing with a complex text. Cueing via an informative priming text and an informative title facilitates the understanding of an ambiguous text.
4. When dealing with figurative language in a text, it is important to

know the hierarchy of figurative words (i.e., metonymies are easier to learn than metaphors). MET/MEI can be an effective strategy for teaching metaphors, especially if graphic visual aids are incorporated into the intervention. Cueing can facilitate the comprehension of homographs.

5. It is important to identify whether the reader with HFASD also has a language impairment and to select strategies accordingly.

STRATEGIES TARGETING WRITING

Many accommodations and interventions are available for students with HFASD who have difficulties in writing. These can include using a keyboard, a word processor, and other assistive technology for written work. Furthermore, in many classes (especially in the elementary grades), the teacher can reduce the writing requirements, modify tests and assignments, and, if necessary, provide the student with class notes and outlines. This section reviews structured writing strategies that were found to be successful for writers with HFASD.

Both in TYP and ASD, early intervention in writing is more effective than later intervention; therefore, if writing proficiency seems to be delayed, it is important to start interventions in the early elementary school years (Troia & Graham, 2003). Four studies examined the written composition ability of children and adolescents with HFASD by training them in self-regulating strategies, which provide organization and scaffolding based on the use of mnemonics. This self-regulated strategy development (SRSD) was designed to teach students how to: (1) plan their writing by aid of direct instruction; (2) set goals and develop self-reinforcement and self-monitoring; and (3) develop specific motivational aspects such as self-efficacy. All four studies utilized a general writing strategy developed by Graham and Harris (1993), which was used successfully to improve the writing of children with learning disabilities, emotional and behavioral disorders, and ADHD (Lane, Graham, Harris, & Weisenbach, 2006; Reid & Lienemann, 2006). Graham and Harris (1993) recommended that when using SRSD, teachers should follow six stages of instruction, modified to meet students' needs: (1) development and activation of background knowledge, (2) discussion of the strategy, (3) modeling of the strategy and self-instructions, (4) memorization of the strategy, (5) support and collaborative practice, and (6) independent practice (see also Harris, Graham, & Mason, n.d.).

These research results demonstrated that utilizing SRSD during the instruction and planning of composition improved the quantitative and qualitative measures of participants' story writing (Asaro & Saddler, 2009; Asaro-Saddler & Saddler, 2010; Delano, 2007b) and essay writing (Delano, 2007a). All participants showed quantitative gains, such as an increase in the average number of words per essay (Asaro & Saddler, 2009; Asaro-Saddler & Saddler, 2010; Delano, 2007a, 2007b), specifically in the use of action words and describing words (Delano, 2007b), as well as an increase in functional essay elements (i.e., topic sentences and reasons; Delano, 2007a) and in story elements (Asaro & Saddler, 2009). Furthermore, an increase also emerged on qualitative measures such as enhanced revision ability (Delano, 2007b), incorporation of learned mnemonics during story writing (Asaro & Saddler, 2009), and spontaneous use of self-regulatory behaviors (Asaro-Saddler & Saddler, 2010).

Delano (2007a) added self-modeling by aid of video to the SRSD approach. Participants watched themselves modeling self-regulatory strategies as follows: (1) Students received a script instructing them of the strategy; (2) they were videotaped modeling that strategy (e.g., counting the number of words in their essays, noting the amount on a bar chart, checking whether they met their goals, setting new goals); and (3) at the beginning of each intervention session, participants watched their videos related to the strategy to be learned. According to Delano (2007a), the participants improved their writing. However, the video modeling strategy was not evaluated in isolation; hence the author could not determine the influence of each strategy separately.

According to Harbinson and Alexander (2009), one of the crucial problems facing English-speaking students with HFASD is the creative, imaginative demands of the English curriculum. These authors examined the efficacy of a generic creative writing intervention that included a graphic framework aimed at developing creative writing skills among high school students with HFASD. The 16-week intervention included 8 weeks of learning in the whole classroom and then 8 weeks of learning in small work groups. To assist students in writing an imaginary text, they learned how to use a graphic framework consisting of a grid with five subheadings—Who? When? Where? What? Why?—which was supplemented by visual cues. Interestingly, Harbinson and Alexander (2009) were pessimistic about the intervention's outcomes, asserting that for some students with HFASD "it is perhaps an insurmountable task to ask them to think imaginatively. To write an imaginative short story . . . may be, not just too difficult, but perhaps impossible" (p. 18). The authors concluded that the most important factor that led to some degree of success was the use of small groups as opposed to the general classroom setting.

Nevertheless, a recent study examining the efficacy of computer-mediated story construction in children with HFASD (mean CA = 8.96 years; mean verbal MA = 8.4 years) in comparison with their matched peers with TYP (mean CA = 8.60 years; mean verbal MA = 9.07 years) demonstrated more promising results for creative writing (Dillon & Underwood, 2012). Each child with HFASD was paired with a child with TYP, and each dyad was asked to create a reality-based story about friends visiting each other's houses after school, as well as a fantasy-based story about aliens living on an unknown planet, via "Bubble Dialogue" software (Cunningham, McMahon, & O'Neill, 1992). Children learned the difference between thought and speech bubbles, and then each child in the dyad received a computerized comic character through which to enact the stories via role play with the partner's character. The dyad was instructed to role-play the two cartoon characters by typing texts at each turn of the conversation (in the character's thought bubble, speech bubble, or both) in response to the partner's bubbles, thereby developing a narrative for each of the two stories. Role play ended when the children stated that they had finished their story or when they were off-task for a certain amount of time. Scoring included individual measures such as appropriate or inappropriate use of bubbles, coherence of narrative, ability to elaborate, and so on.

The authors found that the children with HFASD were as able as the children with TYP to engage in the creation of stories, whether reality or fantasy based. No difference emerged between the groups regarding story length, elaboration, or, somewhat surprisingly, use of emotional-state terms. Both groups elaborated more in the reality-based than in the fantasy-based stories, and both groups did better in logically sequencing the fantasy stories. Despite these quantitative similarities, some qualitative differences emerged, especially concerning the use of thought bubbles: Children with HFASD made errors by trying to make their cartoon character act upon wishes stated by their partner's cartoon character in a thought bubble, although characters should not have been privy to the others' thinking.

In a comparative study that investigated nonfiction narrative and expository writing ability (intending to explain or clarify actions or facts) among adults with HFASD (mean CA = 25.75 years) and adults with TYP (mean CA = 26.56 years), Brown and Klein (2011) found that the HFASD group wrote lower-quality texts of both types and shorter narratives but not shorter expository texts. The study was comparative and not specific to strategy use; therefore, it yielded few educational implications. Nonetheless, Brown and Klein suggested that a possible reason that the two groups wrote expository texts of similar lengths was that both groups wrote according to a traditional five-paragraph structure taught in secondary school. If this was the case, indeed it underscores the importance of a graphic organizer in enhancing writing abilities.

In summary, when implementing writing strategies, the following should be considered:

1. It is important to enable accommodations for general writing disabilities.
2. Self-regulated strategies were found to facilitate writing in HFASD. Mnemonics assisted in implementing the various components of such strategies.
3. Video modeling and computer software may be advantageous in implementing writing strategies.

4. Graphic organizers can assist in developing relevant outlines for writing assignments.
5. Instruction in small groups facilitates writing instruction.

STRATEGIES TARGETING MATHEMATICS

As stated in Chapter 5 in relation to mathematics ability in ASD and HFASD, studies are sparse; therefore, this section, as opposed to the previous one, describes mathematical strategies recommended for students with ASD rather than evidence-based practices. Donaldson and Zager (2010), in their article "Mathematics Interventions for Students with High-Functioning Autism/Asperger's Syndrome," recommended a number of general strategies that enhance mathematical abilities for learners with TYP and with learning disabilities. These recommended strategies include, among others: (1) self-regulation strategies (similar to those recommended for writing interventions), in which students learn to complete a checklist as they perform calculations and computations, thus increasing the accuracy of their answers; (2) goal structure, in which students set goals for themselves and are rewarded accordingly; (3) a "concrete–representational–abstract" strategy for teaching the abstract concept of fractions, in which students first learn the concrete concept (i.e., half a pizza), then learn the representational concept (i.e., a picture of two halves of a shape), and finally learn the abstract concept (the writing of the fraction itself). This strategy was also found to be efficient for teaching mathematical word problems to children with learning disabilities.

In an exploratory study aimed at assessing the efficacy of systematic instruction of mathematical concepts (supported by Project MIND [Math Is Not Difficult®]; Su, 2002), Su, Lai, and Rivera (2010) examined the acquisition of math skills in preschoolers with HFASD and peers with TYP. The math curriculum used in this study was a multisensory-based approach (implementing the use of various senses) via direct or embedded instruction. In the direct-instruction approach, teachers led 15-minute daily learning sessions. In the embedded approach, the mathematical instruction was embedded into various preschool activities such as music, movement, art, cooking, circle time, transition activities, and outdoor play. Su et al. (2010) reported that both of these systematic approaches to teaching mathematics—direct and embedded instruction—yielded mathematical gains.

In summary, when teaching mathematics, it is important to note the following:

1. Self-regulatory strategies and individual goal setting can enhance mathematical abilities and increase accuracy in computation.
2. A "concrete–representational–abstract" strategy can facilitate the understanding of abstract mathematical concepts.

3. Embedded and direct instruction can foster mathematical performance.
4. Systematic teaching based on a multisensory approach can advance mathematical gains.

SELECTING APPROPRIATE STRATEGIES

Although various strategies can be effective for learners with HFASD, as described throughout this chapter, one of the major difficulties that teachers face is choosing the most appropriate strategy to meet the needs of the particular student's disability and at the same time to fit the task requirements. Furthermore, when selecting various strategies, it is important to take into consideration the degree of executive function deficit in individuals with HFASD. One study that examined the ability of children with HFASD to choose and apply an appropriate strategy themselves (for enhancing memory abilities) pinpointed these children's difficulty in applying the appropriate strategy for a given task (Bebko & Ricciuti, 2000). Difficulties in planning and choosing appropriate strategies according to the task at hand, followed by the necessity to monitor and evaluate of the chosen strategy's effectiveness and its alteration when necessary, may all be related to their difficulties in executive functioning (see Chapter 5). This necessitates a more active role on the part of the teacher in determining which strategies to implement, when, and how.

SUMMARY AND CONCLUSIONS

It is important to accentuate that the interventions and strategies described in this chapter are, for the most part, evidence based, relying on research that investigated groups or utilized single-study designs. Yet, in many cases, no follow-up studies were performed to widen and substantiate the findings, and many of these evidence-based studies included very small numbers of participants. Nonetheless, the current research literature does offer many important findings that can assist in developing appropriate strategies for the learner with ASD or HFASD. Throughout the majority of the studies described, one can see that pupils with ASD and HFASD do benefit from specific cognitive instruction using appropriate strategies to foster academic competencies. It is crucial that the strategies and skills be taught explicitly. The instructor (whether teacher, teaching assistant, or parent) should recognize the child's individual cognitive profile and implement the appropriate academic strategy or intervention accordingly. Application of appropriate strategies and accommodations can foster learning both in special and regular educational settings. Once the pupil learns to use the relevant strategy, it is important for the educator to help the pupil generalize and maintain use of the strategy. Other than structured teaching, which is specific to ASD, one of the most prominent and efficient general strategies shown to enhance learning is cueing, whether pictorial, verbal, or textual. The teacher's role in recognizing the appropriate cue and implementing it externally at the relevant time is crucial to students' success.

Due to a paucity of research in all of the fields related to academic strategies for students with ASD and HFASD, it is imperative to continue studying this domain. According to Mesibov and Shea (2011), small studies should be developed to identify specific effective strategies, rather than focusing on studies of "brand name" programs. The findings of these specific studies could be much more useful for teachers and educators, who are in constant need of evidence-based knowledge.

TABLE 8.1. Glossary of Professional Terms for Academic Interventions

Term	Relevant intervention area	Definition
Anaphoric cueing	Reading comprehension	A semantic cueing tool in which words refer to other words that appear antecedently (i.e., relating pronouns to antecedent nouns)
Cloze tasks	Reading comprehension	A task consisting of a text with blanks to denote missing words in which participants fill in the missing words
Collateral skills	Behavioral intervention	When children acquire a specific, targeted, pivotal skill that is taught, they are expected to generalize and expand to additional nontargeted collateral skills that go beyond that learned skill.
Color-coded organizers	Structured teaching	A structured system for organizing information by use of different colors
Concept mapping	Structured teaching Reading comprehension	A structured diagram that shows the relationships among concepts
Concrete–representational–abstract strategy	Mathematics intervention	The learning of an abstract concept via a concrete and then a representational example
Contextual cueing	Reading comprehension Cueing strategy	When encountering an unknown word, readers can make use of pictures or information surrounding the word in order to determine its meaning.

(*continued*)

TABLE 8.1. (*continued*)

Term	Relevant intervention area	Definition
Cueing strategies	Reading comprehension Memory intervention Question-asking strategy	The ability to use various cues (verbal, textual, or pictorial) to understand or remember a concept or concepts
Decoding skills	Reading intervention	The skills necessary to analyze and interpret the graphic symbols that make up a word, including the ability to recognize basic sounds and phonemes and blend them together
Embedded instruction	General strategy	Instructional procedures and learning activities that are implemented during regular, ongoing activities
Emergent literacy		Preliminary skills and knowledge needed for the foundation of literacy, such as phonological processing, awareness of print, vocabulary
External cueing	Memory strategy Question-asking strategy	Cues supplied by the educator to enhance academic and cognitive performance
Factual knowledge	Knowledge	Knowledge related to facts
Flowchart	Structured teaching Reading comprehension Question-asking strategy Writing intervention	A structured diagram that represents a process, showing the various stages with arrows
Graphic maps	Structured teaching Reading comprehension Writing intervention	A structured graphic representation of an item, a process, an idea, etc., that can be used before an assignment to organize it or after an assignment to summarize it
Graphic organizers	Structured teaching Reading comprehension Writing intervention	A structured organizer that assists in organizing ideas, concepts, and knowledge using a graphic presentation (e.g., graphic maps, story maps, concept maps, flowcharts)
Inferential knowledge	Knowledge	Knowledge concerning information that is not directly stated
Intrinsic reinforcers	Motivation	Reinforcement that is given internally
Mental imagery	Memory strategy	The forming of an abstract mental image of a word, thus visualizing it mentally

TABLE 8.1. (*continued*)

Term	Relevant intervention area	Definition
Mnemonics	Memory strategy	Learning techniques that aid memory, most commonly using a short word, acronym, or poem to remember a list, but can also be a visual aid
Multisensory approach	General learning approach	Teaching simultaneously via various senses (auditory and/or visual and/or kinesthetic-tactile). The optimal use is the engagement of all three modalities simultaneously.
Natural environment	Learning	Settings that are natural or normal for the child's same-age peers who have no disabilities, excluding specific places that a child with a disability attends (therapies, etc.)
Pictorial cues	Structured teaching Cueing strategy	Structured external visual clues that aid the child
Pivotal response training (PRT)	Behavioral intervention	When certain behaviors (i.e., pivotal responses) are learned, additional nontargeted collateral behaviors also begin to emerge.
Pivotal skills	Behavioral intervention	Specific skills targeted for learning
Prompt	Behavioral intervention	External assistance to aid the child, which may include gestures (such as pointing) or visual or verbal reminders
Recall task	Memory	A method of measuring memory, comprising three types: free recall, cued recall, and serial recall
Rehearsal	Memory strategy	Repetition of a given word list at the encoding stage until memorized
Repeated storybook-reading technique	Literacy skills Language intervention	Use of storybooks as a context for presenting instructional strategies to promote language and literacy skills
Retrieval stage	Memory	Memory includes encoding, storage, and retrieval; the retrieval stage is the accessing stage, and a retrieval cue is used to trigger the retrieval of stored information.

(*continued*)

TABLE 8.1. (*continued*)

Term	Relevant intervention area	Definition
Rhyming strategy	Memory strategy	A strategy that aids recall by clustering words according to their ending sound (blue–flew; dog–fog)
Scaffolding strategies	General strategy	Specialized instructional supports to facilitate learning
Self-regulating strategy	General strategy Writing intervention Mathematics intervention	A strategy that assists children to regulate learning as they set goals and develop self-reinforcement
Semantic clustering strategy	Memory strategy	An organizational strategy that aids recall by clustering words according to meaning
Story map	Structured teaching Reading comprehension	A graphic organizer that helps identify key elements in a story (characters, setting, events, problem, and solution)
Thematic intervention	Reading comprehension	An approach that provides repeated opportunities for interaction and systematic support while a theme links specific skills to meaningful information; themed intervention often links basic disciplines
Verbal cue	Cueing strategy	A verbal clue (e.g., "Look for the 'wh-' question") directing the child about what to do in an activity
Visual cue	Cueing strategy	A visual clue (e.g., picture, icon) that shows the child where to respond
Visual cue card	Structured teaching Cueing strategy	A series of visual directions that assist the child throughout an activity
Visual schedules	Structured teaching	A visual schedule (with words or pictures) that shows the child a sequence of things to do (hourly, daily, or weekly)
Whole-word (language) approach	Reading intervention	A method to teach reading by introducing words as whole units without analysis of their subword parts (phonemes, letters, etc.)
Word grouping	Memory strategy	A strategy that aids recall by clustering words according to categories (colors, animals, furniture, etc.)

CONCLUSION

Chapter 9

Where Are We Now and Where Do We Want to Go?

This concluding chapter reviews where we are now and where we want to go in terms of understanding the social and academic abilities of the population of children with HFASD and providing treatment. I first summarize where we are now regarding major issues in the social realm, followed by the cognitive-academic domain, and I touch upon areas in need of additional exploration in each of these fields. In the final section of this chapter, I pinpoint three important general issues—neurobiology, sex differences, and language—that have not been comprehensively covered in this book but that provide important complementary information to the understanding of the social and cognitive-academic realms. As I discuss at the end of this chapter, the rich and complex areas of neurobiological and genetic, as well as linguistic, issues in HFASD are beyond the scope of the current book and deserve considerable future discussion, whereas sex differences in HFASD were less a focus in the current volume due to the paucity of research examining gender issues.

THE SOCIAL REALM

As seen throughout this book, social functioning—more specifically, the ability to create and maintain peer relations (as seen in Chapter 3) and the social-cognitive understanding of social situations and emotional states (as seen in Chapter 2)—is a struggle for individuals with HFASD from early development and over the lifespan (Chapter 4), despite their relatively high cognitive capabilities. Their lifelong, continuing struggle with the social-emotional world places these individuals with HFASD at risk for specific vulnerabilities. On the one hand, they express a desire to take part in their social milieu, and indeed they show active participation in social interactions and friendships with peers (Chapter 3), but on the other hand, they lack some necessary prerequisite skills for comprehending those social and emotional situations (Chapter 2) and for performing age-appropriate social behaviors in those interactions (such as conversation skills or coregulation of collaborative acts; Chapter 3). These deficits in social cognition, emotional competence, and social-communicative behavior impair the efficacy of these children's active social participation and heighten their risk for developing comorbid affective difficulties such as depression and anxiety (Chapter 6), as well as for experiencing bullying, ridicule, and social isolation (Chapter 3).

The multidimensional social deficit characterizing individuals with HFASD, which encompasses the threesome of difficulties in social-cognitive skills, emotional competencies, and age-appropriate social-interactive behaviors, calls for a multidimensional orientation toward social treatments for HFASD. Indeed, as presented in Chapter 7, CBT-based models of treatment are proliferating that aim to improve individuals' social-cognitive, emotional, and social-interactive capabilities. The next section summarizes where we are now regarding the main topics discussed in this book for the social realm and also identifies areas calling for future scrutiny.

Social-Cognitive Capabilities

The social-cognitive deficit of children with HFASD already appears at the most basic stage of information processing, where children exhibit difficulties in merely paying **attention to social stimuli,** specifically to dynamic rather than static social stimuli. While observing a dynamic interactive social scenario, children with HFASD tend to look less at the emotionally expressive eye region but more at the mouth or other body region compared with their peers with TYP (e.g., when watching scenes from the film *Who's Afraid of Virginia Woolf?;* see Chapter 2). But this does not mean that people or human faces are not a focus of social interest in HFASD; indeed, as seen in Chapter 2, studies on social attention have consistently demonstrated that individuals with HFASD show a tendency to orient toward people before objects, or to orient visual attention toward human faces at a rate resembling counterparts with TYP. Nevertheless, children with HFASD were slower to look at people, looked less often, and mentioned fewer people in their verbal descriptions of social scenarios compared with peers with TYP.

Clearly, social attention is not an all-or-nothing phenomenon in HFASD, and a fuller understanding of this process is recommended (see Chapter 2) using more naturalistic social-interaction scenarios. Other suggestions that were provided in Chapter 2 for future studies in social attention include the need to examine children's own qualitative reflections on their attention processes during social-interactive situations (what did they look at, and why?), as well as to investigate how attentional processes may differ as a function of the social stimuli's relevance to the child (e.g., interaction with a significant other vs. an interaction with a stranger/experimenter). The vast majority of the available studies on attention (as described in Chapter 2) probed attention to strangers or strangers' faces; thus the role played by the human-social-stimulus relevancy remains unclear.

Social information processing (SIP) and **problem solving** were also thoroughly discussed in Chapter 2. Three main findings emerged for HFASD. First, difficulties were evident in these children's encoding of social information gleaned from observed social scenarios, such as a tendency to encode nonexistent, irrelevant, or peripheral information or the need for more prompts in order to recall details. Second, problems also emerged in social understanding, specifically children's difficulties in generating their own active, social, assertive solutions to various social scenarios and in accurately evaluating various solutions' social appropriateness. Third, children with HFASD perceived themselves as less capable of performing social-assertive behavior in various situations, compared with their peers with TYP. Taken altogether, studies on SIP and problem solving revealed deficits in social understanding and social-knowledge processes, which are essential for efficient social interactions with peers.

Future research should identify individual differences in SIP (e.g., the influence of the child's sensory-temperamental profile), while also looking at SIP correlates and predictors such as central coherence capabilities, executive function, and ToM (see Chapter 1) and exploring their relative contributions to the understanding of SIP processes in HFASD. Difficulties in SIP may be related to children's rigid cognitive shifting capabilities (executive function), overfocus on scenarios' nonsocial details (central coherence weakness), and/or lack of understanding of the role played by others in various situations (ToM). General deficits in social understanding and a narrow "social bank of knowledge" comprising norms and concepts might also explain these difficulties. Due to the high prevalence of comorbidities in HFASD (see Chapter 6), it is important to examine how comorbid conditions such as attention problems and anxiety may affect SIP in HFASD. Children's belief that assertive solutions are less viable for them may stem from their anxiety, and difficulties in the encoding of social stimuli can also be a result of comorbid attention problems. The identification of individual differences in the correlates and predictors of SIP may be very helpful in directing intervention goals.

Emotional Competence

Anomalies in the emotional system were first identified long ago by Kanner (1943) and by the affective theory's explanation for ASD (see Chapter 1). Chapter 2 discussed emotional competence with regard to children's capabilities for emotional understanding and recognition, as well as with regard to children's emotional expressiveness and responsiveness to emotional input.

Despite inconsistencies in findings for the **recognition of basic emotions in others** and for **facial processing**, it may be carefully concluded that children with HFASD show intact visual recognition of prototypical basic emotions such as happiness, sadness, anger, fear, or disgust, as well as recognizing emotions based on vocal intonation. When the emotional stimuli is less straightforward or when more complex elements of social interaction need to be taken into consideration (i.e., nonverbal gestures), then youngsters show slower and less accurate rates of emotion recognition. Lastly, unlike in TYP, children with HFASD fail to show improvement in emotional recognition with development (see Chapter 2).

As seen in Chapter 2 children with HFASD seem to go beyond emotion recognition problems to a more general deficit in **emotion understanding processes**. This deficit encompasses, first, problems in discerning emotions in oneself, especially negative ones, and difficulties in providing narrations for complex emotions requiring an audience, such as embarrassment and pride, or for emotions related to interpersonal relationships, such as jealousy and loneliness. Second, a major difficulty emerges in these youngsters' higher emotion understanding processes, such as comprehending complex emotions in others and in social situations, acknowledging the multifaceted emotion reactions characterizing social situations, and learning rules for how and why people display and hide feelings. Higher-order emotion understanding processes are specifically linked with other areas of difficulty characterizing the social deficit in HFASD. For example, a grasp of complex and hidden emotions requires ToM capabilities and an appreciation of social norms and diverse social situations; moreover, mastery of multifaceted concurrent emotional reactions requires cognitive flexibility—an executive function skill. Thus these children's deficit in emotional understanding is linked with their deficit in social understanding as presented previously, which underscores the multidimensional nature of the social-affective deficit in HFASD.

The manifestations of **emotional expressiveness and responsiveness** in HFASD seem to differ qualitatively from those in TYP, mainly in their communicative quality and clarity of expressions. Clear evidence has been provided (see Chapter 2) that these youngsters can indeed express various emotions, even social emotions such as jealousy and loneliness that are directly related to interpersonal relationships; however, their facial expressions may show mixed emotions, the quality of the expression may seem less mature than that of agemates with TYP, and eye contact to denote communicative intent may be missing. Also, some evidence points to the fact that IQ contributes to better emotional responsiveness skills such as empathy, thereby furnishing support for the cognitive compensation hypothesis (see Chapter 1).

Considering affective issues altogether, individuals with HFASD exhibit an emotional deficit that encompasses both the understanding and the expression of feelings. Nevertheless, they do express and experience various emotions, even social emotions, and they reveal an understanding of some emotional concepts. Due to the importance of emotion in social interaction, this is an important area to be addressed in social intervention planning. Indeed, affective education is a frequent CBT technique used in intervention models for HFASD (see Chapter 7), showing positive results overall in improving these youngsters' emotional recognition and understanding capabilities. Much less is known about treatment effectiveness in rendering change in the way emotions are expressed than in how they are understood; indeed, intervention studies appear to focus to a much lesser extent on treating emotional expression and responsiveness. In this vein, critical questions for future exploration may include, for example: Can interventionists promote a change in children's mechanical intonation, increasing its expressiveness and its fit to the social situation? Can treatment enhance children's capacities to show more cohesive, communicative facial expressions that incorporate eye contact during peer interactions? What is the link between treatments geared toward an increased understanding and awareness of one's own emotional states on the one hand and one's emotional expression and responsiveness capabilities on the other hand? That is, does teaching of emotions through affective education cause a corollary change in children's actual experiencing of such feelings and in children's capabilities for reflecting on these feelings? Beyond IQ, what other areas may lead to progress in emotional responsiveness?

Emotions are important building blocks underlying every social-interactive process. In child–adult interactions, adults can supply important scaffolding for emotional and social exchanges, often within a supportive environment. Yet peer relations comprise a greater challenge for children with HFASD, especially relations with children with TYP. Peer relations encompass children's capabilities for interacting efficiently with peers and, at the pinnacle, the ability to develop friendship. A summary of peer relationships in HFASD is described next.

Peer Relations: Interactions and Friendships

The description of **peer social-interaction processes** in Chapter 3 highlighted several important conclusions. Youngsters with HFASD participate in social interactions with peers but to a lesser degree and while demonstrating a lower quality of social behavior compared with their agemates with TYP. Children with HFASD seem to seek out ways to interact with peers, but, overall, they go about doing this in unusual and socially inadequate ways that reflect their key difficulties in mastering the basics of peer interaction. Conversation with peers and social play are limited, and a specific difficulty emerges in the ability to initiate spontaneous interactions with peers; in addition, during an interaction, these youngsters reveal more passive and low-level social behaviors and fewer active interactive behaviors (see Chapter 3).

Their lower quality of social-interactive behaviors, together with these children's evident desire to take part in such social interactions, places these children at risk for experiencing bullying and victimization from their peers. Indeed, findings indicate that children and adolescents with HFASD encounter victimization and ridicule more often than do their counterparts with TYP (Chapter 3).

However, research outcomes have also shown that exposure to peers with TYP is important in helping these youngsters develop more complex, cooperative, adaptive social behaviors. Thus this integration of HFASD and TYP in inclusive settings seems to be highly important but should be carefully monitored. Other findings show that interaction with another child with a disability (more specifically another child with HFASD) is also beneficial for these youngsters' sense of worth and ease in interaction.

The features of the social environment in which interactions take place also contribute to children's level of social participation. Recess time and free play on the playground—the least structured environments—pose a heightened challenge for these youngsters, requiring them to create social activity with peers. Dyadic interactions in a one-on-one setting are easier for them than triadic or group interactions. The empirical examination of individual differences in interactive skills is currently at its preliminary stages, but researchers suggest that those youngsters with less severe social deficiencies or with better cognitive and verbal skills show more adequate social-interaction skills. However, familial characteristics also appear to contribute to children's social participation, such as parents' own social involvement levels. Altogether, cumulative data on peer interactions in HFASD indeed support the notion that this is an area of great difficulty, requiring careful consideration of the "goodness of fit" between the individual child's characteristics and the social environment's characteristics. Some environments and some social partners will extract a higher level of social participation from the child with HFASD, whereas others will impede the child's ability to take part in interpersonal interactions and may even ostracize the child.

Future investigations of interactive skills in HFASD should be twofold. On the one hand, we need to learn more about individual differences in the social-interaction capabilities of children with HFASD beyond the afore-mentioned variables examined thus far: social severity and cognitive and language skills. Issues such as sex differences in interaction style; personality characteristics such as internalizing or externalizing behavioral tendencies; executive functions beyond abstract reasoning, such as generativity skills, cognitive shifting, and problem solving, as well as ToM capabilities, may all contribute to individual differences in these target children's social-interactive skills. On the other hand, perhaps of equal importance is the need to develop better understanding of the peers who may support social involvement and participation in the child with HFASD. Peers with different characteristics—friends and nonfriends, peers with TYP, and peers with HFASD—may play complementary roles for the child with HFASD. For example, interactions with peers with TYP may challenge children to achieve higher levels of social-interaction behaviors and play, whereas interactions with peers with HFASD may enable more relaxing interactions and opportunities to act as leader instead of follower. The possible impact of the peers' disability or friend status is a very important yet much neglected area of research. Lastly, we should also learn more about the optimal social environment for increasing social participation in HFASD, as well as the roles that staff and parents may play in such environments. For example, research has shown that a one-on-one aide's presence may limit social participation with peers and that peer mediation or support is highly important in increasing participation. Lastly, models of efficient peer modeling and support should be more carefully examined. Thus future studies would do well in striving to explore these individual and familial–environmental factors.

Harsh predictions about the ability to develop **friendship** among youngsters with HFASD based on affective and intersubjectivity theories, as well as on ToM theory (see Chapter 1) notwithstanding, findings have demonstrated that durable and stable friendship is a feasible experience in HFASD, most likely with a same-age and same-sex partner, either with TYP or with a disability. Furthermore, friendship is important for children with HFASD, as shown by the more complex, reciprocal, and close quality of interaction with a friend than with a peer who is not a friend (Chapters 3 and 4). This is not to say that the quality of friendship in HFASD is similar to friendship in TYP. As seen in Chapter 3, friendship differs in many ways and even develops differently (probably requiring much more external support from significant others in the child's environment vs. friendship in TYP). Nevertheless, peer friendship appears to play an important role in the social-emotional world of individuals with HFASD.

Although we know that friendship is not a frequent experience in HFASD, its exact rates are ambiguous. Two types of studies have examined friendship: Studies that screened the whole autism spectrum for friendship presented low friendship rates, whereas other research focused only on children and adolescents who have friends (mainly in HFASD), thereby precluding collection of data on friendship rates across HFASD. Yet the available studies seem to indicate that individuals at older ages (especially in young adulthood) have the lowest number of friendship experiences. Another crucial issue that merits deeper empirical scrutiny relates to how friendship in HFASD is formed beyond parents' and professionals' support. In a like manner, who are those children with HFASD who are able to form friendships? The answers to these questions remain unclear. For example, as seen in Chapter 3, in TYP attachment security was shown to be related to friendship qualities, whereas in HFASD attachment security was found to contribute to friendship through its link with ToM. Thus researchers should continue to ask what characteristics may contribute to children's ability to form friendship beyond ToM, security of attachment, IQ, and verbal IQ.

In my Behavioral Research Laboratory, we are currently exploring the role played by children's ability to experience social emotions such as jealousy at early ages (toddlerhood) in predicting later friendship relationships with peers. Also, individual differences in sensory profile, temperament, and self-regulation were found to predict social competence in HFASD (see Chapter 3); therefore, their relevancy for friendship development should be examined. Likewise, researchers have yet to uncover what else beyond language capabilities differentiates between those children with HFASD who form a friendship with a peer with TYP versus those children with HFASD who form a friendship with an atypical peer (mixed versus non-mixed friendships). Lastly, studies on friendships of different kinds have indicated that social intervention should be more directly focused on teaching individuals how to develop relationships with peers across the lifespan while promoting the necessary skills leading to the formation of relationships rather than mere interactions.

Taken altogether, the difficulties in the **social realm** for individuals with HFASD are multifaceted, encompassing input processes in social cognition and emotional processing, as well as output processes, including overt social-interactive behaviors and friendships with peers. The design of multidimensional social interventions is needed to capture this complexity and to provide treatments targeting both the input and the output processes. The next section focuses on social interventions in HFASD based on the review and guidelines presented in Chapter 7 of the book.

Social Interventions

Theoretical principles, basic techniques, and content domains for social intervention were discussed extensively throughout Chapter 7. Multimodal CBT-based interventions were suggested as a valuable theoretical framework for enhancing integrative social competence in HFASD and for helping these youngsters utilize their relatively high cognitive capabilities in efficient ways to make sense of their social world. Ecological models that implement the treatment in a setting that resembles the child's natural, "real" life as closely as possible (e.g., school) and includes the child's main social agents (e.g., peers with TYP, teachers, parents, siblings) were also recommended. In line with the aim to produce a change in children's understanding of peers and interactions with peers, both cognitive and behavioral techniques were shown to be helpful. Domains and topics for intervention were also introduced, which incorporate treatments addressing these individuals' known difficulties in both social-cognitive skills and social-interactive skills, as well as in friendship and self-regulation. All are extensively discussed throughout Chapter 7.

Important progress has transpired in the understanding of treatment needs and procedures in the field, but vital areas remain to be explored. As described before, in Chapter 7, recommendations were made to implement multifaceted interventions that facilitate both understanding and behavior and that enhance transfer and generalization by incorporating real-life settings and change agents. Related to this integrative curriculum is the need to capture all of these social-functioning complexities in a developmentally appropriate manner to address toddlers', children's, adolescents', and adults' changing needs. Researchers should examine these multidimensional, ecological, developmentally oriented treatments with ever-increasing sample sizes and various age groups. An additional extension recommended for intervention design is to feature the important topic of treating these individuals' frequent comorbid affective difficulties in addition to anxiety, such as depression, OCD, and specific phobias, as well as introducing such affective domains as anger management and emotional self-regulation (see Chapter 6 for a description of comorbid conditions in HFASD). The very few empirical examinations that explored these areas suggested promising initial results, but further empirical inquiry is needed.

Careful differential investigations of the efficacy of specific intervention techniques for various ages may also be helpful. An important direction for further research is to expand on the development of psychometrically sound ecological observational measures for evaluating children's "real life" ongoing interactions with peers in addition to the existing parent- and self-reports. In this book, the tables in Appendix C offer a useful list of available social assessment measures in the social realm, but psychometric qualities should be more carefully scrutinized for some of the measures.

Another important direction for expanding social intervention in HFASD is to examine the role of other social agents in addition to peers with TYP, such as children's siblings. Due to the fact that siblings offer natural, intrinsic opportunities for social experience among individuals with HFASD, their potential role as change agents should be explored further, perhaps utilizing peer-mediation techniques that were found effective for nonsiblings. All in all, the main take-home message for educators, researchers, policymakers, and interventionists for youngsters with HFASD is the need to find ways to help them translate their faulty theoretical knowledge about social-emotional interactions into more fruitful, productive, pragmatically adjusted social peer interactions.

THE COGNITIVE-ACADEMIC REALM

As described in Chapter 5, individuals with HFASD display a wide variance in cognitive abilities alongside a broad range of academic skills, from cognitive impairment to academic giftedness. Knowledge concerning cognitive ability is crucial for education and intervention planning, yet general agreement is lacking concerning the appropriate assessment and testing battery for this population. An important avenue for further study is to deepen knowledge of the various **IQ profiles** in HFASD (i.e., Verbal < Performance; Verbal = Performance; Verbal > Performance IQs) and how they may relate to academic achievement. To date, research indicates that adaptive behavior scores lag behind IQ scores, especially in HFASD, as do memory scores and in some instances academic achievement scores.

The academic profile in HFASD regarding the reading, writing, and mathematics domains generally delineates higher **reading decoding abilities** in comparison with lower **reading comprehension** and **written language skills**, alongside overall variance in **mathematics** capabilities, with areas such as computational skills seeming more intact than areas such as mathematics problem solving. All in all, underachievement is noted in these children when academic tasks are more complex and more heavily linked with other important domains that are deficient in HFASD (see Chapter 1 on the link between cognitive-academic difficulties and cognitive theories). For example, reading comprehension is strongly connected with ToM capabilities, which are deficient in HFASD, and mathematical problem solving is heavily related to deficient executive function skills such as planning.

However, it is not only in the academic domain but also in the cognitive domain that individuals with HFASD demonstrate difficulties—in areas such as **memory, information processing** (the ability to store, retrieve, and even transform concepts and schemas), and **concept formation** (the ability to classify objects, events, or ideas). As seen in Chapter 5, most aspects of memory performance (verbal, nonverbal, and autobiographical) are lower in children with HFASD than in their peers with TYP. A possible reason for their uneven memory abilities may be low information-processing abilities. For the most part, as task and information loads increase, individuals with HFASD show decreased memory abilities and tend not to make use of relational information to enhance recall. Yet appropriate concept formation intervention can enhance memory in general, which can assist individuals with HFASD in improving their ability to retain and recall information.

Cognitive-Academic Interventions

Although the body of literature concerning cognitive and academic abilities in HFASD is growing, much has yet to be learned. Specifically lacking is research exploring mathematical capabilities in HFASD. Furthermore, in comparison with the relative spread of interventions in the social realm, the development of HFASD-oriented intervention techniques and teaching strategies in the academic realm is lagging (as described in Chapter 8). This lag may be due to the fact that academic difficulties are not considered a core deficit, whereas social difficulties are. Or perhaps stakeholders have assumed that due to their relatively high cognitive capabilities, students with HFASD will manage to cope with school requirements. However, as seen throughout Chapter 5, even though many of these children present strengths in the cognitive and academic realm, their functioning is mixed and inconsistent, with limitations and shortcomings in specific areas. This uneven performance accentuates the importance of providing relevant and appropriate teaching strategies and interventions. Various academic strategies were presented throughout Chapter 8, including general strategies such as structured teaching, embedded instruction, cueing strategies, and specific strategies that target various cognitive, as well as academic, skills such as memory, language, reading, writing, and mathematics.

Among the most extensively used and effective teaching strategies for children with HFASD are the visually based interventions, which take advantage of many of these students' **visual learning** preferences. For example, the structured teaching paradigm discussed in Chapter 8 makes extensive use of visual cues (e.g., visual organizers) to help students manage their classroom and school environments as well as academic tasks. These strategies aim to increase students' autonomy in various settings and when coping with diverse school assignments. Interestingly, as seen in Chapter 7 and in Appendix A, visual aids are also frequently employed in social interventions for HFASD in line with the same principle—that many of these students are visual learners.

Other beneficial techniques fall under a general category of **scaffolding** and **cueing** (e.g., semantic, pictorial, textual), which all aim to provide children with the necessary information to redress their inadequate understanding of conceptual information or academic tasks. Scaffolding and cueing intervention strategies correspond well with the cognitive reconstructing and concept clarification techniques that were presented in Chapter 7 for social impairment.

A third group of techniques include more specific rather than general strategies to enhance both cognitive and academic capabilities. A detailed description is given in Chapter 8, but some important take-home points should be noted. For example, rehearsal appears to be a fruitful technique for enhancing children's confidence about a newly learned topic and skills. Hierarchical, developmental, sequential construction of tasks for learning was also mentioned as an important strategy. For example, to teach "wh=" questions such as *What? When? How?* or *Why?*, it was recommended to focus on only one "wh-" question at a time, while gradually building up the child's more general ability to ask questions. Also, when dealing with figurative language in a text, it is important to know the hierarchy of figurative words and to teach them accordingly. It should be noted that the principle of gradually building up children's academic and cognitive knowledge and skills coincides well with the recommendation to build social curricula in hierarchical order, from the least complex levels of understanding (basic, simple emotions) and behavior (one-on-one dyadic interactions) to the most complex levels (higher-order emotional skills and group interactions). In addition, Chapter 8 emphasized the value of trying to connect the learned skills and children's intrinsic motivation (e.g., in selecting texts for reading comprehension practice). Likewise, in social interventions, as part of cognitive reconstruction, we try to help children understand why certain social skills (such as listening or conversing with friends) are important. Also, in both the social and cognitive-academic domains, through the teaching process, abstract concepts become more concrete by providing children with a set of rules and with cues to help figure out the meaning. Moreover, children with HFASD reveal difficulties in solving mathematical problems similar to their problems in solving social problems; hence future researchers may do well to examine whether cognitive techniques directly addressing problem solving may be helpful in both arenas.

Finally, as accentuated in Chapter 8, no discussion of cognitive and academic interventions would be complete without clarifying the need to develop and evaluate **accommodations** in order to "level the playing field" for students as they cope with challenging academic tasks and requirements. For example, students with HFASD might benefit immensely from the use of a keyboard or word processor to address their difficulties in writing. An important topic for future study is to develop a set of accommodations specifically oriented to the unique needs of students with HFASD, as well as to design a set of guidelines determining when accommodation is the best choice versus treatment or remediation of the deficient skill. For example, when should teachers let children use a calculator instead of insisting that they study the multiplication table? As mentioned, research on the area of mathematics is very scarce, and efforts should be focused greatly in this domain.

To sum up, discernible correspondences exist between the cognitive-academic and the social-emotional realms, in terms of many suggested principles and some intervention techniques. Even if the two domains (social and academic) may seem conceptually distant from each other, in actual fact they both share the goal of helping children improve how they perceive the world's stimuli and how they interact with that world; hence the parallels that emerged in this book regarding theoretical, interventional, and empirical recommendations are not so surprising. Again, a multidimensional understanding of the cognitive and academic profile, as well as the complex social deficits of students with HFASD, can facilitate more optimal teaching strategies, interventions, and accommodations. Endeavors to link the cognitive and social deficits may permit the development of unique strategy sets and intervention models to best fit these youngsters' multifaceted needs. A better appreciation of the strengths and weaknesses in each domain and the links between the two domains can help professionals generate wide-ranging, comprehensive interventions that can facilitate caregivers' and professionals' enhancement of youngsters' abilities in both the social and academic realms.

GENERAL FUTURE DIRECTIONS
AND CONCLUDING REMARKS

Overall, in this book, I adapted a psychoeducational perspective, extensively describing psychological and neuropsychological characteristics of individuals with HFASD along the social and cognitive-academic realms, with an emphasis on the periods from childhood through adolescence. The discussion of etiologies for HFASD was outside the current focus of this book. However, it is important to note that emerging data coming from the fields of neuroscience, neurobiology, and genetics hold promise in providing important supplementary information on the causes and possibly also effective treatments for ASD (see excellent reviews in Dawson, Sterling, & Faja, 2009; Neuhaus, Beauchaine, & Bernier, 2010; Schroeder, Desrocher, Bebko, & Cappadocia, 2010).

For example, Dawson et al. (2009) suggested an etiological model in which early autism risk factors such as genetics (e.g., autism is considered polygenic based on multiple genes interacting epistatically, with 2–10 possibly contributing loci) and environment (e.g., prenatal influences of alcohol, thalidomide, and intrauterine exposure to viruses) lead to risk processes (i.e., alternation of patterns of child × environment interaction, based on the atypical child's perception of and responses to the social environment), which in turn result in abnormalities of brain development/neural circuitry and full emergence of autism symptoms. The correspondence between genetic–environmental factors and the development of autism assumed by the presented model is not one-to-one; rather, Dawson et al. (2009) suggest that autism emerges as a result of the interaction between early risk factors and the context in which the child develops.

In their review of neurological findings for ASD, Schroeder et al. (2010) presented some interesting links between brain regions and the cognitive deficits in ASD (see WCC and ToM in Chapter 1), suggesting that each of these deficiencies may be supported by neurological influences. Based on their review of the literature, they suggested that the cerebellum and frontal lobes may be implicated in both ToM and WCC and that ToM might also be associated with the temporal lobe and with the mirror neuron system (which enables imitation of actions performed by others). Also, Schroeder et al. (2010) suggested that both ToM and the mirror neuron systems involve the inferior frontal gyrus and the superior temporal sulcus.

In a different review, Neuhaus et al. (2010) focused on neurobiological correlates of social functioning in autism. They noted that several of the potential mechanisms of social behavioral deficit in ASD are those that involve neural networks including the amygdala, the mesocorticolimbic system, and the oxytocin system, with specific emphasis on those models that integrate mechanisms across biological systems, such as those linking dopamine and oxytocin with brain regions critical to reward processing. Neuhaus et al. (2010) suggested three conclusions that have specific implications for the study of the more cognitively able individuals with HFASD on whom the present book focuses. First, they concluded that insights from neurobiological studies highlight the heterogeneity in ASD, which may potentially provide valuable information for early detection, as well as for understanding individual differences in response to treatment, and may assist in identifying subgroups within ASD. For example, individuals who approach normal mirror neuron EEG responses during imitation tasks may benefit more from observational learning procedures than individuals with atypical EEG responses. Due to the fact that participants in most of the neurobiological studies were of mixed functioning levels (low and high), it is difficult to draw conclusions about specific implications for the more able children on the spectrum. Future studies would do well to pinpoint the links between individual biological differences and children's cognitive profiles. However, importantly, the heterogeneity found to characterize the biological and neurological systems of individuals with ASD appears to substantiate the subgroups identified through the psychological studies described throughout this book, presenting higher social functioning for the more able children versus those with LFA.

Second, Neuhaus et al. (2010) emphasized that some neurobiological processes are dynamic, continuing to change throughout development, such as the amygdala and the processes regulating serotonin synthesis. Thus neurological plasticity and biological amenability suggest that treatment efforts may continue throughout adolescence and into adulthood. This conclusion holds promise for the possible effectiveness of intervention studies in the social and academic realms when performed with older adolescents and young adults with HFASD. Third, these researchers concluded that neurobiological studies furnish support for efforts to implement more comprehensive interventions that target integrative concepts of social functioning rather than those treating isolated skills, that are generalizable across contexts, and that are performed in children's real-life settings. The last recommendation coincides well with the recommendations for treatment that have been presented throughout this book based on the perspectives of psychoeducational studies. Future psychoeducational research combined with biological research may be the key to identifying treatment domains and to recognizing individual differences in responses to intervention, thereby enabling the design of individualized treatment models based on each child's psychological–biological profile.

Another topic that was less specifically discussed throughout the book involves individual differences based on gender. Findings for ASD support male predominance, which appears even more at the high-functioning level. According to the Centers for Disease Control and Prevention (2012), the ratio of males to females in ASD is 54 to 252 (a male:female ratio of 2.5 to 4.1). However, the most consistently reported sex difference is that girls are more likely to have comorbid intellectual deficit than boys (Centers for Disease Control and Prevention, 2007; Lord & Schopler, 1985; Lord,

Schopler, & Revicki, 1982; Volkmar, Szatmari, & Sparrow, 1993). Given this marked sex discrepancy, research on individuals with HFASD has predominantly sampled male participants, and if girls did participate, they were usually too few to enable conclusive remarks based on sex.

Yet several recently published studies did present informative findings on females with HFASD. For example, Solomon et al. (2012) explored autism symptoms and internalizing characteristics among girls with HFASD (CA = 8–18 years) versus boys with HFASD, as well as versus girls and boys with TYP. Symptoms of autism were not found to differ between boys and girls with HFASD; however, internalizing symptoms (a composite of anxiety, depression, and somatization items) did—in adolescence (CA = 12–18 years). During the whole age range (8–18 years), girls with HFASD showed higher levels of internalizing symptoms than girls with TYP. Adolescent girls with HFASD (12–18 years) also differed from adolescent girls with TYP in depression levels, but not from adolescent boys with HFASD. Altogether, based on this study, girls who are high functioning are not more likely to show autistic symptoms than boys who are high functioning, but they may be at greater risk of developing internalizing psychopathologies than boys with HFASD (based on self-reported measures), especially during adolescence.

Two studies presented sex differences in young toddlers with ASD of mixed IQ levels. Carter et al. (2007) reported that boys (CA = 1.7–2.8 years) demonstrated a different developmental and cognitive profile from girls. Female toddlers showed better visual reception, whereas male toddlers revealed more developed language and fine motor skills, as well as more advanced social functioning. In Hartley and Sikora (2009), female toddlers (CA = 1.5–3.9 years) showed higher levels of impaired communication skills (based on the ADOS; Lord et al., 2000), as well as more sleep and affective problems (anxiety, depression) than males. Boys exhibited more stereotyped and repetitive behaviors than girls.

Interestingly, Lai et al. (2011) found similarities between adult males and females with HFASD (CA = 18–45 years) on self-reported empathy, anxiety, depression, and obsessive–compulsive symptoms. Yet females showed more lifetime sensory symptoms, fewer current social-communicative difficulties, and more self-reported autistic traits than males. In a different study (McLennan, Lord, & Schopler, 1993) examining a very wide age range (CA = 6–36 years, IQ > 60), females had fewer friendships based on the ADI parent report (Rutter et al., 2003). Thus, altogether, it seems that gender issues in HFASD pose an important yet overlooked area, which holds implications for both the social and the cognitive-academic realms, thereby calling for extensive future research.

Before closing the book, I would like to underscore the importance of language to both the social and the academic realms for youngsters with HFASD. Indeed, language in its own right was not a main focus of this book, but linguistic issues were discussed in various contexts due to their close relevance to both the social-emotional and cognitive-academic domains. For example, language was emphasized as an important predictor of better social functioning (mainly in Chapters 3 and 4); children's descriptions of social conversation reflected difficulties in pragmatics (Chapter 3); children's narrative abilities, as well as the importance of language skills to academic functioning, were discussed throughout Chapter 5; and Chapter 8 reviewed intervention techniques to improve academic functioning, including language capabilities such as strategies for teaching the skills of question asking and answering as well as strategies to facilitate the comprehension of figurative words and phrases. Language is a major domain in the understanding of HFASD, and, as such, deserves a thorough discussion in a book of its own, containing elaborated and thorough descriptions of these children's linguistic characteristics, their assessment, and optimal intervention models customized to individual differences in language. Interested readers who would like to gain more comprehensive information about language in ASD and HFASD may refer to two excellent recent reviews in this area (Boucher, 2012; Stefanatos & Baron, 2011).

Throughout this summary chapter, I touched upon some of the major domains explored in this book regarding the social and academic abilities of youngsters with HFASD, highlighted various practical implications for effective treatments, and pinpointed some crucial areas still in need of further empirical exploration. As seen throughout this book, individuals with HFASD comprise an important and unique subgroup within the autism spectrum who reveal capabilities for potentially high social and academic functioning. However, by the same token, these individuals are at risk for developing specific difficulties in light of their inadequate social and academic understanding and performance on the one hand and their enhanced recognition of the gaps between themselves and their peers with TYP on the other hand. My hope is that the present book will serve educators, empiricists, policy makers, other specialized mental health professionals, and parents as they work to achieve a more efficacious and productive social and academic life for these individuals.

Cognitive-Behavioral Therapy Techniques and Settings

TABLE A1. Definitions of Major CBT-Based Cognitive and   234
Behavioral Techniques for HFASD, with Examples
(Derived from Literature and Especially from Bauminger's
C-B-E Interventions)

TABLE A2. Role Description of Main Change Agents   240
in Interventions

FIGURE A1. CBT-based social intervention techniques   241
and settings. Cognitive and behavioral techniques based
on CBT and treatment settings focusing on various change
agents (Beelmann et al., 1994; Bierman & Welsh, 2000;
Dobson & Dobson, 2009; Ronen, 1998; Spence, 2003).

TABLE A1. Definitions of Major CBT-Based Cognitive and Behavioral Techniques for HFASD, with Examples (Derived from Literature and Especially from Bauminger's C-B-E Interventions)

Technique	Definition/aim	Examples
		Cognitive techniques: Enhancing social-cognition capabilities
Cognitive reconstruction and concept clarification	*Cognitive reconstruction:* • Corrects distorted or deficient conceptualizations of the social world • Teaches social norms and standards • Explains social constructs • Concretizes (makes explicit) the reality of social situations *Concept clarification:* • Clarifies basic social concepts • Emphasizes their importance *Joint aims:* • Builds up social-emotional knowledge, awareness, and understanding of what X social construct is, why X is important in social interaction, and how X should be manifested (see reviews in Anderson & Morris, 2006; Attwood, 2003, 2004; Krasny et al., 2003)	Examples taken from Bauminger's (2002, 2007a, 2007b) CBE intervention unit targeting the ability to focus attention on social and emotional stimuli ("Social listening inside and outside"): *Concept clarification:* • *What is social listening?* Directing my focus of attention in social situations toward verbal and nonverbal social cues. • *What are verbal and nonverbal social cues?* Nonverbal: smiles, change in intonation, body gestures; Verbal: invitation to play, declaring about emotional state, e.g., "I'm happy." *Cognitive reconstruction:* • *Why is social listening important?* It is a way to know my friends' feelings and areas of interest, a way to become friends. • *How do I listen to a friend?* Look into his eyes, read her facial expression, listen to his tone of voice, try to remember her words, pay attention to his body language. • *How do I identify listening barriers?* Identify inner thoughts, overly crowded places, distractions such as computer games. • *How do I get to know my social attention process?* Identify people and situations that are easy/hard for me to listen to and why. • *How do I overcome listening barriers?* Identify actions or thoughts that may help me cope with such barriers. • *How do I listen inside?* Listen to my own inner world and identify my feelings, desires, preferences, difficulties, and strengths.

Self-instruction and self-talk	*Self-instruction/self-talk* (see reviews in Luria, 1961[a]; Vygotsky, 1962):
	• Internal talk that guides cognitive processes and overt behavior, usually in problem-solving processes
	• In CBT, change agents (adults, peers) usually state problem-solving stages aloud while gradually aiming for child to develop internal talk that will include "saying the stages to myself" in various social situations inside and outside the treatment setting.
		Self-instruction example from Beaumont and Sofronoff (2008):
		The **DECODE** formula to solve social problems:
		  Define the problem/task.
		  Explore solutions.
		  Consider consequences and choose a solution.
		  Organize a plan.
		  Do it.
		  Evaluate how it went.
		Self-instruction example from Bauminger (2002, 2007b):
		1. What is the problem?
		2. How do I and they (problem partners) feel?
		3. What can be done?
		4. What will happen if . . . ?
		5. What is/are the best solution(s)? Why?
		6. How do I apply the chosen solution?

Problem solving	*Problem solving* (see reviews in Spivack & Shure, 1974[a]; Shure, 1981[a]): • Provides a social schema to enable perception and processing of various social situations through presentation of short social vignettes, comprising several stages: 1. Identifying the social task/problem 2. Finding alternative solutions 3. Considering solutions' consequences 4. Choosing the most efficient solution that best meets the social task's demands.	Examples of brief vignettes for applying these problem-solving stages are taken from Bauminger (2002, 2007b): • *Initiating a conversation:* "John went out at recess time and saw his friend Steve sitting alone. John would like to start a conversation with Steve, but he doesn't know how." • *Inviting a friend to play:* "Jill likes to play cards very much. It is recess time now and Jill cannot play alone. What can she do?" • *Negotiating and persuading:* "Joel and Bob want to go see a movie together. Joel wants to see X and Bob wants to see Y. It is hard for them to decide which movie to watch. What can they do?" • *Joining a friend's activity:* "Mark and Ben are playing cards during recess. Johnny would really love to join them, but he does not know how. What can he do?"

(continued)

235

TABLE A1. (*continued*)

Technique	Definition/aim	Examples
		• *Sharing experiences:* "Yuval went skiing with her parents this weekend and had a lot of fun. The teacher asked the children to tell about an experience they had over the weekend, and all the children shared with the class, except for Yuval. The children asked Yuval: "What did you do over the weekend?" What should Yuval do now?
Affective education	*Affective education* (see reviews in Attwood, 2003, 2004; and see Kam, Greenberg, & Kusche, 2004)[a]: • Helps us understand, name, and recognize emotions in ourselves, in others, and in various social situations • Explains why emotions are important • Expands emotional repertoire • Helps regulate emotions.	*Emotion dictionary* (Bauminger, 2007a) asks children to provide a pragmatic definition of each emotion, for example: • *Embarrassment:* When an unpleasant event happens to me while others are watching • *Pride:* When I accomplish something that I worked hard on • *Loneliness:* When I am alone but do not want to be • *Disappointment:* (1) When I expect something that I want to happen but it does not happen; (2) When I fail at something I really want; (3) When someone who promises me something lets me down. *Four categories of cues for emotion recognition* (Bauminger, 2002, 2007a, 2007b): • Facial expressions and body gestures (a smile, a cry, hands stretched overhead for pride, pointing finger for threat) • Verbal cues ("I'm happy," "I'm so bored") • Situational cues (when someone is losing a race and other children are laughing at him, he probably feels embarrassed) • Internal cues ("Where do I feel my emotions?"—awareness of inner sensations that accompany different emotional experiences) *Emotional tool box* (Attwood, 2004, review; Scarpa & Reyes, 2011): • Relaxation tools such as painting, drawing, reading, and listening to music

- Physical tools such as a hammer to release tension
- Social tools to find supportive social activities that are enjoyable
- Thinking tools—a manual that includes positive self-statements and puts events in perspective, as well as guidance for cue-controlled relaxation

Comic strip conversations (Gray, 1998, review):

- In this procedure, figures are drawn to depict a social situation. Thought and speech bubbles identify what people are doing, thinking, and feeling. Different colors identify emotional content and clarify children's interpretation of events and rationale for thoughts and responses. Alternative thoughts can be drawn to explore how these will affect other participants' thoughts, feelings, and actions.

Social stories	*Social stories* (see reviews in Gray, 1998, 2000; Kokina & Kern, 2010; Reynhout & Carter, 2006): • Describe the salient aspects of a specific social situation(s) • Explain the likely reactions of others • Help children understand and read various social situations • Provide information about appropriate behavioral responses. Example of typical social story structure, usually containing four main sentence types (Gray, 1998, 2000): • A descriptive *factual statement* ("Children play many different types of games") • A *directive*, which suggests how to behave ("Before you start to play with your friends, be sure to learn game rules") • A *perspective*, which describes a person's thoughts and feelings ("Before you start to play with your friends, ask them about their preferred game—because different children may like to play different things") • An *affirmative*, which provides reassurance ("It's okay to feel sad when your friend refuses to play with you")

Behavioral techniques: Practicing social-interactive behaviors

Modeling	*Modeling* (Ronen, 1998,[a] review): • Demonstrates how to perform a particular social behavior Modeling can be performed through: • Live human mediation by adults or peers (Bauminger, 2002, 2007a, 2007b) • Other modalities, such as video modeling

(*continued*)

TABLE A1. (continued)

Technique	Definition/aim	Examples
Behavioral rehearsal	*Behavioral rehearsal* (Ronen, 1998,[a] review): • Enables practice and experience of the skills learned through cognitive techniques in a safe, controllable environment • Helps transform theoretical knowledge into more pragmatic knowledge • Enables practice of "bad" alternatives, too, to improve understanding of their consequences	Examples of behavioral rehearsal through role play in dyads and in small groups (Bauminger, 2002, 2007a, 2007b): • Role play focusing on rehearsal of various skills: initiating a conversation with a friend, cooperating with a friend on a construction game, negotiating, persuading, behaving flexibly, entering a group conversation or activity • Role play focusing on one main skill (e.g., negotiating) in different social scenarios • Role play for practicing a whole continuing scenario (e.g., group entry into a conversation) using the problem-solving stages described above and exploring consequences of behavioral choices (e.g., asking: Did children cooperate with my initiation or not? Then what should I do next?)
Feedback and reinforcement	*Reinforcement:* • Positively reinforces behaviors to increase appropriate response strategies *Feedback:* • Provides feedback about performance during behavioral rehearsals or role play, either by an adult mediator, other group members, or the children themselves *Joint aims:* • Helps child understand what went well and why and what went wrong and why, to promote internalization of this self-evaluation process to be generalized to future social experiences (Ronen, 1998,[a] review)	Examples from Bauminger (2002, 2007a, 2007b): • Taping children's talk during social conversation session and listening to tapes together with the children while providing immediate feedback on the conversation's quality and flow (e.g., Social? Informational? Interview? Lecture? Level of reciprocity? Consideration of other's point of view?) • Reinforcing children in various ways, such as providing a compliment; providing a privilege such as having more computer time; or providing a statement about the child's strengths and abilities (e.g., when children make a phone call to the peer aide as part of the homework in a session on social conversation, they receive a statement of "great job" and the privilege of more computer time).

238

Homework	*Homework* (Ronen, 1998,[a] review): • Practice learned skills in other settings (home, school) • Practice learned skills with various people (parents, peers, siblings)	Examples from Bauminger (2002, 2007a, 2007b): • Making a phone call to a friend from the group • Recording parents' and siblings' social conversations • Observing other children's conversations or activities during recess time at school
Relaxation and exposure	*Relaxation* (Davis, Eshelman, & McKay, 2000[a]; Dobson & Dobson, 2009[a]): • Teaches awareness and control over physiological and muscular reactions to anxiety through systematic tension-releasing exercises *Exposure* (Dobson & Dobson, 2009[a]): • Reduces avoidant reactions and builds new reactions to anxiety-provoking stimuli through gradual, controlled systematic exposure to that feared stimuli • Causes habituation of physiological anxiety, extinction of fears, and provision of opportunities for new learning to occur	Examples of relaxation skills: • Breathing exercises and muscle relaxation techniques (e.g., Sung et al., 2011) • Visualization exercises, such as imagining walking on the beach (Davis et al., 2000[a]) • "Relaxation tools" that lower the heart rate, such as listening to music or reading a book (Sofronoff, Attwood, & Hinton, 2005) Examples of exposure (Wood, Drahota, Sze, Har, et al., 2009): • Repeatedly exposing children in vivo to feared situations while using coping skills that have been learned and remaining in the situations until habituation occurs • Creating a "fear situation" hierarchy in which feared situations are ordered from the least to most distressing; children work their way up the hierarchy and are rewarded as they attempt increasingly fear-invoking activities

[a]Literature related to CBT in general, not to ASD in particular.

TABLE A2. Role Description of Main Change Agents in Interventions

Adult–child mediation
(e.g., Paul, 2003, review)

- Plays a major role in teaching the social task according to the perception that social competence can be learned
- Scaffolds social activities during dyadic and small-group social skill training
- Supports peers with TYP during peer mediation program
- Provides efficient mediation mode during the learning stage

Dyadic peer mediation
(e.g., Bass & Mulick, 2007, review; Rogers, 2000, review; Kasari, Rotheram-Fuller, Locke, & Gulsrud, 2012; Owen-DeSchryver et al., 2008)

- Develop, support, and increase the level of social interaction that children with HFASD experience with their peers with TYP in a setting as close as possible to naturalistic social environment (e.g., classroom, playground)
- Furnish an adult mediator to scaffold social activities and support the partner with TYP
- Provide an efficient mediation mode during the experiencing stage, when dyadic skills require naturalistic practice with a partner

Small social group
(e.g., Barry et al., 2003; Bauminger, 2007a)

- Offers opportunities to practice newly learned skills in a relatively naturalistic semistructured social environment that may promote spontaneous interaction with other children
- Furnishes an adult mediator to scaffold social activities and support peers with TYP
- Provides an efficient mediation mode during the experiencing stage, when small-group skills require naturalistic practice

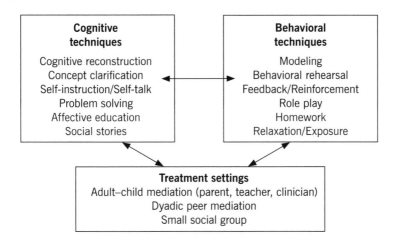

FIGURE A1. CBT-based social intervention techniques and settings. Cognitive and behavioral techniques based on CBT and treatment settings focusing on various change agents (Beelmann et al., 1994; Bierman & Welsh, 2000; Dobson & Dobson, 2009; Ronen, 1998; Spence, 2003).

Multimodal Cognitive-Behavioral-Ecological Interventions

TABLE B1. Main Curriculum Topics for CBE   244
    Dyadic Intervention

TABLE B2. Main Curricular Topics for CBE   245
    Small-Group Intervention

TABLE B3. Criteria for Selection of Peer Aide   246
    with TYP in CBE Treatments

FIGURE B1. CBE intervention model   247

FIGURE B2. Excerpts from a sample CBE curriculum unit   248
    for combining both learning and experiencing
    of social conversation

TABLE B1. Main Curriculum Topics for CBE Dyadic Intervention (Bauminger, 2002, 2007b)

Curricular topic	Examples of targets	Comments
1. Social understanding	Instruction in prerequisite language concepts that should form the basis for more efficient problem-solving processes and discussions, such as: • *Weighing alternatives* (i.e., X or Y; X and Y; X and not Y; not X and not Y) • *Time-related words* (i.e., now, later, all the time, part of the time, before, after) • *Words to reflect my and others' preferences* (I like X; X likes Y) • *Sequence and causality* (what will happen if . . . ; it happened because of . . .) • *Doubting words* (i.e., maybe, not sure, possible)	Other concepts that were taught as prerequisite social concepts to the problem-solving stage: • What is a friend? • In what ways am I like or different from my friends? • What is social listening and why it is important?
2. Emotional understanding and recognition	• Simple emotions (sad, happy, afraid, angry), taught by describing the rule for each emotion • How to identify the emotion in myself and in others through the recognition of facial expressions, gestures, and vocalizations • How to identify emotions in social situations	Affective education was also combined with the social-interpersonal problem-solving model in Topic 3 below: Teachers asked children to think of the emotions that might be elicited in each of the social situations described in the social-problem vignettes.
3. Social-interpersonal problem solving	Targeted social and prosocial interaction skills: • Initiating a conversation with a friend (dyadic conversation) • Inviting a friend to play • Cooperating with a friend • Expressing an interest in a friend • Asking a friend questions • Sharing experiences, thoughts, and feelings with a friend • Joining a friend's activity • Comforting a friend • Encouraging a friend • Asking for help and suggesting help • Negotiating and persuading a friend	Children were trained on these target skills via three short social vignettes each (see examples in Appendix A, Table A1)

TABLE B2. Main Curriculum Topics for CBE Small-Group Intervention (Bauminger, 2007a)

Curricular topic	Example of targets
1. Instruction in prerequisite concepts for group involvement	• What is a group? • What activities can be held in a group? What are group rules of behavior, such as how to listen and take turns?
2. Affective education focusing on higher processes of emotional understanding	• Identifying each of the complex and basic emotions • Comprehending verbal and nonverbal social-emotional and behavioral markers of complex emotions (i.e., disappointment, jealousy, embarrassment, pride, insult, guilt, and loneliness) • Identifying ways to cope with negative emotions • Grasping rules for displaying emotions • Understanding hidden emotions and mixed emotions
3. Group conversation skills	• (See expansion in Figure B2)
4. Cooperative skills	• Definition of cooperation as mutual planning, mutual choosing, and shared implementation of different social tasks and activities • Focus on the separate prosocial skills necessary for effective cooperation (e.g., compromising, encouraging, comforting, sharing, providing help, asking for forgiveness)
5. Higher-order social-emotional understanding	• Understanding double-message issues (e.g., recognizing cynicism, irony, sarcasm, white lies) • Understanding humor
6. Coping with group stress situations	• Group pressure • Social rejection

TABLE B3. Criteria for Selection of Peer Aide with TYP in CBE Treatments

Criteria	Treatment mode	
	Dyadic	Group
Age	Peer is considered a cotherapist; therefore, based on our clinical experience, the preferable age of the peer aide is fourth grade and up (depending on the target child's CA)	Peers serve as equal partners for social activities; thus they should be equal in age to the target child with HFASD
Sex	Same-sex peer enables role modeling for gender-appropriate social behaviors	At least one of the two peers with TYP should be the same sex as the target child with HFASD
Social competence level	Adequate level of social competence; excluding children with TYP who have attention or behavioral difficulties or other disabilities	
Profile	Age-appropriate emotional maturity according to teacher's or other school professional's recommendation; consistent and reliable; having a natural prosocial inclination, meaning that giving and helping form an intrinsic motivation for the child with TYP	

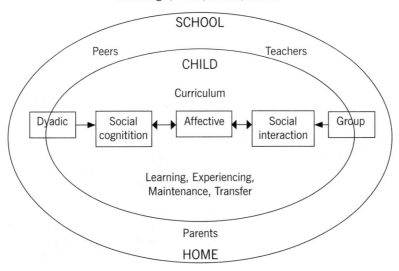

FIGURE B1. CBE intervention model. From Bauminger-Zviely (2011). Reprinted with permission of the author.

Introduction to mediator for the social conversation unit

When we teach social conversation to children with HFASD, we will use cognitive reconstruction through concept clarification and through problem solving in the learning stage, and we will use role play, behavioral rehearsals, feedback, and reinforcement in the experiencing stage; in addition, we will use different games and activities to practice the learned concepts. Learning and experiencing will be interlinked throughout the whole teaching process, following the CBE manual.

A. Introductory lessons: Understanding what social conversation is and why it is important

Concept clarification: Define social conversation:
- Provide written, visually presented, pragmatic rules for social conversation.
  - *Example:* "Social conversation can help me become friends with a peer and to get to know him or her better, and it is based on mutual sharing of my own and his or her experiences, thoughts, and feelings."

Cognitive reconstruction of social conversation:
- Teach how social conversation differs from other forms of conversation such as functional/informational conversation (i.e., aims to provide and obtain information), interview (i.e., a series of questions and replies), and lecture (i.e., a monologue, not dialogue, on a specific topic).
  - *Example:* Give children preprepared recorded and written examples of different short conversational types and ask them to identify the differences between these types. Next, ask children to role-play types of conversation (with teacher, one peer, or group). Audio-record the role playing and then listen together to the conversations and identify their types (using feedback, self-evaluation). Combine other activities, such as a memory game or bingo, that include examples of conversation types that children need to identify. Discuss social importance and significance of social conversation (i.e., to eliminate loneliness, be part of the peer group).
- Discuss differences between dyadic conversation and group conversation (i.e., more complex listening skills in groups vs. more responsibility for promoting dyadic interaction).
- Recognize topics for conversation with friends (i.e., experiences, preferred activities, games, hobbies, TV programs and computer games, pets, suggesting and planning a shared activity, school, movies, sports, music, family, siblings, etc.).
- Discuss ways to recognize whether the topic is of interest to my friends (i.e., they are listening to me; they answer my questions; they ask me about the topic; they share about the topic).

Affective education:
- Discuss the feelings accompanying social conversation (e.g., anxiety).

Problem solving and affective education:
- Use problem-solving technique to discuss ways to cope with feelings related to social conversation.
  - *Example*: Give short vignette about X who feels anxious about starting a conversation and follow the problem-solving process's different stages to find the most appropriate solution to help the child cope with anxiety during social conversation. Practice it through role play.

B. Learning and experiencing conversation stages
- Explore the three stages:

FIGURE B2. Excerpts from a sample CBE curriculum unit for combining both learning and experiencing of social conversation (Bauminger 2002, 2007a, 2007b). Various aspects are applicable to adult–child, peer-dyadic, and peer-group settings.

1. *How do I start a conversation?* Provide children with written pragmatic rules for conversation initiation (e.g., ask my friend something about himself or herself or tell him or her something interesting about myself). Provide written examples of initiating sentences for different topics.
2. *How do I proceed and develop a conversation?* Discuss ways to maintain a conversation (e.g., remember what my friend just said and try to learn more about his or her experience—expansion; tell my friend about something similar that happened to me—sharing).
   - *How do I switch between topics?* Teach why switching topics is important; discuss how to recognize junctions for topic exchanges as a way to expand the conversation length. Provide sentences to be used to change topic (e.g., the new topic should be related somehow to the previous one).
3. *How do I end a conversation?* Provide the children with ending sentences (e.g.,"I have to go to class now, talk to you later").
   - Provide children with the *RELIEVE(F)* summary rule for social conversation: *RE*—reciprocity; *LI*—listening; *EV*—expansion and variation; *E*—eliminate interview or lecture; *F*—focus on what was said.

C. Practicing social conversation (executed simultaneously with section B, while learning the conversational stages)
- Practice each of the conversational stages in the dyad or group or with the teacher. Record children's conversation at each stage. Collect feedback from teacher, peers, and the child him- or herself about whether or not a social conversation developed and what made the conversation social.
- Incorporate different games into the learning and experiencing processes, to make the intervention more entertaining and enjoyable and to enhance variety and interest (especially important due to this topic's difficulty for most children).
   - *Examples*: Create competitions such as who can make a longer conversation. Give points to the first child who suggests initiating sentences. Provide children with a basket of topics that they need to "fish out" and use to start the talking process.

D. Teaching group conversation entry
- Devote a unique lesson to rules for making entry into a group conversation:
   - Stand in close proximity to the group or dyad.
   - Watch and listen to their conversation or activity.
   - Find out the conversation topic.
   - Wait your turn.
   - Make up an initiating sentence.
   - Refer it to a specific child.
   - Look into his or her eyes.
   - Say something relevant to the conversation topic or activity.
   - Talk loud enough.
   - Don't give up after the first try.

Then practice children's entry into an ongoing conversation in the group. Collect feedback about performance from teacher, peers, and the child, using the written pragmatic rules.

E. Homework
- Assign several homework tasks. Discuss homework performance in the dyad or group and collect feedback from teacher, peers, and the child.
   - *Examples*: Make social conversation with parents and siblings at home; make a phone call to the assigned peer in the dyadic training or to one of the children in the small group; listen to social peer conversations during school recess and at home.

FIGURE B2. (*continued*)

Assessment Measures to Evaluate Social Characteristics and Intervention Outcomes for School-Age Children and/or Adolescents with High-Functioning Autism Spectrum Disorders

TABLE C1. Measures of Attachment   252

TABLE C2. Measures of Emotional Expressiveness   253
and Responsiveness

TABLE C3. Measures of Emotional Understanding   255
and Recognition

TABLE C4. Measures of Executive Function   258

TABLE C5. Measures of Friendship   260

TABLE C6. Measures of Social Cognition: Problem Solving   263

TABLE C7. Measures of Social Cognition: ToM   265

TABLE C8. Measures of Social Competence   267
and Social Adjustment

TABLE C9. Measures of Social Interaction   272

TABLE C1. Measures of Attachment

Tool name	Assessment procedure	Tool aim	Reference	Description
Kerns Security Scale (KSS)	Self-report	Assesses children's perceptions (in middle childhood and early adolescence) of security in mother–child and father–child relationships	Kerns, K. A., Klepac, L., & Cole, A. K. (1996). Peer relationships and preadolescents' perceptions of security in the child–mother relationships. *Developmental Psychology, 32,* 457–466.	Perceptions of security in parent–child relationships include availability, reliance, and open communication with the parent. 15-item forced-choice self-report measure providing a continuous security score, with higher scores indicating more secure attachment. A cutoff score of 45 was suggested for secure–insecure differentiation.
Inventory of Parent and Peer Attachment (IPPA)	Adolescent and parent report	Assesses parents' and adolescents' (12–20 years) perception of the positive and negative affective–cognitive qualities of their relationships	Armsden, G. C., & Greenberg, M. T. (1987). The inventory of parent and peer attachment: Individual differences and their relationship to psychological well-being in adolescence. *Journal of Youth and Adolescence, 16,* 427–454.	25-item questionnaire yielding an overall score and three broad relationship qualities: (1) mutual trust, (2) quality of communication, (3) extent of anger and alienation.

TABLE C2. Measures of Emotional Expressiveness and Responsiveness

Tool name	Assessment procedure	Tool aim	Reference	Description
Children's Depression Inventory (CDI)	Self-report	Assesses depressive symptoms in school-age children and adolescents (7–17 years)	Kovacs, M. (1992). *Children's Depression Inventory manual.* North Tonawanda, NY: Multi-Health Systems.	27 groups of three items describing different aspects of child mood, interpersonal problems, feelings of effectiveness, physical symptoms, and self-esteem. Children are instructed to select the statement from each group that best describes them for the last 2 weeks. Scores over 18 are considered to be in the above-average range for boys ages 7–12 years.
Empathy Quotient (EQ-C) and Systemizing Quotient (SQ-C)—Child version (combined)	Parent report	Assesses the extent to which children (4–11 years) empathize and systemize	Auyeung, B, Wheelwright, S., Allison, C., Atkinson, M., Samarawickrema, N., & Baron-Cohen, S. (2009). The children's empathy quotient and systemizing quotient: Sex differences in typical development and in autism spectrum conditions. *Journal of Autism and Developmental Disorders, 39,* 1509–1521.	55 items, with 4 alternatives for each question. Parents indicate how strongly they agree with each statement. Two main scores are derived: (1) child's level of empathic responses (e.g., "My child often doesn't understand why some things upset other people so much"; 27 items), and (2) child's tendency for systemizing ("My child enjoys arranging things precisely; e.g., flowers, books, music collections"; 28 items).

(continued)

253

TABLE C2. (continued)

Tool name	Assessment procedure	Tool aim	Reference	Description
Index of Empathy for Children and Adolescents (IECA)	Self-report	Assesses dispositional affective empathy or emotional responsiveness (in children 6 years and older)	Bryant, B. K. (1982). An index of empathy for children and adolescents. *Child Development,* 53, 413–425.	22 statements of affective reactions: empathy, sympathy, and personal distress (e.g., "It makes me sad to see a boy/girl who can't find anyone to play with"; "I get upset when I see a boy/girl being hurt"). Children can answer either *Yes, like me* or *No, not like me.*
Loneliness Rating Scale	Self-report	Assesses children's feelings of loneliness (elementary school age)	Asher, S. R., Hymel, S., & Renshaw, P. D. (1984). Loneliness in children. *Child Development,* 55, 1456–1464.	24 items rated on a 5-point scale, including 16 items focusing on feelings of loneliness and social dissatisfaction (e.g. "I have nobody to talk to in class"; "I don't have any friends in class") and 8 filler items covering hobbies, interests, and school subject preferences. Children obtain a total loneliness score.
UCLA Loneliness Scale	Self-report	Assesses feelings of loneliness (in adolescence)	Russell, D. (1996). The UCLA loneliness scale (Version 3): Reliability, validity, and factor structure. *Journal of Personality Assessment,* 66, 20–40.	20-item questionnaire (11 items positive, 9 items negative), rated on a 4-point Likert-type scale describing subjective feelings of loneliness without specific reference to loneliness (e.g., "How often do you feel part of a group of friends?" and "How often do you feel that you lack companionship?").

TABLE C3. Measures of Emotional Understanding and Recognition

Tool name	Assessment procedure	Tool aim	Reference	Description
Affective Matching Measure	Picture task	Assesses children's ability to identify emotions from their social context	Adapted from Feshbach, N. (1993). *The Affective Matching Measure.* Unpublished manuscript, University of California at Los Angeles. Bauminger, N., Schorr-Edelsztein, H., & Morash, J. (2005). Social information processing and emotional understanding in children with learning disabilities. *Journal of Learning Disabilities, 38,* 45–61.	12 different pictures depicting social scenarios of basic emotions (1 picture each of happiness, fear, anger, and sadness) and complex emotions (2 pictures each of loneliness, pride, embarrassment, and guilt), in which one of the depicted figures is without facial expression. Social context should provide the clues for participants' identification of the appropriate emotion.
Cambridge Mindreading Face-Voice Battery—Children Version (CAM-C)	Video and audio task	Assesses recognition of complex emotions and mental states in social contexts (in school-age children)	Golan, O., & Baron-Cohen, S. (2006). The Cambridge Mindreading Face-Voice Battery for Children (CAM-C): Testing basic and complex emotion recognition in children with and without autism spectrum conditions. *Journal of Autism and Developmental Disorders, 36,* 169–183.	20 emotions with two tasks: emotion recognition in the face and emotion recognition in the voice. Children are asked to choose the word that best describes how the person is feeling.

(continued)

TABLE C3. (*continued*)

Tool name	Assessment procedure	Tool aim	Reference	Description
Child and Adolescent Social Perception Measure (CASP)	Standardized, individually administered, videotaped social scenes	Assesses social perception and emotional recognition (in children 6–15 years)	Magill-Evans, J., Koning, C., Cameron-Sadava, A., & Manyk, K. (1995). The child and adolescent social perception measure. *Journal of Nonverbal Behavior, 19,* 151–169.	10 unrelated videotaped scenes depicting social interactions, which are audio filtered so that meaning must be derived from nonverbal and situational cues. Children are asked to describe what happened in the sequence, how each character felt, and how they knew the character felt that way. Yields an emotion score (based on identification of feelings) and a nonverbal cues score (based on ability to correctly interpret facial, body, or voice cues).
Diagnostic Analysis of Non-Verbal Accuracy–2, Adult Facial Expressions (DANVA-2-AF) and Child Facial Expressions (DANVA 2-CF)	Picture task	Assesses facial expression recognition (both the DANVA-2-AF and the DANVA 2-CF have acceptable internal consistency for school-age children, but norms are available for ages 3–99 years)	Nowicki, S., & Carton, J. (1993). The measurement of emotional intensity from facial expressions. *Journal of Social Psychology, 133,* 749–750.	DANVA-2-AF contains 24 photographs of an equal number of men and women making happy, sad, angry, and fearful facial expressions of both low and high intensity. DANVA 2-CF is similar, but pictures depict children ages 6–12. Participants are asked to select which one of the four emotional labels corresponds to the photo.

Measure	Type	Construct	Description	Reference
Emotion Inventory	Interview with the child	Assesses emotional knowledge via definitions and emotional experiences via personal accounts (in middle childhood and early adolescence)	Children are given a list of 5 simple emotions (happy, sad, angry, afraid, and disgusted), 3 complex emotions (curious, disappointed, and surprised), 4 complex self-conscious emotions (proud, embarrassed, guilty, and ashamed), as well as 2 nonemotions (tired and sick) presented in random order. They are asked to define each and then tell the experimenter about a time at which they felt that way.	Adapted from Seidner, L. B., Stipek, D., & Feshbach, N. (1988). A developmental analysis of elementary school-aged children's concepts of pride and embarrassment. *Child Development, 59,* 367–377. Losh, M., & Capps, L. (2003). Narrative ability in high functioning children with autism or Asperger's syndrome. *Journal of Autism and Developmental Disorders, 33,* 239–251.
Pictures of Facial Affect System	Picture task	Assesses recognition of facial expressions of basic emotions (extensively used with various ages, including children and adolescents)	Stimulus consists of six monochrome photographs of adult Caucasian male and female faces arranged on a card, each presenting one of six basic emotions: happiness, sadness, fear, anger, surprise, and disgust. The experimenter reads the name of an emotion aloud, and participants are asked to point to the appropriate face on the card.	Ekman, P., & Friesen, W. V. (1976). *Pictures of facial affect.* Palo Alto, CA: Consulting Psychologists Press.
Reading the Mind in Films—Child Version (RMF-C)	Video task	Assesses recognition of complex emotions in social contexts (in middle childhood)	22 scenes involving social-emotional interactions among 1–4 classmates and the expression of complex emotions (relieved, guilty, lonely). Children are asked to identify the emotion expressed in the video from a choice of four visually presented emotions.	Golan, O., Golan-Cohen, S., & Golan, Y. (2008). The "Reading the Mind in Films" Task [Child Version]: Complex emotion and mental state recognition in children with and without autism spectrum conditions. *Journal of Autism and Developmental Disorders, 38,* 1534–1541.

TABLE C4. Measures of Executive Function

Tool name	Assessment procedure	Tool aim	Reference	Description
Behavior Rating Inventory of Executive Function (BRIEF)	Teacher–parent questionnaire	Assesses impairment of executive function (ages 5–18 years)	Gioia, G. A., Isquith, P. K., Guy, S. C., & Kenworthy, L. (2000). *Behavior Rating Inventory of Executive Functioning: Professional manual.* Lutz, FL: Psychological Assessment Resources.	Eight subscales (Inhibit, Shift, Emotional Control, Initiate, Working Memory, Plan/Organize, Organization of Materials, and Monitor) that can be combined to create two broad indexes: (1) Behavior Regulation (inhibition, shifting, emotional control) and (2) Metacognition (initiations, working memory, planning/organization of material). Also provides global executive composite score (GEC).
Delis Kaplan Executive Function System (D-KEFS)	Test battery	Assesses vital executive functions in both the verbal and spatial modalities (ages 8–89 years)	Delis, D. C., Kaplan, E., & Kramer, J. H. (2001). *D-KEFS: Examiners manual.* San Antonio, TX: Psychological Corporation.	Nine subtests that can stand alone (e.g., Verbal and Design Fluency, Color–Word Interference, Sorting, Visual–Motor, and Twenty Questions to assess deduction and logical thinking), which tap executive functions such as flexibility of thinking, inhibition, problem solving, planning, impulse control, concept formation, abstract thinking, and creativity.
Junior Hayling Test	Cloze task	Assesses response initiation and inhibition (ages 8–17 years)	Shallice, T, Marzocchi, G. M, Coser, S., Savio, M. D., Meuter, F. R., & Rumiati, R. I. (2002). Executive function profile of children with attention deficit hyperactivity disorder. *Developmental Neuropsychology, 21,* 43–71.	Two sets of 15 sentences each with the last word missing. For the first set, the examiner reads each sentence aloud, and participants are simply asked to complete the sentences. For the second set, participants are asked to complete each sentence with an incorrect ending word.

| Tower of Hanoi | Performance task | Assesses executive functioning specifically to detect deficits in planning and problem solving (in school-age children) | Borys, S. V., Spitz, H. H., & Dorans, B. A. (1982). Tower of Hanoi performance of retarded young adults and nonretarded children as a function of solution length and goal state. *Journal of Experimental Child Psychology, 33*, 87–110. | Participants are presented with a tower of disks in consecutive sizes on one of three pegs. The goal is to move the tower from one peg to another designated peg. The rules are that only one disk can be moved at a time and that placing a larger disk over a smaller one is not permitted. |
| Wisconsin Card Sorting Test (WCST) | Task and computer version | Assesses perseveration and abstract reasoning measures of executive function (in children and adolescents) | Heaton, R. K., Chelune, G. J., Talley, J. L., Kay, G. G., & Curtiss, G. (1993). *Wisconsin Card Sorting Test manual: Revised and expanded.* Odessa, FL: Psychological Assessment Resources. | Participants are asked to sort four stimulus cards that vary along three dimensions (color, shape, and number). Participants are given 128 cards that vary along the same dimensions and are asked to match each card in the deck with one of the four stimulus cards. |

TABLE C5. Measures of Friendship

Tool name	Assessment procedure	Tool aim	Reference	Description
Dyadic Relationships Q-Set (DRQ)	Q-set Observation	Assesses the quality of observed dyadic peer interactions and friendships (at various ages from preschool up to early adolescence)	Park, K. A., & Waters, E. (1989). Security of attachment and preschool friendships. *Child Development, 60,* 1076–1081.	The observer of the dyad's interaction sorts the 55 DRQ items into a forced-choice format from the least characteristic behavior (pile 1) to the most characteristic behavior (pile 7) for each dyad. The sorted items then provide seven dyadic relationship-quality dimensions: positive social orientation, cohesiveness, harmony, coordinated play, responsiveness, control, and self-disclosure.
Early Childhood Friendship Survey	Survey for parents or professionals such as teachers	Assesses nature, development, and maintenance of friendship in children with TYP or atypical development (originally designed for preschoolers but was adapted for school age)	Buysse, V. (1991). *Early Childhood Friendship Survey for Parents and Caregivers.* Chapel Hill, NC: University of North Carolina, Frank Porter Graham Child Development Center.	19 closed- and open-ended questions addressing the child's: (1) mutual friendships (e.g. "Does your child currently have one friend who, in turn, thinks of your child as a friend?" Yes/No); (2) unilateral friendships in which the target child initiates interactions with a peer who does not reciprocate; (3) unilateral friendships in which the target child does not reciprocate toward a peer who initiates.

Friendship Observation Scale (FOS)	Observation of friendship interaction	Assesses friendship manifestations in the target child during interaction with a friend (in preadolescent)	Baumiger, N., Rogers, S. J., Aviezer, A., & Solomon, M. (2005). *The Friendship Observation Scale (FOS)*. Unpublished manual, Bar Ilan University, Israel, and University of California, Davis.	Includes minute-by-minute and global evaluations of friendship manifestations in the target child during an interaction with a friend, including behaviors, verbalizations, and affects identified as indicators of friendship. Coding consists of two main scales: (1) Positive Social Interaction comprises 21 indices in seven main categories: goal-directed behavior; sharing behaviors; prosocial behavior; conversation; nonverbal interaction; affect; and play (parallel, social, and coordinated play, unoccupied). (2) Global Evaluation Scale includes child's role as leader or follower, conversational skills and flow, shared fun, and affective closeness.
Friendship Nominations and Peer Acceptance	Sociometric evaluation—self-report by class members	Assesses friendship reciprocity and social network–peer acceptance scores (in school-age children)	Adapted from Cairns, R. B., & Cairns, B. D. (1994). *Social networks and the function of friendships*. New York: Cambridge University Press. Chamberlain, B., Kasari, C., & Rotheram-Fuller, E. (2007). Involvement or isolation?: The social networks of children with autism in regular classrooms. *Journal of Autism and Developmental Disorders, 37,* 230–242.	For reciprocal friendship nomination: The child is instructed to circle the names of three closest friends in the class ("Top 3") and to put a star by the name of one "best friend" in the classroom. For peer acceptance: Children are instructed to sort the classmates into two piles: Those with whom they like to "hang out" and those with whom they do not.

(continued)

TABLE C5. (*continued*)

Tool name	Assessment procedure	Tool aim	Reference	Description
Friendship Qualities Scale (FQS)	Self-report	Assesses perceived qualities of friendship with a best friend (in children and adolescents)	Bukowski, W. M., Hoza, B., & Boivin, M. (1994). Measuring friendship quality during pre and early adolescence: The development and psychometric properties of the Friendship Qualities Scale. *Journal of Social and Personal Relationships, 11,* 471–484.	23 items assessing five friendship quality dimensions—companionship, conflict, help, security, and closeness—rated on a 5-point Likert-type scale. Prior to completing the questionnaire, children are asked to identify their best friend.
Social Support Scale for Children (SSSC)	Self-report	Assesses children's perceived level of support from significant others	Harter, S. (1985). *Manual for the Social Support Scale for Children.* Denver, CO: University of Denver.	24 items yielding four subscales assessing the perceived support and positive regard that a child gets from parents, teachers, classmates, and close friends. Children are asked to rate the extent to which they experience support from their peers, friends, teachers, and parents on a 4-point Likert-type scale (*Never true* to *Always true*).

TABLE C6. Measures of Social Cognition: Problem Solving

Tool name	Assessment procedure	Tool aim	Reference	Description
Problem-Solving Measure (PSM)	Paper–pencil task	Assesses children's social understanding of social scenarios through problem-solving skills	Lochman, J. E., & Lampron, L. B. (1986). Situational social problem-solving skills and self-esteem of aggressive and nonaggressive boys. *Journal of Abnormal Psychology, 14,* 605–661.	Nine hypothetical social problems (e.g., initiating a conversation and play with a friend, coping with teasing), each containing a beginning and an end. Children are asked to compose possible solutions to the given problem.
Test of Problem Solving–3 (TOPS-3)	Photograph task	Assesses reasoning, problem solving, and critical thinking, as well as several important executive function capabilities such as impulse control and inhibition (ages 6–11 years)	Bowers, L., Huisingh, R., & LoGiudice, C. (2005). *Test of problem solving 3 Elementary.* East Moline, IL: Linguisystems.	14 stimulus pictures depicting various scenarios that entail social problems (e.g., a new child in class wants to make friends). Children are asked to identify the overall gist of a social situation (planning); to generate feasible solutions to social problems (set maintenance, organized search, and cognitive flexibility); and to select between them (impulse control, inhibition of prepotent but irrelevant responses). Scoring penalizes for misinterpreting questions; for providing vague, inadequate, perseverative, irrelevant, concrete, or tangential responses; for failing to provide context for responses; and for the inability to generate responses.

(continued)

TABLE C6. (continued)

Tool name	Assessment procedure	Tool aim	Reference	Description
Video vignettes	Video task	Assesses social information and attribution processing (in school-age children)	Dodge, K. A., Petit, G. S., Bates, J. E., & Valente, E. (1995). Social information-processing patterns partially mediate the effect of early physical abuse on later conduct problems. *Journal of Abnormal Psychology, 104,* 632–643.	24 videotaped vignettes (themes such as peer group entry, friendship initiation, peer rebuff, and object acquisition) followed by questions designed to elicit attributions regarding the "peer" behavior witnessed in the vignette, as well as information-processing patterns related to attributions.
Why Kids Do Things (WKDT)	Interview	Assesses social information and attribution processing (in school-age children)	Crick, N. R., & Dodge, K. A. (1994). A review and reformulation of social information-processing mechanisms in children's social adjustment. *Psychological Bulletin, 115,* 74–101.	10 vignettes on various provocative social situations. Children are asked to describe reasons for the provocation, to determine whether characters were "trying to be mean" or "not trying to be mean," and to rate feelings of distress if the story were to happen to them.

TABLE C7. Measures of Social Cognition: ToM

Tool name	Assessment procedure	Tool aim	Reference	Description
Faux Pas Stories	Story task	Assesses advanced perspective-taking skills (ages 6–11 years)	Baron-Cohen, S., O'Riordan, M., Stone, V., Jones, R., & Plaisted, K. (1999). A new test of social sensitivity: Detection of faux pas in normal children and children with Asperger syndrome. *Journal of Autism and Development Disorders*, 29, 407–418.	10 short narrative stories, each containing a faux pas (i.e., a speaker says something without considering whether the listener might not want to hear or know it, which typically has negative consequences that the speaker never intended). Children are told that in several stories, someone will say something that he or she was not supposed to say. Four questions follow each story. The first two involve detecting the faux pas; the third is a control question designed to see whether children understand a critical element of the story; and the fourth is a probe to see whether children understand why the faux pas was committed.
John and Mary Ice-Cream Van Story	Story task	Assesses children's second-order false belief (ToM)	Adapted from Perner, J., & Wimmer, H. (1985). "John thinks that Mary thinks that . . .": Attribution of second-order beliefs by 5- to 10-year-old children. *Journal of Experimental Child Psychology*, 39, 437–471.	After hearing a story about John and Mary, children are asked: (1) a belief question—to predict the thoughts of one child based on the thoughts of the other (i.e., what Mary believes about John's whereabouts) and (2) to provide a justification (i.e., answer "why?").
			Baron-Cohen, S. (1989). The autistic child's theory of mind: A case of specific developmental delay. *Journal of Child Psychology and Psychiatry*, 30, 285–297.	

(continued)

265

TABLE C7. (continued)

Tool name	Assessment procedure	Tool aim	Reference	Description
Reading Mind in the Eyes Test—Child Revised Version	Picture task	Assesses ability to attribute a mental state to another person by viewing only the person's eyes (ages 8–14 years)	Baron-Cohen, S., Wheelwright, S., Scahill, V., Lawson, J., & Spong, A. (2001). Are intuitive physics and intuitive psychology independent?: A test with children with Asperger syndrome. *Journal of Developmental and Learning Disorders, 5,* 47–78.	28 pictures of eyes. For each, participants are instructed to choose which one of four words best describes what the person in the picture is thinking or feeling (e.g., a choice between playful, comforting, irritated, and bored) and to identify person's sex.
Real and Deceptive Emotion Task	Story task	Assesses advanced ToM identification of real and deceptive emotions (ages 6–8 years)	Harris, P. L., Donnel, Y. K., Guz, G. R., & Pitt-Watson, R. (1986). Children's understanding of the distinction between real and apparent emotion. *Child Development, 57,* 895–909.	10 short narratives, each with a vignette describing why a hypothetical character, Terry, would feel one way inside but show a facial emotion that was different. Participants listen to the stories and judge how Terry looks on her or his face and how he or she feels inside. Instructions stress that Terry's face might look one way but he or she may feel a different way inside. Within each narrative, story valence is either positive or negative.
Strange story measure	Story task	Assesses understanding of another person's motivation to make utterances that are not literally true (ages 8–45 years)	Happé, F. G. E. (1994). An advanced test of theory of mind: Understanding of story characters' thoughts and feelings by able autistic, mentally handicapped, and normal children and adults. *Journal of Autism and Developmental Disorders, 24,* 129–154.	24 short vignettes, each including two sets of questions: comprehension questions ("Was it true what X said?") and justification questions ("Why did X say that?"). 12 stories include various social topics and relate to mental states (e.g., pretend, joke, lie, white lie, persuade, double bluff, hiding emotions); 6 stories are physical, not involving mental states; and 4 stories are examples, 2 of each story type (mental states and physical).

TABLE C8. Measures of Social Competence and Social Adjustment

Tool name	Assessment procedure	Tool aim	Reference	Description
Autism Diagnostic Interview—Revised (ADI-R)	Semistructured parent interview	Diagnoses ASD based on the DSM-IV (1994) and the ICD-10 (World Health Organization, 1993) (from age 2+ across the lifespan)	Lord, C., Rutter, M., & Le Couteur, A. (1994). Autism Diagnostic Interview—Revised: A revised version of a diagnostic interview for caregivers of individuals with possible pervasive developmental disorders. *Journal of Autism and Developmental Disorders, 24,* 659–685.	A diagnostic interview focusing on developmental history and current presentation of core symptoms of ASD. Provides scores in the areas of reciprocal social interaction, language/communication, and restricted, repetitive, and stereotyped patterns of behavior, as well as overall score indicating diagnosis of autism.
Autism Diagnostic Observation Schedule (ADOS)	Standardized behavioral observation and coding	Assesses and diagnoses autism and ASD across ages, developmental levels, and language skills	Lord, C., Risi, S., Lambrecht, L., Cook, E. H., Leventhal, B. L., DiLavore, P. C., et al. (2000). The Autism Diagnostic Observational Schedule-Generic: A standard measure of social and communication deficits associated with the spectrum of autism. *Journal of Autism and Developmental Disorders, 30,* 205–223.	Semistructured observational assessment focusing on core symptoms of ASD, including the areas of communication, reciprocal social interaction, imagination/creativity, and stereotyped behaviors and restricted interests. Provides a diagnosis based on communicational activity, tasks, and conversation with a clinician.

(continued)

TABLE C8. (continued)

Tool name	Assessment procedure	Tool aim	Reference	Description
Behavior Assessment System for Children (BASC-2 PRS)	Parent and teacher questionnaire and a student observation system	Assesses emotional and behavioral problems in addition to adaptive and social skills (for three age spans: 2–5, 6–11, and 12–21 years)	Reynolds, C. R., & Kamphaus, R. W. (2004). *Behavior assessment system for children* (2nd ed.). Circle Pines, MN: American Guidance Service.	System comprising teacher and parent behavior-rating scales (PRS); a self-reported personality inventory; a structured developmental history form (SRP); and a method for observing student behaviors. The PRS lists varied numbers of items for different age groups (preschooler, 134 items; child, 160 items; adolescent, 150 items). The parent or teacher rates the occurrence of each item (behavior) on a 4-point scale ranging from *Never* to *Almost always*. Altogether, it provides results for eight "clinical" scales (i.e., Hyperactivity, Aggression, Anxiety, Depression, Somatization, Atypicality, Withdrawal, and Attention Problems) and for four "adaptive" scales (i.e., Adaptability, Social Skills, Activities of Daily Living, and Functional Communication). Also provides scores for four composite domains (i.e., Externalizing Problems, Internalizing Problems, Adaptive Skills, and the Behavioral Symptoms Index).

Measure	Informant	Purpose	Reference	Description
Child Behavior Checklist (CBCL)	Parent, teacher, or self-report	Assesses externalizing and internalizing behaviors and psychiatric conditions (ages 6–18 years)	Achenbach, T. M., & Rescorla, L. A. (2001). *Manual for the ASEBA school-age forms and profiles*. Burlington: University of Vermont, Research Center for Children, Youth, and Families.	113 items covering diverse behavioral and emotional problems in children and adolescents, rated along three response options. Yields eight subdomains: Withdrawn, Somatic Complaints, Anxious/Depression, Aggression, Social Problems, Thought Problems, Attention Problems, Delinquency, and Aggressive Behavior. These subscales further yield two broad behavior-problem scales: the Internalizing scale and Externalizing scale.
Self-Perception Profile for Children (SPPC)	Self-report	Assesses self-perceptions (in middle childhood and early adolescence)	Harter, S. (1985). *Manual of the Self-Perception Profile for Children*. Denver, CO: University of Denver.	36 items tapping children's domain-specific judgments of their competence, as well as a global perception of their worth as a person or self-esteem. Contains six separate subscales consisting of five specific domains: (1) Scholastic Competence, (2) Social Acceptance, (3) Athletic Competence, (4) Physical Appearance, and (5) Behavioral Conduct, as well as a general domain of Global Self-Worth.
Social Communication Questionnaire (SCQ) (formerly known as the Autism Screening Questionnaire—ASQ)	Parent or other primary caregiver report	Diagnoses autism (from MA of 2+ years across the lifespan)	Rutter, M., Bailey, A., & Lord, C. (2003). *Social Communication Questionnaire*. Los Angeles: Western Psychological Services.	Brief screening instrument designed to identify ASD characteristics (e.g., communication skills, social functioning, and repetitive behaviors) in individuals across the lifespan. Based on the ADI-R (see above).

(*continued*)

TABLE C8. (continued)

Tool name	Assessment procedure	Tool aim	Reference	Description
Social Competence Inventory (SCI)	Parent–teacher questionnaire	Assesses social functioning (ages 7–10 years)	Rydell, A. M., Hagekull, B., & Bohlin, G. (1997). Measurement of two social competence aspects in middle childhood. *Developmental Psychology, 33*, 824–833.	25 items measuring behavioral aspects of social competence, scored on a 5-point scale comprising two subscales: the Prosocial Orientation (PO) index, which assesses children's ability to behave appropriately in normal and problematic social situations with peers, and the Social Initiative (SI) index, which captures children's capacity to initiate social interactions.
Social Responsiveness Scale (SRS)	Parent–teacher questionnaire	Assesses social impairments associated with autism (ages 4–18 years)	Constantino, J. N., & Gruber, C. P. (2005). *Social Responsiveness Scale (SRS).* Los Angeles: Western Psychological Services.	65 items rated on a 4-point scale from *Not true* to *Almost always true* based on child's behavior over the past 6 months. Provides an overall score and five treatment subscales that can be used for program planning: Social Awareness, Social Cognition, Social Communication, Social Motivation, and Autistic Mannerisms.
Social Skills Rating Scale (SSRS)	Teacher, parent, and student questionnaires	Assesses social behaviors (ages 3–18 years).	Gresham, F. M., & Elliott, S. N. (1990). *Social skills rating system.* Circle Pines, MN: American Guidance Service	An estimation of the frequency with which a variety of specific social skills are displayed (e.g. interest in others, initiating conversations) on three scales: (1) Social Skills Scale (cooperation, assertion, responsibility, empathy, and self-control), (2) Problem Behaviors Scale (externalizing problems, internalizing problems, and hyperactivity), and (3) Academic Competence Scale.

Teacher Perception Measure	Teacher report	Assesses teachers' perceptions of students' social skills and classroom conduct (ages 6–11 years)	Kasari, C., Locke, J., Gulsrud, A., & Rotheram-Fuller, E. (2011). Social networks and friendships at school: Comparing children with and without ASD. *Journal of Autism and Developmental Disorders, 41*, 533–544.	26 items regarding teachers' perceptions of students' social skills or strengths (e.g., adaptability to the school classroom and environment, quality of interactions with peers) and of students' classroom conduct or problems (e.g., disruptive, impulsive, withdrawn).
Vineland Adaptive Behavior Scale (VABS)	Parent–professional interview/survey	Assesses adaptive capabilities (birth to adulthood)	Sparrow, S., Balla, D. A., & Cicchetti, D. V. (1984). *Vineland Adaptive Behavior Scales.* Circle Pines, MN: American Guidance Services. Sparrow, S., Cicchetti, D., & Balla, D. (2005). *Vineland Adaptive Behavior Scales* (2nd ed.). Minneapolis, MN: Pearson Assessment.	Semistructured standardized interview (or survey version) that provides a general assessment of adaptive behavior (composite score) and four main domain scores: Communication, Daily Living Skills, Socialization, and Motor Skills. Also includes questions to assess abnormal maladaptive behavior.
Walker–McConnell Scale of Social Competence and School Adjustment (WMS)	Teacher questionnaire	Assesses social competence and school adjustment (children in grades 7–12)	Walker, H. M., & McConnell, S. R. (1995). *The Walker–McConnell Scale of Social Competence and School Adjustment: Elementary version.* San Diego, CA: Singular.	43 items comprising three subscales (Teacher-Preferred Social Behavior, Peer-Preferred Social Behavior, School Adjustment Behavior) and a total scale score. Social competence is defined as the development of effective interpersonal relationships with peers and adults, and school adjustment is defined as satisfactorily meeting the behavioral and academic standards of teachers within instructional settings.

TABLE C9. Measures of Social Interaction

Tool name	Assessment procedure	Tool aim	Reference	Description
Peer Interaction Observation Schedule (PIOS)	Observation scale	Assesses the type, duration, and frequency of the interaction behaviors between a focal student and peers (in mainstreamed secondary schools)	Adapted from Pellegrini, A. D., & Bartini, M. (2000). A longitudinal study of bullying, victimization, and peer affiliation during the transition from primary to middle school. *American Educational Research Journal, 37,* 699–725. Humphrey, N., & Symes, W. (2011). Peer interaction patterns among adolescents with autistic spectrum disorders (ASDs) in mainstream school settings. *Autism, 15,* 397–415.	22 observable behavior codes: 15 referring to behaviors exhibited by the focal student (e.g., social initiation, cooperative interaction, games) and 7 referring to peers' behaviors (e.g., acceptance of social initiation by focal student; reactive aggression).
Playground Observation of Peer Engagement (POPE)	Observation scale	Assesses engagement with peers on playground and frequency of initiations and responses (ages 6–11, grades 1–5)	Kasari, C., Rotheram-Fuller, & Locke. J., (2005). *The development of the Playground Observation of Peer Engagement (POPE) measure.* Unpublished manuscript, University of California, Los Angeles.	Taps child's engagement behaviors with peers on the playground (e.g., solitary, proximately, parallel, parallel-aware, involved in games with rules, and jointly engaged with peers) and initiations toward other children. Codes successful initiations as well as peer responses with a nonverbal gesture or verbal language. Also codes failed initiation attempts.

Pragmatic Rating Scale (PRS) Coding	Observation scale	Assesses pragmatic behaviors during conversation (originally developed for parents; used with youth 12–18 years)	Landa, R., Piven, J., Wzorek, M., Gayle, J., Chase, G., & Folstein, S. (1992). Social language use in parents of autistic individuals. *Psychological Medicine, 22,* 245–254.	30 items identifying pragmatic behaviors reflecting abnormalities reported to be typical of autism, categorized into three major groupings: (1) pragmatic behaviors, which focus primarily on topic management and reciprocity (e.g., items such as "overly talkative," "unresponsive," and "vague"); (2) speech and prosodic behaviors, which concern the form of speaker production (e.g., "indistinct speech," "intonation is unusual," and "unusual rhythm"); and (3) paralinguistic behaviors, which include the physical behaviors that accompany speech (e.g., "gestures," "facial expression," "physical distance," and "gaze").
Social Interaction Observation Scale	Observation scale	Assesses children's spontaneous initiations and responses during peer interactions (7–18 years)	Bauminger, N. (2002). The facilitation of social-emotional understanding and social interaction in high-functioning children with autism: Intervention outcomes. *Journal of Autism and Developmental Disorders, 32,* 283–298. Bauminger, N., Shulman, C., & Agam, G. (2003). Peer interaction and loneliness in high-functioning children with autism. *Journal of Autism and Developmental Disorders, 33,* 489–507.	Minute-by-minute observation coding scale assessing children's interactive behaviors with their peers, during semistructured (lunch time) or nonstructured (school recess) social interaction, according to three main categories: (1) positive interaction (e.g., eye contact, smile); (2) low-level interaction (e.g., looking, close proximity); and (3) negative social interaction (e.g., physical/verbal aggression, avoidance).

(continued)

TABLE C9. (continued)

Tool name	Assessment procedure	Tool aim	Reference	Description
Quality of Play Questionnaire (QPQ)	Parent–adolescent questionnaire	Assesses the frequency of adolescents' get-togethers with peers and the level of conflict during these get-togethers	Frankel, F., Gorospe, C., Chang, Y., & Catherine, S. (2011). Mothers' reports of play dates and observation of school playground behavior of children having high-functioning autism spectrum disorders. *Journal of Child Psychology and Psychiatry, 52*, 571–579.	12-item conflict scale rating peer conflict (e.g., "criticized or teased each other") and estimation of the number of invited and hosted get-togethers the adolescent has had over the previous month.

274

References

Achenbach, T. M., & Rescorla, L. A. (2001). *Manual for the ASEBA school-age forms and profiles*. Burlington, VT: University of Vermont, Research Center for Children, Youth, and Families.

Adachi, T., Koeda, T., Hirabayashi, S., Maeoka, Y., Shiota, M., Wright, E. C., et al. (2004). The metaphor and sarcasm scenario test: A new instrument to help differentiate high functioning pervasive developmental disorder from attention deficit/hyperactivity disorder. *Brain and Development, 26,* 301–306.

Adamson, L. B., Deckner, D. F., & Bakeman, R. (2010). Early interests and joint engagement in typical development, autism, and Down syndrome. *Journal of Autism and Developmental Disorders, 40,* 665–676.

Ainsworth, M. D. S. (1989). Attachments beyond infancy. *American Psychologist, 44,* 709–716.

Ainsworth, M. D. S., Blehar, M. C., Waters, E., & Wall, S. (1978). *Patterns of attachment: A psychological study of the Strange Situation.* Hillsdale, NJ: Erlbaum.

Alberto, P. A., Frederick, L., Hughes, M., McIntosh, L., & Cihak, D. (2007). Components of visual literacy: Teaching logos. *Focus on Autism and Other Developmental Disabilities, 22,* 234–243.

Alderson-Day, B., & McGonigle-Chalmers, M. (2011). Is it a bird? Is it a plane?: Category use in problem-solving in children with autism spectrum disorders. *Journal of Autism and Developmental Disorders, 41,* 555–565.

Altemeier, L., Jones, J., Abbott, R., & Berninger, V. (2006). Executive factors in becoming writing-readers and reading-writers: Note-taking and report writing in third and fifth graders. *Developmental Neuropsychology, 29,* 161–173.

American Psychiatric Association. (1994). *Diagnostic and statistical manual of mental disorders* (4th ed.). Washington, DC: Author.

American Psychiatric Association. (2000). *Diagnostic and statistical manual of mental disorders* (4th ed., text rev.). Washington, DC: Author.

American Psychiatric Association. (2013). *Diagnostic and statistical manual of mental disorders* (5th ed.). Washington, DC: Author.

Ames, C., & Fletcher-Watson, S. (2010). A review of methods in the study of attention in autism. *Developmental Review, 30,* 2–73.

Anderson, D., Lord, C., Risi, S., DiLavore, P., Shulman, C., Thurm, A., et al. (2007). Patterns of growth in verbal abilities among children with autism spectrum disorder. *Journal of Consulting and Clinical Psychology, 75,* 594–604

Anderson, S., & Morris, J. (2006). Cognitive behaviour therapy for people with Asperger syndrome. *Behavioural and Cognitive Psychotherapy, 34,* 293–303.

Asaro, K., & Saddler, B. (2009). Effects of planning instruction on a young writer with Asperger syndrome. *Intervention in School and Clinic, 44,* 268–275.

Asaro-Saddler, K., & Saddler, B. (2010). Planning instruction and self-regulation training: Effects on writers with autism spectrum disorders. *Council for Exceptional Children, 77,* 107–124.

Asberg, J., & Sandberg, A. D. (2010). Discourse comprehension intervention for high-functioning students with autism spectrum disorders: Preliminary findings from a school-based study. *Journal of Research in Special Educational Needs, 10,* 91–98.

Asperger, H. (1991). Autistic psychopathy in childhood. In U. Frith (Trans., & Annot.), *Autism and Asperger syndrome* (pp. 37–92). Cambridge, UK: Cambridge University Press. (Original work published 1944)

Astington, J. W. (2003). Sometimes necessary, never sufficient: False belief and social competence. In B. Repacholi & V. Slaughter (Eds.), *Individual differences in theory of mind: Implications for typical and atypical development* (Macquarie Monographs in Cognitive Science, pp. 13–38). New York: Psychology Press.

Attwood, T. (2003). Frameworks for behavioral interventions. *Child and Adolescent Psychiatric Clinics, 12,* 65–86.

Attwood, T. (2004). Cognitive behaviour therapy for children and adults with Asperger's syndrome. *Behaviour Change, 21,* 147–161.

Bacon, A. L., Fein, D., Morris, R., Waterhouse, L., & Allen, D. (1998). The responses of autistic children to the distress of others. *Journal of Autism and Developmental Disorders, 28,* 129–142.

Baker, K., Montgomery, A., & Abramson, R. (2010). Brief report: Perception and lateralization of spoken emotion by youths with high-functioning forms of autism. *Journal of Autism and Developmental Disorders, 40,* 123–129.

Baker-Ward, L., Hess, T. M., & Flannagan, D. A. (1990). The effects of involvement on children's memory for events. *Cognitive Development, 5,* 55–69.

Baldwin, D. A. (1995). Understanding the link between joint attention and language. In C. Moore & P. J. Dunham (Eds.), *Joint attention: Its origins and role in development* (pp. 131–158). Hillsdale, NJ: Erlbaum.

Barbaro, J., & Dissanayake, C. (2007). A comparative study of the use and understanding of self-presentational display rules in children with high-functioning autism and Asperger's disorder. *Journal of Autism and Developmental Disorders, 37,* 1235–1246.

Barnhill, G., Hagiwara, T., Smith Myles, B., & Simpson, R. L. (2000). Asperger syndrome: A study of the cognitive profiles of 37 children and adolescents. *Focus on Autism and Other Developmental Disabilities, 15,* 146–153.

Barnhill, G. P., & Smith Myles, B. (2001). Attributional style and depression in adolescents with Asperger syndrome. *Journal of Positive Behavior Interventions, 3,* 175–182.

Baron-Cohen, S. (2000). Theory of mind and autism: A fifteen-year review. In S. Baron-Cohen, H. H. Tager-Flusberg, & D. J. Cohen (Eds.), *Understanding other minds: Perspectives from developmental cognitive neuroscience* (pp. 3–20). Oxford, UK: Oxford University Press.

Baron-Cohen, S., Leslie, A. M., & Frith, U. (1985). Does the autistic child have a "theory of mind"? *Cognition, 21,* 37–46.

Baron-Cohen, S., & Wheelwright, S. (2003). The Friendship Questionnaire: An investigation of adults with Asperger syndrome or high-functioning autism, and normal sex differences. *Journal of Autism and Developmental Disorders, 33,* 509–517.

Baron-Cohen, S., & Wheelwright, S. (2004). The Empathy Quotient: An investigation of adults with Asperger syndrome or high-functioning autism, and normal sex differences. *Journal of Autism and Developmental Disorders, 34,* 163–175.

Barry, T. D., Grofer-Klinger, L., Lee, J. M., Palardy, N., Gilmore, T., & Douglas-Bodin, S. D. (2003). Examining the effectiveness of an outpatient clinic-based social skills group for high-functioning children with autism. *Journal of Autism and Developmental Disorders, 33*, 685–701.

Basil, C., & Reyes, S. (2003). Acquisition of literacy skills by children with severe disability. *Child Language Teaching and Therapy, 19*, 27–48.

Bass, J. D., & Mulick, J. A. (2007). Social play skill enhancement of children with autism using peers and siblings as therapists. *Psychology in the Schools, 44*, 727–735.

Basso, M. R., Schefft, B. K., Ris, M. D., & Dember, W. N. (1996). Mood and global–local visual processing. *Journal of the International Neuropsychological Society, 2*, 249–255.

Bauminger, N. (2002). The facilitation of social-emotional understanding and social interaction in high-functioning children with autism: Intervention outcomes. *Journal of Autism and Developmental Disorders, 32*, 283–298.

Bauminger, N. (2004). The expression and understanding of jealousy in children with autism. *Development and Psychopathology, 16*, 157–177.

Bauminger, N. (2007a). Group social-multimodal intervention for HFASD. *Journal of Autism and Developmental Disorders, 37*, 1605–1615.

Bauminger, N. (2007b). Individual social-multimodal intervention for HFASD. *Journal of Autism and Developmental Disorders, 37*, 1593–1604.

Bauminger, N., Chomsky-Smolkin, L., Orbach-Caspi, E., Zachor, D., & Levy-Shiff, R. (2008). Jealousy and emotional responsiveness in young children with ASD. *Cognition and Emotion, 22*, 595–619.

Bauminger, N., & Cohen, L. (2000). *Social interaction in HFASD and social context.* Unpublished master's thesis, Bar-Ilan University, Ramat-Gan, Israel.

Bauminger, N., & Kasari, C. (2000). Loneliness and friendship in high-functioning children with autism. *Child Development, 71*, 447–456

Bauminger, N., & Shoham Kugelmas, D. (2013). Mother–stranger comparisons of social attention in a jealousy context and attachment in HFASD and typical preschoolers. *Journal of Abnormal Child Psychology, 41*(2), 253–264.

Bauminger, N., & Shulman, C. (2003). The development and maintenance of friendship in high-functioning children with autism: Maternal perception. *Autism: International Journal of Research and Practice, 7*, 81–97.

Bauminger, N., Shulman, C., & Agam, G. (2003). Peer interaction and loneliness in high-functioning children with autism. *Journal of Autism and Developmental Disorders, 33*, 489–507.

Bauminger, N., Shulman, C., & Agam, G. (2004). The link between the perception of self and of social relationships in high-functioning children with autism. *Journal of Development and Physical Disabilities, 16*, 193–214.

Bauminger, N., Solomon, M., Aviezer, A., Heung, K., Brown, J., & Rogers, S. (2008). Friendship in high-functioning children with ASD: Mixed and non-mixed dyads. *Journal of Autism and Developmental Disorders, 38*, 1121–1229.

Bauminger, N., Solomon, M., Aviezer, A., Heung, K., Gazit, L., Brown, J., & Rogers, S. (2008). Friendship manifestations, dyadic qualities of friendship, and friendship perception in high-functioning preadolescents with autism spectrum disorder. *Journal of Abnormal Child Psychology, 36*, 135–150.

Bauminger, N., Solomon, M., & Rogers, S. J. (2010). Predicting friendship quality in autism spectrum disorders and typical development. *Journal of Autism and Developmental Disorders, 40*, 751–761.

Bauminger-Zviely, N. (2011, May). *School-based CBT approach for HFASD social cognition, emotion, and social interaction: Study synthesis and future directions.* Paper presented at the International Meeting for Autism Research (IMFAR), San Diego, CA.

Bauminger-Zviely, N., & Agam Ben-Artzi, G. (2012). *Young friendship in HFASD and typical development: Friend vs. non-friend comparisons.* Manuscript in preparation.

Beaumont, R., & Newcombe, P. (2006). Theory of mind and central coherence in adults with high-functioning autism or Asperger syndrome. *Autism, 10,* 365–382.

Beaumont, R., & Sofronoff, K. (2008). A multi-component social skills intervention for children with Asperger syndrome: The Junior Detective Training Program. *Journal of Child Psychology and Psychiatry, 49,* 743–753.

Bebko, J. M., & Ricciuti, C. (2000). Executive functioning and memory strategy use in children with autism: The influence of task constraints on spontaneous rehearsal. *Autism, 4,* 299–320.

Beelmann, A., Pfingsten, U., & Losel, F. (1994). Effects of training social competence in children: A meta-analysis of recent evaluation studies. *Journal of Clinical Child Psychology, 23,* 260–271.

Beer, J. S., & Ochsner, K. N. (2006). Social cognition: A multilevel analysis. *Brain Research, 1079,* 98–105.

Begeer, S., Gevers, C., Clifford, P., Verhoeve, M., Kat, K., & Hoddenbach, E. (2011). Theory of mind training in children with autism: A randomized controlled trial. *Journal of Autism and Developmental Disorders, 41,* 997–1006.

Begeer, S., Koot, H. M., Rieffe, C., Terwogt, M., & Stegge, H. (2008). Emotional competence in children with autism: Diagnostic criteria and empirical evidence. *Developmental Review, 28,* 342–369.

Begeer, S., Terwogt, M., Rieffe, C., Stegge, H., & Koot, J. M. (2007). Do children with autism acknowledge the influence of mood on behaviour? *Autism, 11,* 503–521.

Bellini, S. (2004). Social skill deficits and anxiety in high-functioning adolescents with autism spectrum disorders. *Focus on Autism and Other Developmental Disabilities, 19,* 78–86.

Bellon, M. L., Ogletree, B. T., & Harn, W. E. (2000). Repeated storybook reading as a language intervention for children with autism: A case study on the application of scaffolding. *Focus on Autism and Other Developmental Disabilities, 15,* 52–58.

Belmonte, M. K. (2009). What's the story behind "theory of mind" and autism? *Journal of Consciousness Studies, 16,* 118–139.

Bennetto, L., Pennington, B. F., & Rogers, S. J. (1996). Intact and impaired memory functions in autism. *Child Development, 67,* 1816–1835.

Ben-Sasson, A., Hen, L., Fluss, L., Cermak, S.A., Engel-Yeger, B., & Gal, E. (2009). A meta-analysis of sensory modulation symptoms in individuals with autism spectrum disorders. *Journal of Autism and Developmental Disorders, 39,* 1–11.

Ben Shalom, D., Mostofsky, S. H., Hazlett, R. L., Goldberg, M. C., Landa, R. J., Faran, Y., et al. (2006). Normal physiological emotions but differences in expression of conscious feelings in children with high-functioning autism. *Journal of Autism and Developmental Disorders, 36,* 395–400.

Berger, H., Aerts, F., van Spaendonck, K. Cools, A., & Teunisse, J.-P. (2003). Central coherence and cognitive shifting in relation to social improvement in high-functioning young adults with autism. *Journal of Clinical and Experimental Neuropsychology, 25,* 502–511.

Best, J. R., Miller, P. H., & Jones, L. L. (2009). Executive functions after age 5: Changes and correlates. *Developmental Review, 29,* 180–200.

Bierman, K., & Welsh, J. A. (2000). Assessing social dysfunction: The contributions of laboratory and performance-based measures. *Journal of Clinical Child Psychology, 29,* 526–539.

Blakemore, S. J., & Choudhury, S. (2006). Development of the adolescent brain: Implications for executive function and social cognition. *Journal of Child Psychiatry and Psychology, 47,* 296–312.

Boggs, K. M., & Gross, A.M. (2010). Cue salience in face processing by high-functioning individuals with autism spectrum disorders. *Journal of Development and Physical Disabilities, 22,* 595–613.

Bolte, S., Dziobek, I., & Poustka, F. (2009). Brief report: The level and nature of autistic intelligence revisited. *Journal of Autism and Developmental Disorders, 39,* 678–682.

Booth-LaForce, C., & Kerns, K. A. (2009). Child–parent attachment relationships, peer relationships, and peer-group functioning. In K. H. Rubin, W. Bukowski, & B. Laursen (Eds.), *Handbook of peer interactions, relationships, and groups* (pp. 490–507). New York: Guilford Press.

Boucher, J. (2012). Research review: Structural language in autistic spectrum disorder: Characteristics and causes. *Journal of Child Psychology and Psychiatry, 53,* 219–233.

Boudreau, D. M., & Hedburg, N. L. (1999). A comparison of early literacy skills in children with specific language impairment and their typically developing peers. *American Journal of Speech–Language Pathology, 8,* 249–260.

Bowlby, J. (1982). *Attachment and loss: Vol. 1. Attachment.* New York: Basic Books. (Original work published 1969)

Bowler, D. M. (1992). "Theory of mind" in Asperger syndrome. *Journal of Child Psychology and Psychiatry, 33,* 877–895.

Bowler, D. M., Limoges, E., & Mottron, L. (2009). Different verbal learning strategies in autism spectrum disorder: Evidence from the Rey Auditory Verbal Learning Test. *Journal of Autism and Developmental Disorders, 39,* 910–915.

Boyd, B. A., McBee, M., Holtzclaw, T., Baranek, G. T., & Bodfish, J. W. (2009). Relationships among repetitive behaviors, sensory features, and executive functions in high-functioning autism. *Research in Autism Spectrum Disorders, 3,* 959–966.

Brock, J., Norbury, C., Einav, S., & Nation, K. (2008). Do individuals with autism process words in context? Evidence from language-mediated eye movements. *Cognition, 108,* 896–904.

Bronfenbrenner, U. (1979). *The ecology of human development: Experiment in nature and design.* Cambridge, MA: Harvard University Press.

Bronfenbrenner, U. (1992). Ecological systems theory. In R. Vasta (Ed.), *Annals of child development: Six theories of child development: Revised formulations and current issues* (pp. 178–249). London: Kingsley.

Broun, L. (2004). Teaching students with autistic spectrum disorders to read. *Teaching Exceptional Children, 36,* 36–40.

Brown, H. M., & Klein, P. D. (2011). Writing, Asperger syndrome and theory of mind. *Journal of Autism and Developmental Disorders, 41,* 1464–1474.

Brown, N. B., & Dunn, W. (2010). Relationship between context and sensory processing in children with autism. *American Journal of Occupational Therapy, 64,* 474–483.

Bruck, M., London, K., Landa, R., & Goodman, J. (2007). Autobiographical memory and suggestibility in children with autism spectrum disorder. *Developmental Psychopathology, 19,* 73–95.

Bryan, L. C., & Gast, D. L. (2000). Teaching on-task and on-schedule behaviors to high-functioning children with autism via picture activity schedules. *Journal of Autism and Developmental Disorders, 30,* 553–567.

Buitelaar, J. K. (1995). Attachment and social withdrawal in autism: Hypotheses and findings. *Behavior, 132,* 319–350.

Bukowski, W. M., Motzoi, C., & Meyer, F. (2009). Friendship as process, function, and outcome. In K. H. Rubin, W. Bukowski, & B. Laursen (Eds.), *Handbook of peer interactions, relationships, and groups* (pp. 100–117). New York: Guilford Press.

Bull, R., & Scerif, G. (2001). Executive functioning as a predictor of children's mathematical ability: Inhibition, switching and working memory. *Developmental Neuropsychology, 19,* 273–293.

Burnette, C. P., Mundy, P. C., Meyer, J. A., Sutton, S. K., Vaughan, A. E., & Charak, D. (2005). Weak central coherence and its relations to theory of mind and anxiety in autism. *Journal of Autism and Developmental Disorders, 35,* 63–73.

Campbell, J. M., & Marino, C. A. (2009). Brief report: Sociometric status and behavioral characteristics of peer-nominated buddies for a child with autism. *Journal of Autism and Developmental Disorders, 39,* 1359–1363.

Cappadocia, M. C., Weiss, J. A., & Pepler, D. (2012). Bullying experiences among children and youth with autism spectrum disorders. *Journal of Autism and Developmental Disorders, 42,* 266–277.

Capps, L., Kasari, C., Yirmiya, N., & Sigman, M. (1993). Parental perception of emotional expressiveness in children with autism. *Journal of Consulting and Clinical Psychology, 61,* 475–484.

Capps, L., Kehres, J., & Sigman, M. (1998). Conversational abilities among children with autism and children with developmental delays. *Autism, 2,* 325–344.

Capps, L., Losh, M., & Thurber, C. (2000). "The frog ate the bug and made his mouth sad": Narrative competence in children with autism. *Journal of Abnormal Child Psychology, 28,* 193–204.

Capps, L., Sigman, M., & Mundy, P. (1994). Attachment security in children with autism. *Developmental Psychopathology, 6,* 249–261.

Capps, L., Yirmiya, N., & Sigman, M. (1992). Understanding of simple and complex emotions in nonretarded children with autism. *Journal of Child Psychology and Psychiatry, 33,* 1169–1182.

Cardoso-Martins, C., & da Silva, J. R. (2010). Cognitive and language correlates of hyperlexia: Evidence from children with autism spectrum disorders. *Reading and Writing, 23,* 129–145.

Carnahan, C., Williamson, P., & Haydon, T. (2009). Matching literacy profiles with instruction for students on the spectrum: Making reading instruction meaningful. *Beyond Behavior, 19,* 10–16.

Carter, S. (2009). Bullying of students with Asperger syndrome. *Issues in Comprehensive Pediatric Nursing, 32,* 145–154.

Carter, A. S., Black, D. O., Tewani, S., Connolly, C. E., Kadlec, M. B., & Tager-Flusberg, H. (2007). Sex differences in toddlers with autism spectrum disorders. *Journal of Autism and Developmental Disorders, 37,* 86–97.

Cartwright, K. B. (2006). Fostering flexibility and comprehension in elementary students. *The Reading Teacher, 59,* 628–634.

Cederlund, M., Hagberg, B., Billstedt, I., Gillberg, C., & Gillberg, C. (2008). Asperger syndrome and autism: A comparative longitudinal follow-up study more than 5 years after original diagnosis. *Journal of Autism and Developmental Disorders, 38,* 72–85.

Cederlund, M., Hagberg, B., & Gillberg, C. (2010). Asperger syndrome in adolescent and young adult males: Interview, self-, and parent assessment of social, emotional, and cognitive problems. *Research in Developmental Disabilities, 31,* 287–298.

Centers for Disease Control and Prevention. (2007). *Prevalence of autism spectrum disorders: Autism and Developmental Disabilities Monitoring Network, 14 sites, United States, 2002* (Surveilance Summary 56 [No. SS-1], 12–28). Retrieved from *www.cdc.gov/mmwr/preview/mmwrhtml/ss5601a2.htm.*

Centers for Disease Control and Prevention. (2012). *Prevalence of autism spectrum disorders (ASDs) among multiple areas of the United States in 2008* (Community report from the Autism and Developmental Disabilities Monitoring [ADDM] Network). Retrieved from *www.cdc.gov/ncbddd/autism/documents/ADDM-2012–Community-Report.pdf.*

Chalfant, A. M., Rapee, R., & Carroll, L. (2007). Treating anxiety disorders in children with high-functioning autism spectrum disorders: A controlled trial. *Journal of Autism and Developmental Disorders, 37,* 1842–1857.

References

281

Chamberlain, B., Kasari, C., & Rotheram-Fuller, E. (2007). Involvement or isolation?: The social networks of children with autism in regular classrooms. *Journal of Autism and Developmental Disorders, 37*, 230–242.

Channon, S., Charman, T., Heap, J., Crawford, S., & Rios, P. (2001). Real-life-type problem solving in Asperger's syndrome. *Journal of Autism and Developmental Disorders, 31*, 451–469.

Charlop-Christy, M. H., & Kelso, S. E. (2003). Teaching children with autism conversational speech using a cue card/written script program. *Education and Treatment of Children, 26*, 108–127.

Charman, T. (2003). Why is joint attention a pivotal skill in autism? *Philosophical Transactions of the Royal Society of London B-Biological Science, 358*, 315–324.

Charman, T. (2011). Development from preschool through school age. In D. G. Amaral, G. Dawson, & D. H. Geschwind (Eds.), *Autism spectrum disorders* (pp. 229–240). New York: Oxford University Press.

Charman, T., Pickles, A., Simonoff, E., Chandler, S., Loucas, T., & Baird, G. (2010). IQ in children with autism spectrum disorders: Data from the Special Needs and Autism Project (SNAP). *Psychological Medicine, 41*, 619–627.

Charman, T., Swettenham, J., Baron-Cohen, S., Cox, A., Baird, G., & Drew, A. (1997). Infants with autism: An investigation of empathy, pretend play, joint attention and imitation. *Developmental Psychology, 33*, 781–789.

Charman, T., Taylor, E., Drew, A., Cockerill, H., Brown, J., & Baird, G. (2005). Outcome at 7 years of children diagnosed with autism at age 2: Predictive validity of assessments conducted at 2 and 3 years of age and pattern of symptom change over time. *Journal of Child Psychology and Psychiatry, 46*, 500–513.

Chawarska, K., Klin, A., Paul, R., & Volkmar, F. (2007). Autism spectrum disorder in the second year: Stability and change in syndrome expression. *Journal of Child Psychology and Psychiatry, 48*, 128–138.

Chiang, H. M., & Carter, M. (2008). Spontaneity of communication in individuals with autism. *Journal of Autism and Developmental Disorders, 38*, 693–705.

Chiang, H. M., & Lin, Y. H. (2007). Mathematical ability of students with Asperger syndrome and high-functioning autism: A review of literature. *Autism, 11*, 547–556.

Chin, H. Y., & Bernard-Opitz, V. (2000). Teaching conversational skills to children with autism: Effect on the development of a theory of mind. *Journal of Autism and Developmental Disorders, 30*, 569–583.

Church, C., Alinsanski, S., & Amanullah, S. (2000). The social, behavioural, and academic experiences of children with Asperger syndrome. *Focus on Autism and Other Developmental Disabilities, 15*, 12–20.

Cihak, D. F., & Foust, J. L. (2008). Comparing number lines and touch points to teach addition facts to students with autism. *Focus on Autism and Other Developmental Disabilities, 23*, 131–137.

Cirino, P. T., Morris, M. K., & Morris, R. D. (2002). Neuropsychological concomitants of calculation skills in college students referred for learning difficulties. *Developmental Neuropsychology, 21*, 201–218.

Clifford, S., & Dissanayake, C. (2008). The early development of joint attention in infants with autistic disorder using home video observations and parental interview. *Journal of Autism and Developmental Disorders, 38*, 791–805.

Clifford, S., Hudry, K., Brown, L., Pasco, G., & Charman, T. (2010). The Modified-Classroom Observation Schedule to Measure Intentional Communication (M-COSMIC): Evaluation of reliability and validity. *Research in Autism Spectrum Disorders, 4*, 509–525.

Colasent, R., & Griffith, P. L. (1998). Autism and literacy: Looking into the classroom with rabbit stories. *The Reading Teacher, 51*, 414–420.

Conners, K. C. (2008). *Conners 3rd edition.* Toronto, Ontario, Canada: Multi-Health Systems.

Connor, C. M., Morrison, F. J., Fishman, B., Giuliani, S., Luck, M., Underwood, P. S., et al. (2011). Testing the impact of child characteristics × instruction interactions on third graders' reading comprehension by differentiating literacy instruction. *Reading Research Quarterly, 46*, 189–221.

Constantino, J. N., & Gruber, C. P. (2005). *Social Responsiveness Scale (SRS) manual.* Los Angeles, CA: Western Psychological Services.

Cooper, C. R. (1980). Development of collaborative problem solving among preschool children. *Developmental Psychology, 16*, 433–440.

Coplan, R. J., & Arbeau, K. A. (2009). Peer interaction and play in early childhood. In K. H. Rubin, W. M. Bukowski, & B. Laursen (Eds.), *Handbook of peer interaction, relationships, and groups* (pp. 143–161). New York: Guilford Press.

Corona, R., Dissanayake, C., Arbelle, S., Wellington, P., & Sigman, M. (1998). Is affect aversive to young children with autism? Behavioral and cardiac responses to experimenter distress. *Child Development, 69*, 1494–1502.

Craig, J., & Baron-Cohen, S. (2000). Story-telling ability in children with autism or Asperger syndrome: A window into the imagination. *Israel Journal of Psychiatry and Related Sciences, 37*, 64–70.

Crane, L., & Goddard, L. (2008). Episodic and semantic autobiographical memory in adults with autism spectrum disorders. *Journal of Autism and Developmental Disorders, 38*, 498–506.

Crick, N. R., & Dodge, K. A. (1994). A review and reformulation of social information-processing mechanisms in children's social adjustment. *Psychological Bulletin, 115*, 74–101.

Crooke, P. J., Hendrix, R. E., & Rachman, J. Y. (2008). Measuring the effectiveness of teaching social thinking to children with Asperger syndrome (AS) and high-functioning autism (HFA). *Journal of Autism and Developmental Disorders, 38*, 581–591.

Cunningham, D., McMahon, H., & O'Neill, B. (1992). Bubble dialogue: A new tool for instruction and assessment. *Educational Technology Research and Development, 40*, 59–67.

Cutting, L. E., Materek, A., Cole, C. A. S., Levine, T. M., & Mahone, E. M. (2009). Effects of fluency, oral language, and executive function on reading comprehension performance. *Annals of Dyslexia, 59*, 34–54.

Dahlgren, S. O., & Trillingsgaard, A. (1996). Theory of mind in nonretarded children with autism and Asperger's syndrome: A research note. *Journal of Child Psychology and Psychiatry, 37*, 759–763.

Daniel, L. S., & Billingsley, B. S. (2010). What boys with an autism spectrum disorder say about establishing and maintaining friendships. *Focus on Autism and Other Developmental Disabilities, 25*, 220–229.

Davis, M., Eshelman, E. R., & McKay, M. (2000). *The relaxation and stress reduction workbook* (5th ed.). Oakland, CA: New Harbinger Press.

Dawson, G., Meltzoff, A. N., Osterling, J., Rinaldi, J., & Brown, E. (1998). Children with autism fail to orient to naturally occurring social stimuli. *Journal of Autism and Developmental Disorders, 28*, 479–485.

Dawson, G., Sterling, L., & Faja, S. (2009). Autism, risk factors, risk processes, and outcome. In M. de Haan & M. R. Gunnar (Eds.), *Handbook of social neuroscience* (pp. 435–458). New York: Guilford Press.

Dawson, G., Toth, K., Abbott, R., Osterling, J., Munson, J., Estes, A., et al. (2004). Early social attention impairments in autism: Social orienting, joint attention, and attention in autism. *Developmental Psychology, 40*, 271–283.

de Bruin, E. I., Ferdinand, R. F., Meester, S., de Nijs, P. F., & Verheij, F. (2007). High rates of psychiatric co-morbidity in PDD-NOS. *Journal of Autism and Developmental Disorders, 37*, 877–886.

Delano, M. E. (2007a). Improving written language performance of adolescents with Asperger syndrome. *Journal of Applied Behavior Analysis, 40,* 345–351.

Delano, M. E. (2007b). Use of strategy instruction to improve the story writing skills of a student with Asperger syndrome. *Focus on Autism and Other Developmental Disabilities, 22,* 252–258.

Delinicolas, E. K., & Young, R. L. (2007). Joint attention, language, social relating, and stereotypical behaviours in children with autistic disorder. *Autism, 11,* 425–436.

Delis, D. C., Kramer, J. H., Kaplan, E., & Ober, B. A. (1994). *California Verbal Learning Test—Children's Version.* San Antonio, TX: Psychological Assessment Resources.

Denham, S. A. (1998). *Emotional development in young children.* New York: Guilford Press.

Dennett, D. (1978). *Brainstorms: Philosophical essay on mind and psychology.* Montgomery, UK: Harvester Press.

Dennis, M., Lockyer, L., & Lazenby, A. L. (2000). How high-functioning children with autism understand real and deceptive emotion. *Autism, 4,* 370–381.

Diehl, J. J., Bennetto, L., & Young, E. C. (2006). Story recall and narrative coherence of high-functioning children with autism spectrum disorders. *Journal of Abnormal Child Psychology, 34,* 87–102.

Dillon, G., & Underwood, J. (2012). Computer-mediated imaginative storytelling in children with autism. *International Journal of Human-Computer Studies, 70,* 169–178.

Dissanayake, C., & Crossley, S. A. (1996). Proximity and sociable behaviors in autism: Evidence for attachment. *Journal of Child Psychology and Psychiatry, 37,* 149–156.

Dissanayake, C., & Crossley, S. A. (1997). Autistic children's response to separation and reunion with their mothers. *Journal of Autism and Developmental Disorders, 27,* 295–312.

Dissanayake, C., & Sigman, M. (2001). Attachment and emotional responsiveness in children with autism. *International Review of Research in Mental Retardation, 23,* 239–266.

Dissanayake, C., Sigman, M., & Kasari, C. (1996). Long-term stability of individual differences in the emotional responsiveness of children with autism. *Journal of Child Psychology and Psychiatry, 37,* 461–467.

Dobson, D., & Dobson, K. (2009). *Evidence-based practice of cognitive behavioral therapy.* New York: Guilford Press.

Dodge, K. A. (1986). A social information-processing model of social competence in children. In M. Perlmutter (Ed.), *Minnesota Symposium in Child Psychology* (Vol. 18, pp. 77–125). Hillsdale, NJ: Erlbaum.

Donaldson, J. B., & Zager, D. (2010). Mathematics interventions for students with high-functioning autism/Asperger's syndrome. *Teaching Exceptional Children, 42,* 40–46.

Drahota, A., Wood, J. J., Sze, K. M., & Van Dyke, M. (2011). Effects of cognitive behavioral therapy on daily living skills in children with high-functioning autism and concurrent anxiety disorders. *Journal of Autism and Developmental Disorders, 41,* 257–265.

Duarte, C. S., Bordin, I. A. S., de Oliveira, A., & Bird, H. (2003). The CBCL and the identification of children with autism and related conditions in Brazil: Pilot findings. *Journal of Autism and Developmental Disorders, 33,* 703–707.

Duncan, A. M., & Klinger, L. G. (2010). Autism spectrum disorders: Building social skills in group, school, and community settings. *Social Work with Groups, 33,* 175–193.

Duncan, J. (1986). Disorganization of behavior after frontal lobe damage. *Cognitive Neuropsychology, 3,* 271–290.

Dunn, L. M., & Dunn, L. M. (1997). *Examiner's manual for the Peabody Picture Vocabulary Test Third Edition*. Circle Pines, MN: American Guidance Service.

Eaves, L. C., & Ho, H. H. (2008). Young adult outcome of autism spectrum disorders. *Journal of Autism and Developmental Disorders, 38*, 739–747.

Eigsti, I. M., Bennetto, L., & Dadlani, M. B. (2007). Beyond pragmatics: Morphosyntactic development in autism. *Journal of Autism and Developmental Disorders, 37*, 1007–1023.

Eigsti, I. M., de Marchena, A. B., Shuh, J. M., & Kelley, E. (2011). Language acquisition in autism spectrum disorders: A developmental review. *Research in Autism Spectrum Disorders, 5*, 681–691.

Elison, J. T., Sasson, N. J., Turner-Brown, L. M., Dichter, G. S., & Bodfish, J. W. (2012). Age trends in visual exploration of social and nonsocial information in children with autism. *Research in Autism Spectrum Disorders, 6*, 842–851.

Embregts, P., & van Nieuwenhuijzen, M. (2009). Social information processing in boys with autistic spectrum disorder and mild to borderline intellectual disabilities. *Journal of Intellectual Disability Research, 35*, 922–931.

Engström, I., Ekström, L., & Emilsson, B. (2003). Psychosocial functioning in a group of Swedish adults with Asperger syndrome or high-functioning autism. *Autism, 7*, 99–110.

Esbensen, A. J., Seltzer, M. M., Lam, K. S. L., & Bodfish, J. W. (2009). Age-related differences in restricted repetitive behaviors in autism spectrum disorders. *Journal of Autism and Developmental Disorders, 39*, 57–66.

Espy, K. A., McDiarmid, M. M., Cwik, M. F., Stalets, M. M., Hamby, A., & Senns, T. E. (2004). The contribution of executive functions to emergent mathematic skills in preschool children. *Developmental Neuropsychology, 26*, 465–486.

Estes, A., Rivera, V., Bryan, M., Cali, P., & Dawson, G. (2011). Discrepancies between academic achievement and intellectual ability in higher-functioning school-aged children with autism spectrum disorder. *Journal of Autism and Developmental Disorders, 41*, 1044–1052.

Evans, D., Canavera, K., Kleinpeter, F., Maccubbin, E., & Taga, K. (2005). The fears, phobias, and anxieties of children with autism spectrum disorders and Down syndrome: Comparisons with developmentally and chronologically age-matched children. *Child Psychiatry and Human Development, 36*, 3–26.

Fabes, R. A., Martin, C. L., & Hanish, L. D. (2009). Children's behavior and interactions with peers. In K. H. Rubin., W. M. Bukowski, & B. Laursen (Eds.), *Handbook of peer interactions, relationships, and groups* (pp. 45–62). New York: Guilford Press.

Farran, E. K., Branson, A., & King, B. J. (2011). Visual search for basic emotional expressions in autism: Impaired processing of anger, fear and sadness, but a typical happy face advantage. *Research in Autism Spectrum Disorders, 5*, 455–462.

Fawcett, L. M., & Garton, A. F. (2005). The effect of peer collaboration on children's problem-solving ability. *British Journal of Educational Psychology, 75*, 157–169.

Fecteau, S., Mottron, L., Berthiaume, C., & Burack, J. A. (2003). Developmental changes of autistic symptoms. *Autism, 7*, 255–268.

Feng, H., Lo, Y., Tsai, S., & Cartledge, G. (2008). The effects of theory-of-mind and social skill training on the social competence of a sixth-grade student with autism. *Journal of Positive Behavior Interventions, 10*, 228–242.

Fisher, N., & Happé, F. (2005). A training study of theory of mind and executive function in children with autistic spectrum disorders. *Journal of Autism and Developmental Disorders, 35*, 757–771.

Flood, A. M., Hare, D. G., & Wallis, P. (2011). An investigation into social information processing in young people with Asperger syndrome. *Autism, 15*, 601–624.

Foley-Nicpon, M., Assouline, S. G., & Stinson, R. D. (2012). Cognitive and academic distinctions between gifted students with autism and Asperger syndrome. *Gifted Child Quarterly, 56,* 77–89.

Frankel, F., Myatt, R., Sugar, C., Whitham, C., Gorospe, C., & Laugeson, E. (2010). A randomized controlled study of parent-assisted children's friendship training with children having autism spectrum disorders. *Journal of Autism and Developmental Disorders, 40,* 827–842.

Freeth, M., Ropar, D., Mitchell, P., Chapman, P., & Loher, S. (2011). Brief report: How adolescents with ASD process social information in complex scenes: Combining evidence from eye movements and verbal descriptions. *Journal of Autism and Developmental Disorders, 41,* 364–371.

Frith, U. (1989). *Autism: Explaining the enigma.* Oxford, UK: Blackwell.

Frith, U. (2004). Emanuel Miller lecture: Confusion and controversies about Asperger syndrome. *Journal of Child Psychology and Psychiatry, 45,* 672–686.

Frith, U., & Happé, F. (1999). Theory of mind and self-consciousness: What is it like to be autistic? *Mind & Language, 14,* 1–22.

Frith, U., & Snowling, M. (1983). Reading for meaning and reading for sound in autistic and dyslexic children. *Journal of Developmental Psychology, 1,* 329–342.

Gabig, C. S. (2008). Verbal working memory and story retelling in school-age children with autism. *Language, Speech and Hearing Services in Schools, 39,* 498–511.

Gabig, C. S. (2010). Phonological awareness and word recognition in reading by children with autism. *Communication Disorders Quarterly, 31,* 67–85.

Gadow, K. D., DeVincent, C. J., Olvet, D. M., Pisarevskaya, V., & Hatchwell, E. (2010). Association of DRD4 polymorphism with severity of oppositional defiant disorder, separation anxiety disorder and repetitive behaviors in children with autism spectrum disorder. *European Journal of Neuroscience, 32,* 1058–1065.

Gadow, K. D., DeVincent, C. J., & Pomeroy, J. (2006). ADHD symptom subtypes in children with pervasive developmental disorder. *Journal of Autism and Developmental Disorders, 36,* 271–283.

Gadow, K.D., DeVincent, C., & Schneider, J. (2008). Predictors of psychiatric symptoms in children with an autism spectrum disorder. *Journal of Autism and Developmental Disorders, 38,* 1710–1720.

Gadow, K. D., & Sprafkin, J. (2002). *Child Symptom Inventory–4 screening and norms manual.* Stony Brook, NY: Checkmate Plus.

Gadow, K. D., & Sprafkin, J. (2009). *The symptom inventories: An annotated bibliography.* Stony Brook, NY: Checkmate Plus.

Gadow, K. D., & Sprafkin, J. (2012). *The Child and Adolescent Symptom Inventory— 4R.* Stony Brook, NY: Checkmate Plus

Gantman, A., Kapp, S. K., Orenski, K., & Laugeson, E. (2012). Social skills training for young adults with high-functioning autism spectrum disorders: A randomized controlled pilot study. *Journal of Autism and Developmental Disorders, 42,* 1094–1103.

Ganz, J. B. (2007). Classroom structuring methods and strategies for children and youth with autism spectrum disorders. *Exceptionality, 15,* 249–260.

Ganz, J. B., Kaylor, M., Bourgeois, B., & Hadden, K. (2008). The impact of social scripts and visual cues on verbal communication in three children with autism spectrum disorders. *Focus on Autism and Other Developmental Disabilities, 23,* 79–94.

Garvey, C. (1977). *Play.* London: Fontana.

Gately, S. (2008). Facilitating reading comprehension for students on the autism spectrum. *Teaching Exceptional Children, 40,* 40–45.

Gevers, C., Clifford, P., Mager, M., & Boer, F. (2006). A theory-of-mind-based social-cognition training program for school-aged children with pervasive developmental disorders: An open study of its effectiveness. *Journal of Autism and Developmental Disorders, 36,* 567–571.

Ghaziuddin, M. (2010). Brief report: Should the DSM-5 drop Asperger syndrome? *Journal of Autism and Developmental Disorders, 40,* 1146–1148.

Ghaziuddin, M., Alessi, N., & Greden, J. (1995). Life events and depression in children with pervasive developmental disorders. *Journal of Autism and Developmental Disorders, 25,* 495–502.

Ghaziuddin, M., Ghaziuddin, N., & Greden, J. (2002). Depression in persons with autism: Implications for research and clinical care. *Journal of Autism and Developmental Disorders, 32,* 299–306.

Ghaziuddin, M., & Greden, J. (1998). Depression in children with autism/pervasive developmental disorders: A case-control family history study. *Journal of Autism and Developmental Disorders, 28,* 111–115.

Ghaziuddin, M., Weidmer-Mikhail, E., & Ghaziuddin, N. (1998). Comorbidity of Asperger syndrome: A preliminary report. *Journal of Intellectual Disability Research, 4,* 279–283.

Gifford-Smith, M. E., & Rabiner, D. L. (2004). Social information processing and children's social adjustment. In J. B. Kupersmidt & K. A. Dodge (Eds.), *Children's peer relations: From development to intervention* (pp. 61–80). Washington, DC: American Psychological Association.

Gillespie-Lynch, K., Sepeta, L., Wang, Y., Marshall, S., Gomez, L., Sigman, M., et al. (2012). Early childhood predictors of the social competence of adults with autism. *Journal of Autism and Developmental Disorders, 42,* 161–174.

Gillott, A., Furniss, F., & Walter, A. (2001). Anxiety in high-functioning children with autism. *Autism, 4,* 117–132.

Gilotty, L., Kenworthy, L., Sirian, L., Black, D., & Wagner, A. (2002). Adaptive skills and executive function in autism spectrum disorders. *Child Neuropsychology, 8,* 241–248.

Goddard, L., Howlin, P., Dritschel, B., & Patel, T. J. (2007). Autobiographical memory and social problem-solving in Asperger syndrome. *Journal of Autism and Developmental Disorders, 37,* 291–300.

Golan, O., Baron-Cohen, S., & Golan, Y. (2008). The "Reading the Mind in Films" Task [Child Version]: Complex emotion and mental state recognition in children with and without autism spectrum conditions. *Journal of Autism and Developmental Disorders, 38,* 1534–1541.

Goldman, S. (2008). Brief report: Narratives of personal events in children with autism and developmental language disorders: Unshared memories. *Journal of Autism and Developmental Disorders, 38,* 1982–1988.

Goldstein, G., Allen, D. N., Minshew, N. J., Williams, D. L., Volkmar, F., Klin, A., et al. (2008). The structure of intelligence in children and adults with high-functioning autism. *Neuropsychology, 22,* 301–312.

Goodman, R. (1997). The Strengths and Difficulties Questionnaire: A research note. *Journal of Child Psychology and Psychiatry, 38,* 581–586.

Gotham, C., Bishop, S. L., & Lord, C. (2011). Diagnosis of autism spectrum disorders. In D. G. Amaral, G. Dawson, & D. H. Geschwind (Eds.), *Autism spectrum disorders* (pp. 30–43). New York: Oxford University Press.

Graham, S., & Harris, K. R. (1993). Self-regulated strategy development: Helping students with learning problems develop as writers. *Elementary School Journal, 94,* 169–181.

Gras-Vincendon, A., Mottron, L., Salame, P., Bursztejn, C., & Danion, J. M. (2007). Temporal context memory in high-functioning autism. *Autism, 11,* 523–534.

Gray, C. A. (1998). Social stories and comic strip conversations with students with Asperger syndrome and high-functioning autism. In E. Schopler, G. Mesibov, & L. Kunce (Eds.), *Asperger syndrome or high-functioning autism* (pp. 167–199). New York: Plenum Press.

Gray, C. (2000). *The new social story book.* Arlington, TX: Future Horizons.

Green, J., Gilchrist, A., Burton, D., & Cox, A. (2000). Social and psychiatric functioning in adolescents with Asperger syndrome compared with conduct disorder. *Journal of Autism and Developmental Disorders, 30,* 279–293.

Greenberg, M. T., Kusche, C. A., Cook, E. T., & Quamma, J. P. (1995). Promoting emotional competence in school-aged children: The effects of the PATHS curriculum. *Development and Psychopathology, 7,* 117–136.

Grigorenko, E. L., Volkmar, F., & Klin, A. (2003). Hyperlexia: Disability or superability? *Journal of Child Psychology and Psychiatry, 44,* 1079–1091.

Griswold, D. E., Barnhill, G. P., Myles, B. S., Hagiwara, T., & Simpson, R. L. (2002). Asperger syndrome and academic achievement. *Focus on Autism and Other Developmental Disabilities, 17,* 94–102.

Gulsrud, A. C., Jahromi, L. B., & Kasari, C. (2010). The co-regulation of emotions between mothers and their children with autism. *Journal of Autism and Developmental Disorders, 40,* 227–237.

Guralnick, M. G., Neville, B., Hammond, M. A., & Connor, R. T. (2007). The friendships of young children with developmental delays: A longitudinal analysis. *Journal of Applied Developmental Psychology, 28,* 64–79.

Hala, S., Rasmussen, C., & Henderson, A. M. E. (2005). Three types of source monitoring by children with and without autism: The role of executive function. *Journal of Autism and Developmental Disorders, 35,* 75–89.

Halberstadt, A. G., Denham, S. A., & Dunsmore, J. C. (2001). Affective social competence. *Social Development, 10,* 79–119.

Hale, C. M., & Tager-Flusberg, H. (2005). Social communication in children with autism: The relationship between theory of mind and discourse development. *Autism, 9,* 157–178.

Ham, H. S., Bartolo, A., Corley, M., Rajendran, G., Szabo, A., & Swanson, S. (2011). Exploring the relationship between gestural recognition and imitation: Evidence of dyspraxia in autism spectrum disorders. *Journal of Autism and Developmental Disorders, 41,* 1–12.

Happé, F. (1993). Communicative competence and theory of mind in autism: A test of relevance theory. *Cognition, 48,* 101–119.

Happé, F. (1997). Central coherence and theory of mind in autism: Reading homographs in context. *British Journal of Developmental Psychology, 15,* 1–12.

Happé, F. (2005). The weak central coherence account of autism. In F. R. Volkmar, R. Paul, A. Klin, & D. Cohen (Eds.), *Handbook of autism and pervasive developmental disorders* (pp. 640–649). Hoboken, NJ: Wiley.

Happé, F., & Frith, U. (2006). The weak coherence account: Detail-focused cognitive style in autism spectrum disorders. *Journal of Autism and Developmental Disorders, 35,* 5–25.

Harbinson, H., & Alexander, J. (2009). Asperger syndrome and the English curriculum: Addressing the challenges. *Support for Learning, 24,* 11–18.

Harris, K., Graham, S., & Mason, L. (n.d.) *Self-regulated strategy development in writing: Story and opinion essay writing for students with disabilities or severe difficulties in the early elementary grades.* University of Maryland, Department of Special Education, Center for Accelerating Student Learning. Retrieved from *http://kc.vanderbilt.edu/casl/srsd.html.*

Harris, P. L. (1989). *Children and emotion: The development of psychological understanding.* Oxford, UK: Basil Blackwell.

Hart, K. J., & Morgan, J. R. (1993). Cognitive behavioral therapy with children: Historical context and current status. In A. J. Finch, W. M. Nelson, & E. S. Ott (Eds.), *Cognitive behavior procedures with children and adolescents: A practical guide* (pp. 1–24). Boston: Allyn & Bacon.

Hartley, S. L., & Sikora, D. M. (2009). Sex differences in autism spectrum disorder: An examination of developmental functioning, autistic symptoms, and coexisting behavior problems in toddlers. *Journal of Autism and Developmental Disorders, 39*, 1715–1722.

Hartup, H. H. (2009). Critical issues and theoretical viewpoint. In K. H. Rubin, W. Bukowski, & B. Laursen (Eds.), *Handbook of peer interactions, relationships, and groups* (pp. 3–19). New York: Guilford Press.

Hauck, M., Fein, D., Waterhouse, L., & Feinstein, C. (1995). Social initiations by autistic children to adults and other children. *Journal of Autism and Developmental Disorders, 25*, 579–595.

Hawkins, E., Kingsdorf, S., Charnock, J., Szabo, M., & Gautreaux, G. (2009). Effects of multiple exemplar instruction on naming. *European Journal of Behavior Analysis, 10*, 265–273.

Hedley, D., & Young, R. (2006). Social comparison processes and depressive symptoms in children and adolescents with Asperger syndrome. *Autism, 10*, 139–153.

Heerey, E. A., Keltner, D., & Capps, L. M. (2003). Making sense of self-conscious emotion: Linking theory of mind and emotion in children with autism. *Emotion, 3*, 394–400.

Hendricks, D. (2010). Employment and adults with autism spectrum disorders: Challenges and strategies for success. *Journal of Vocational Rehabilitation 32*, 125–134.

Hermelin, B., & O'Connor, N. (1985). The logico-affective disorder in autism. In E. Schopler & G. B. Mesibov (Eds.), *Communication problems in autism* (pp. 283–310). New York: Plenum Press.

Hesling, I., Dilharreguy, B., Peppé, S., Amirault, M., Bouvard, M., & Allard, M. (2010). The integration of prosodic speech in high-functioning autism: A preliminary fMRI study. *PLoS ONE, 5*(7), e11571.

Heumer, S. V., & Mann, V. (2010). A comprehensive profile of decoding and comprehension in autism spectrum disorders. *Journal of Autism and Developmental Disorders, 40*, 485–493.

Hileman, C., Henderson, H., Jaime, M., Newell, L., & Mundy, P. (2010, August). *Face processing ability in autism: Developmental and diagnostic effects.* Paper presented at the annual meeting of the American Psychological Association, San Diego, CA.

Hillier, A., & Allinson, L. (2002). Understanding embarrassment among those with autism: Breaking down the complex emotion of embarrassment among those with autism. *Journal of Autism and Developmental Disorders, 32*, 583–592.

Hilton, C., Graver, K., & LaVesser, P. (2007). Relationship between social competence and sensory processing in children with high-functioning autism spectrum disorders. *Research in Autism Spectrum Disorders, 1*, 164–173.

Hilton, C., Harper, J. D., Kueker, R. H., Lang, A., Abbacchi, A. M., Todorov, A., et al. (2010). Sensory responsiveness as a predictor of social severity in children with high-functioning autism spectrum disorders. *Journal of Autism and Developmental Disorders, 40*, 937–945.

Hobson, P. (2002). *The cradle of thought: Exploring the origins of thinking.* London: Macmillan Press.

Hobson, P. (2005). Autism and emotion. In F. R. Volkmar, R. Paul, A. Klin., & D. Cohen (Eds.), *Handbook of autism and pervasive developmental disorders* (pp. 406–422). Hoboken, NJ: Wiley.

Hobson, P., Chidambi, G., Lee, A., & Meyer, J. (2006). Foundations of self-awareness: An exploration through autism. *Monographs of the Society for Research in Child Development, 71*(1, Serial No. 284).

Hobson, R. P., & Hobson, J. A. (2007). Identification: The missing link between joint attention and imitation? *Development and Psychopathology, 19*, 411–431.

Hobson, R. P., Lee, A., & Hobson, J. A. (2009). Qualities of symbolic play among children with autism: A social-developmental perspective. *Journal of Autism and Developmental Disorders, 39*, 12–22.

Hobson, R. P., & Meyer, J. A. (2005). Interpersonal foundations for the self: The case of autism. *Developmental Science, 8*, 481–491.

Honey, E., Leekam, S., Turner, M., & McConachie, H.(2007). Repetitive behavior and play in typically developing children and children with autism spectrum disorders. *Journal of Autism and Developmental Disorders, 37*, 1107–1115.

Hooper, S. R., Swartz, C. W.,Wakely, M. B., de Kruif, R. E., & Montgomery, J. W. (2002). Executive functions in elementary school children with and without problems in written expression. *Journal of Learning Disabilities, 35*, 57–68.

Horn, E., Lieber, J., Li, S., Sandall, S., & Schwartz, I. (2000). Supporting young children's IEP goals in inclusive settings through embedded learning opportunities. *Topics in Early Childhood Special Education, 20*, 208–223.

Howes, C. (1996). *The earliest friendships.* In W. M. Bukowski, A. F. Newcomb, & W. W. Hartup (Eds.), *The company they keep: Friendship in childhood and adolescence* (pp. 66–86). Cambridge, UK: Cambridge University Press.

Howlin, P. (2000). Outcome in adult life for more able individuals with autism or Asperger syndrome. *Autism, 4*, 63–83.

Howlin, P., Goode, S., Hutton, J., & Rutter, M. (2004). Adult outcome for children with autism. *Journal of Child Psychology and Psychiatry 45*, 212–229.

Hubbard, K. M., & Trauner, D. A. (2007). Intonation and emotion in autistic spectrum disorders. *Journal of Psycholinguistic Research, 36*, 159–173.

Hudenko, W. J., Stone, W., & Bachorowski, J. (2009). Laughter differs in children with autism: An acoustic analysis of laughs produced by children with and without the disorder. *Journal of Autism and Developmental Disorders, 39*, 1392–1400.

Hume, K., & Odom, S. (2007). Effects of an individual work system on the independent functioning of students with autism. *Journal of Autism and Developmental Disorders, 37*, 1166–1180.

Humphrey, N., & Symes, W. (2011). Peer interaction patterns among adolescents with autistic spectrum disorders (ASDs) in mainstream school settings. *Autism, 15*, 397–415.

Hundert, J., & van Delft, S. (2009). Teaching children with autism spectrum disorders to answer inferential "why" questions. *Focus on Autism and Other Developmental Disabilities, 24*, 67–76.

Hurlburt, R.T., Happé, F., & Frith, U. (1994). Sampling the form of inner experience in three adults with Asperger syndrome. *Psychological Medicine, 24*, 385–395.

Hurlbutt, K., & Chalmers, L. (2004). Employment and adults with Asperger syndrome. *Focus on Autism and Other Developmental Disabilities, 91*, 215–222.

Ingersoll, B., & Lalonde, K. (2010). The impact of object and gesture imitation training on language use in children with autism spectrum disorder. *Journal of Speech, Language, and Hearing Research, 53*, 1040–1051.

Jacques, S., & Zelazo, P. D. (2001). The Flexible Item Selection Task (FIST): A measure of executive function in preschoolers. *Developmental Neuropsychology, 20*, 573–591.

Jaedicke, S., Storoschuk, S., & Lord, C. (1994). Subjective experience and causes of affect in high-functioning children and adolescents with autism. *Development and Psychopathology, 6*, 273–284.

Jahr, E. (2001). Teaching children with autism to answer novel "wh" questions by utilizing a multiple exemplar strategy. *Research in Developmental Disabilities, 22*, 407–423.

James, I. (2003). Autism in mathematicians. *Mathematical Intelligencer, 25*, 62–65.

James, I. (2010). Autism and mathematical talent. *Mathematical Intelligencer, 32*, 56–58.

Jemel, B., Mottron, L., & Dawson, M. (2006). Impaired face processing in autism: Fact or artifact? *Journal of Autism and Developmental Disorders, 36,* 91–106.

Jennes-Coussens, M., Magill-Evans, J., & Koning, C. (2006). The quality of life of young men with Asperger syndrome: A brief report. *Autism, 10,* 403–414.

Jobe, L. E., & White, S. W. (2007). Loneliness, social relationships, and a broader autism phenotype in college students. *Personality and Individual Differences, 42,* 1479–1489.

Johnson, C. R., & Rakison, D. H. (2006). Early categorization of animate/inanimate concepts in young children with autism. *Journal of Developmental and Physical Disabilities, 18,* 73–89.

Jones, C. R. G., Happé, F., Golden, H., Marsden, A. J., Tregay, J., Simonoff, E., et al. (2009). Reading and arithmetic in adolescents with autism spectrum disorders: Peaks and dips in attainment. *Neuropsychology, 23,* 718–728.

Jones, C. R. G., Happé, F., Pickles, A., Marsden, A. J., Tregay, J., Baird, G., et al. (2011). "Everyday memory" impairments in autism spectrum disorders. *Journal of Autism and Developmental Disorders, 41,* 455–464.

Jones, C., Pickles, A., Falcaro, M., Marsden, A., Happé, F., Scott, S., et al. (2011). A multimodal approach to emotion recognition ability in autism spectrum disorders. *Journal of Child Psychology and Psychiatry, 52,* 275–285.

Jones, C. D., & Schwartz, I. S. (2009). When asking questions is not enough: An observational study of social communication differences in high-functioning children with autism. *Journal of Autism and Developmental Disorders, 39,* 432–443.

Jordan, R. (2003). Social play and autistic spectrum disorders: A perspective on theory, implications and educational approaches. *Autism, 7,* 347–360.

Joseph, R. M., & Tager-Flusberg, H. (2004). The relationship between theory of mind and executive functions to symptom type and severity in children with autism. *Development and Psychopathology, 16,* 137–155.

Joseph, R. M., Tager-Flusberg, H., & Lord, C. (2002). Cognitive profiles and social-communicative functioning in children with autism spectrum disorder. *Journal of Child Psychology and Psychiatry, 43,* 807–821.

Joshi, G., Petty, C., Wozniak, J., Henin, A., Fried, R., Galdo, M., et al. (2010). The heavy burden of psychiatric comorbidity in youth with autism spectrum disorders: A large comparative study of a psychiatrically referred population. *Journal of Autism and Developmental Disorders, 40,* 1361–1370.

Kaland., N. (2011). Brief report: Should Asperger syndrome be excluded from the forthcoming DSM-5? *Research in Autism Spectrum Disorders, 5,* 984–989.

Kam, C. M., Greenberg, M. T., & Kusche, C. A. (2004). Sustained effect of the PATHS curriculum on the social and psychological adjustment of children in special education. *Journal of Emotional and Behavioral Disorders, 12,* 66–78.

Kamio, Y., & Toichi, M. (2000). Dual access to semantics in autism: Is pictorial access superior to verbal access? *Journal of Child Psychology and Psychiatry, 41,* 859–867.

Kamps, D., Leonard, B., Vernon, S., Dugan, E., Delquadri, J., Gershon, B., et al. (1992). Teaching social skills to students with autism to increase peer interactions in an integrated first-grade classroom. *Journal of Applied Behavior Analysis, 25,* 281–288.

Kamps, D., Royer, J., Dugan, E., Kravits, T., Gonzalez-Lopez, A., Garcia, J., et al. (2002). Peer training to facilitate social interaction for elementary students with autism and their peers. *Exceptional Children, 68,* 173–187.

Kanner, L. (1943). Autistic disturbance of affective contact. *Nervous Child, 2,* 217–250.

Kasari, C., Chamberlain, B., & Bauminger, N. (2001). Social emotions and social relationships in autism: Can children with autism compensate? In J. Burack, T.

Charman, N. Yirmiya, & P. Zelazo (Eds.), *Development and autism: Perspectives from theory and research* (pp. 309–323). Hillsdale, NJ: Erlbaum.

Kasari, C., Locke, J., Gulsrud, A., & Rotheram-Fuller, E. (2011). Social networks and friendships at school: Comparing children with and without ASD. *Journal of Autism and Developmental Disorders, 41,* 533–544.

Kasari, C., Rotheram-Fuller, E., Locke, J., & Gulsrud, A. (2012). Making the connection: Randomized controlled trial of social skills at school for children with autism spectrum disorders. *Journal of Child Psychology and Psychiatry, 53,* 431–439.

Kaufman, J., Birmaher, B., Brent, D., Rao, U., Flynn, C., Moreci, P., et al. (1997). Schedule for Affective Disorders and Schizophrenia for School-Age Children—Present and Lifetime Version (K-SADS-PL): Initial reliability and validity data. *Journal of the American Academy Child and Adolescent Psychiatry, 36,* 980–988.

Kessler, R. C., Berglund, P., Demler, O., Jin, R., Koretz, D., Merikangas, K. R., et al. (2003). The epidemiology of major depressive disorder: Results from the national comorbidity survey replication (NCS-R). *Journal of the American Medical Association, 289,* 3095–3105.

Kessler, R. C., Berglund, P., Demler, O., Jin, R., Merikangas, K. R., & Walters, E. E. (2005). Lifetime prevalence and age-of-onset distributions of DSM-IV disorders in the national comorbidity survey replication. *Archives of General Psychiatry, 62,* 593–602.

Kikuchi, Y., Senju, A., Tojo, Y., Osanai, H., & Hasegawa, T. (2009). Faces do not capture special attention in children with autism spectrum disorder: A change blindness study. *Child Development, 80,* 1421–1433.

Kim, J. A., Szatmari, P., Bryson, S. E., Streiner, D. L., & Wilson, F. J. (2000). The prevalence of anxiety and mood problems among children with autism and Asperger syndrome. *Autism, 4,* 117–133.

Kimhi, Y., & Bauminger-Zviely, N. (2012). Collaborative problem solving in preschoolers with HFASD and with typical development. *Journal of Autism and Developmental Disorders, 42,* 1984–1997.

Klin, A. (2000). Attributing social meaning to ambiguous visual stimuli in higher functioning autism and Asperger syndrome: The social attribution task. *Journal of Child Psychology and Psychiatry, 41,* 831–846.

Klin, A. (2011). Asperger's syndrome: From Asperger to modern day. In D. G. Amaral, G. Dawson, & D. H. Geschwind (Eds.), *Autism spectrum disorders* (pp. 44–59). New York: Oxford University Press.

Klin, A., Jones, W., Schultz, R., & Volkmar, F. (2003). The enactive mind or from actions to cognition: Lessons from autism. *Philosophical Transactions of the Royal Society B: Biological Sciences, 358,* 345–360.

Klin, A., Jones, W., Schultz, R., Volkmar, F., & Cohen, D. (2002). Visual fixation patterns during viewing of naturalistic social situations as predictors of social competence in individuals with autism. *Archives of General Psychiatry, 59,* 809–815.

Klin, A., Saulnier, C. A., Sparrow, S. S., Cicchetti, D. V., Volkmar, F. R., & Lord, C. (2007). Social and communication abilities and disabilities in higher functioning individuals with autism spectrum disorders: The Vineland and the ADOS. *Journal of Autism and Developmental Disorders, 42,* 161–174.

Klinger, L. G., & Williams, A. (2009). Cognitive-behavioral interventions for students with autism spectrum disorders. In M. J. Mayer, R. Van Acker, J. E. Lochman, & F. M. Gresham (Eds.), *Cognitive-behavioral interventions for emotional and behavioral disorders: School-based practice* (PP. 328–362). New York: Guilford Press.

Kluth, P., & Darmody-Latham, J. (2003). Beyond sight words: Literacy opportunities for students with autism. *The Reading Teacher, 56,* 532–535.

Koegel, L. K., Koegel, R. L., Green-Hopkins, I., & Barnes, C. C. (2010). Brief report:

Question asking and collateral language acquisition in children with autism. *Journal of Autism and Developmental Disorders, 40,* 509–515.

Koegel, L. K., Koegel, R. L., Harrower, J. K., & Carter, C. M. (1999). Pivotal response intervention: I. Overview of approach. *Journal of the Association for Persons with Severe Handicaps, 24,* 174–185.

Koegel, R. L., Koegel, L. K., & Carter, C. M. (1999). Pivotal teaching interactions for children with autism. *School Psychology Review, 28,* 576–594.

Koegel, R. L., Shirotova, L., & Koegel, L. K. (2009). Brief report: Using individualized orienting cues to facilitate first-word acquisition in non-responders with autism. *Journal of Autism and Developmental Disorders, 39,* 1587–1592.

Kokina, A., & Kern, L. (2010). Social Story interventions for students with autism spectrum disorders: A meta-analysis. *Journal of Autism and Developmental Disorders, 40,* 812–826.

Koning, C., & Magill-Evans, J. (2001). Social and language skills in adolescent boys with Asperger syndrome. *Autism, 5,* 23–36.

Koppenhaver, D. A., & Erickson, K. A. (2003). Natural emergent literacy supports for preschoolers with autism and severe communication impairments. *Topics in Language Disorders, 23*(4), 283–292.

Koren-Karie, N., Oppenheim, D., Dolev, S., & Yirmiya, N. (2009). Mothers of securely attached children with autism spectrum disorder are more sensitive than mothers of insecurely attached children. *Journal of Child Psychology and Psychiatry, 50,* 643–650.

Kovacs, M. (1992). *Children's Depression Inventory manual.* North Tonawanda, NY: Multi-Health Systems.

Krasny, L., Williams, B. J., Provencal, S., & Ozonoff, S. (2003). Social skills interventions for autism spectrum: Essential ingredients and a model curriculum. *Child and Adolescent Psychiatric Clinics, 12,* 107–122.

Krug, D. A., Arik, J., & Almond, P. (1980). Behavior checklist for identifying severely handicapped individuals with high levels of autistic behavior. *Journal of Child Psychology and Psychiatry, 21,* 221–229.

Kumpulainen, K., & Kaartinen, S. (2003). The interpersonal dynamics of collaborative reasoning in peer interactive dyads. *Journal of Experimental Education, 71,* 333–370.

Kuo, M. H., Orsmond, G. I., Cohn, E. S., & Coster, W. J. (2012). Friendship characteristics and activity patterns of adolescents with an autism spectrum disorder. *Autism.* Available at *www.aut.sagepub.com/content/early/2011/11/03/1362361 311416380.*

Kuschner, E. S., Bennetto, L., & Yost, K. (2007). Patterns of nonverbal cognitive functioning in young children with autism spectrum disorders. *Journal of Autism and Developmental Disorders, 37,* 795–807.

Kushki, A., Chau, T., & Anagnostou, E. (2011). Handwriting difficulties in children with autism spectrum disorders: A scoping review. *Journal of Autism and Developmental Disorders, 41,* 1706–1716.

Kuusikko, S., Pollock-Wurman, R., Jussila, K., Carter, A. S., Mattila, M., Ebeling, H., et al. (2008). Social anxiety in high-functioning children and adolescents with autism and Asperger syndrome. *Journal of Autism and Developmental Disorders, 38,* 1697–1709.

Lai, M. C., Lombardo, M. V., Pasco, G., Ruigrok, A. N. V., Wheelwright, S. J., Sadek, S. A., et al. (2011). A behavioral comparison of male and female adults with high-functioning autism spectrum conditions. *PLoS ONE, 6*(6), e20835.

Lainhart, J. E. (1999). Psychiatric problems in individuals with autism, their parents and siblings. *International Review of Psychiatry, 11,* 278–298.

Lam, Y. G., & Yeung, S. S. (2012). Cognitive deficits and symbolic play in preschoolers with autism. *Research in Autism Spectrum Disorders, 6,* 560–564.

Landa, R. (2000). Social language use in Asperger syndrome and in high-functioning autism. In A. Klin, F. R. Volkmar, & S. S. Sparrow (Eds.), *Asperger syndrome* (pp. 121–155). New York: Guilford Press.

Lane, K. L., Graham, S., Harris, K. R., & Weisenbach, J. L. (2006). Teaching writing strategies to young students struggling with writing and at risk for behavior disorders: Self-regulated strategy development. *Teaching Exceptional Children, 39*, 60–64.

Lasgaard, M., Nielsen, A., Eriksen, M. E., & Goossens, L. (2010). Loneliness and social support in adolescent boys with autism spectrum disorders. *Journal of Autism and Developmental Disorders, 40*, 218–226.

Laugeson, E., & Frankel, F. (2010). *Social skills for teenagers with developmental and autism spectrum disorders.* New York: Routledge Press.

Laugeson, E., Frankel, F., Gantman, A., Dillon, A., & Mogil, C. (2012). Evidence-based social skills training for adolescents with autism spectrum disorders: The UCLA PEERS program. *Journal of Autism and Developmental Disorders, 42*, 1025–1036.

Laurent, A. C., & Rubin, E. (2004). Emotional regulation challenges in Asperger syndrome and high-functioning autism. *Topics in Language Disorders, 24*, 286–297.

Lauth, B., Arnkelsson, G. B., Magnússon, P., Skarphéðinsson, G. Á., Ferrari, P., & Pétursson, H. (2010). Validity of K-SADS-PL (Schedule for Affective Disorders and Schizophrenia for School-Age Children—Present and Lifetime Version) depression diagnoses in an adolescent clinical population. *Nordic Journal of Psychiatry, 6*, 409–420.

Lecavalier, L. (2006). Behavioral and emotional problems in young people with pervasive developmental disorders: Relative prevalence, effects of subject characteristics, and empirical classification. *Journal of Autism and Developmental Disorders, 36*, 1101–1114.

Lecavalier, L., Gadow, K. D., DeVincent, C. J., & Edwards, M. C. (2009). Validation of DSM-IV model of psychiatric syndromes in children with autism spectrum disorder. *Journal of Autism and Developmental Disorders, 39*, 278–289.

Lee, D. O., & Ousley, O. Y. (2006). Attention-deficit hyperactivity disorder symptoms in a clinic sample of children and adolescents with pervasive developmental disorders. *Journal of Child and Adolescent Psychopharmacology, 16*, 737–746.

LeGoff, D. B. (2004). Use of LEGO® as a therapeutic medium for improving social competence. *Journal of Autism and Developmental Disorders, 34*, 557–571

Lehman, E. (Producer), & Nichols, M. (Director). (1966). *Who's afraid of Virginia Woolf?* [Motion picture]. United States: Warner Brothers.

Lehmkuhl, H. D., Storch, E. A., Bodfish, J. W., & Geffken, G. R. (2008). Exposure and response prevention for obsessive-compulsive disorders in a 12-year-old with autism. *Journal of Autism and Developmental Disorders, 38*, 977–981.

Lemerise, E. A., & Arsenio, W. F. (2000). An integrated model of emotion processes and cognition in social information processing. *Child Development, 71*, 107–118.

Lemon, J. M., Gargaro, B., Enticott, P. G., & Rinehart, N. J. (2011). Executive functioning in autism spectrum disorders: A gender comparison of response inhibition. *Journal of Autism and Developmental Disorders, 41*, 352–356.

Lewis, M. (1993). The emergence of human emotions. In M. Lewis & J. M. Haviland (Eds.), *Handbook of emotions* (pp. 223–235). New York: Guilford Press.

Leyfer, O. T., Folstein, S. E., Bacalman, S., Davis, N. O., Dinh, E., Morgan, J., et al. (2006). Comorbid psychiatric disorders in children with autism: Interview development and rates of disorders. *Journal of Autism and Developmental Disorders, 36*, 849–861.

Licciardello, C. C., Harchik, A. E., & Luiseli, J. K. (2008). Social skills intervention for children with autism during interactive play at a public elementary school. *Education and Treatment of Children, 31*, 27–37.

Liebal, K., Colombi, C., Rogers, S., Warneken, F., & Tomasello, M. (2008). Cooperative activities in children with autism. *Journal of Autism and Developmental Disorders, 38,* 224–238.

Lind, S. E. (2010). Memory and the self in autism: A review and theoretical framework. *Autism, 14,* 430–456.

Lind, S. E., & Bowler, D. M. (2009). Recognition memory, self–other source memory, and theory of mind in children with autism spectrum disorder. *Journal of Autism and Developmental Disorders, 39,* 1231–1239.

Lind, S. E., & Bowler, D. M. (2010). Episodic memory and episodic future thinking in adults with autism. *Journal of Abnormal Psychology, 119,* 896–905.

Liss, M., Fein, D., Allen, D., Dunn, M., Feistein, C., Norris, R., et al. (2001). Executive functioning in high-functioning children with autism. *Journal of Child Psychology and Psychiatry, 42,* 261–270.

Little, L. (2002). Middle-class mothers' perceptions of peer and sibling victimization among children with Asperger's syndrome and nonverbal learning disorders. *Issues in Comprehensive Pediatric Nursing, 25,* 43–57.

Locke, J., Ishijima, E., Kasari, C., & London, N. (2010). Loneliness, friendship quality and the social networks of adolescents with high-functioning autism in an inclusive school setting. *Journal of Research in Special Educational Needs, 10,* 74–81.

Loftin, R. L., Odom, S. L., & Lantz, J. F. (2008). Social interaction and repetitive motor behaviors. *Journal of Autism and Developmental Disorders, 38,* 1124–1135.

Lombardo, M. V., & Baron-Cohen, S. (2011). The role of the self in mindblindness in autism. *Consciousness and Cognition, 20,* 130–140.

Lopez, B., & Leekam, S. R. (2003). Do children with autism fail to process information in context? *Journal of Child Psychology and Psychiatry, 44,* 285–300.

Lopez, B., Leekam, S. R., & Arts, G. R. J. (2008). How central is central coherence?: Preliminary evidence on the link between conceptual and perceptual processing in children with autism. *Autism, 12,* 159–171.

Lopez, B. R., Lincoln, A. J., Ozonoff, S., & Lai, Z. (2005). Examining the relationship between executive functions and restricted, repetitive symptoms of autistic disorder. *Journal of Autism and Developmental Disorders, 35,* 445–460.

Lord, C. (2010). Autism: From research to practice. *American Psychologist, 65,* 815–826.

Lord, C., Floody, H., Anderson, D., & Pickles, A. (2003). *Social engagement in very young children with autism: Differences across context.* Paper presented at the meeting of the Society for Research in Child Development, Tampa, FL.

Lord, C., & Jones, R. M. (2012). Annual research review: Re-thinking the classification of autism spectrum disorders. *Journal of Child Psychology and Psychiatry, 53,* 490–509.

Lord, C., & Magill-Evans, J. (1995). Peer interactions of autistic children and adolescents. *Development and Psychopathology, 7,* 611–626.

Lord, C., Petkova, E., Hus, V., Gan, W., Lu, F., Martin, D. M., et al. (2012). A multisite study of the clinical diagnosis of different autism spectrum disorders. *Archives of General Psychiatry, 69,* 306–313.

Lord, C., Risi, S., Lambrecht, L., Cook, E. H., Leventhal., B. L., DiLavore, P. C., et al. (2000). The Autism Diagnostic Observational Schedule—Generic: A standard measure of social and communication deficits associated with the spectrum of autism. *Journal of Autism and Developmental Disorders, 30,* 205–223.

Lord, C., Rutter, M., & Le Couteur, A. (1994). Autism Diagnostic Interview—Revised: A revised version of a diagnostic interview for caregivers of individuals with possible pervasive developmental disorders. *Journal of Autism and Developmental Disorders, 24,* 659–685.

Lord, C., & Schopler, E. (1985). Differences in sex ratios in autism as a function of measured intelligence. *Journal of Autism and Developmental Disorders, 15,* 185–193.

Lord, C., Schopler, E., & Revicki, D. (1982). Sex differences in autism. *Journal of Autism and Developmental Disorders, 12,* 317–330.

Lord, C., Wagner, A., Rogers, S., Szatmari, P., Aman, M., Charman, T., et al. (2005). Challenges in evaluating psychosocial interventions for autistic spectrum disorders. *Journal of Autism and Developmental Disorders, 35,* 695–708.

Losh, M., & Capps, L. (2003). Narrative ability in high-functioning children wih autism or Asperger's syndrome. *Journal of Autism and Developmental Disorders, 33,* 239–251.

Losh, M., & Capps, L. (2006). Understanding of emotional experience in autism: Insights from the personal accounts of high-functioning children with autism. *Developmental Psychology, 42,* 809–818.

Loth, E., Gomez, J. C., & Happé, F. (2008). Event schemas in autism spectrum disorders: The role of theory of mind and weak central coherence. *Journal of Autism and Developmental Disorders, 38,* 449–463.

Loveland, K. A., Pearson, D. A., Tunali-Kotoski, B., Ortegon, J., & Gibbs, M. C. (2001). Judgments of social appropriateness by children and adolescents with autism. *Journal of Autism and Developmental Disorders, 31,* 367–376.

Luria, A. R. (1961). *The role of speech and language in the regulation of normal and abnormal behavior.* New York: Macmillan.

Macintosh, K., & Dissanayake, C. (2004). Annotation: The similarities and differences between autistic disorder and Asperger's disorder: A review of empirical evidence. *Journal of Child Psychology and Psychiatry, 45,* 421–434.

Macintosh, K., & Dissanayake, C. (2006). A comparative study of the spontaneous social interactions of children with high-functioning autism and children with Asperger's disorder. *Autism, 10,* 199–220.

Mackay, T., Knott, F., & Dunlop, A. (2007). Developing social interaction and understanding in individuals with autism spectrum disorder: A groupwork intervention. *Journal of Intellectual and Developmental Disability, 32,* 279–290.

Main, M., & Solomon, J. (1986). Discovery of an insecure-disorganized/disoriented attachment pattern. In T. Brazelton & M. W. Yogman (Eds.), *Affective development in infancy* (pp. 95–124). Norwood, NJ: Ablex.

Main, M., & Solomon, J. (1990). Procedures for identifying infants as disorganized/disoriented during the Ainsworth Strange Situation. In M. T. Greenberg, D. Cicchetti, & E. M. Cummings (Eds.), *Attachment in the preschool years: Theory, research and intervention* (pp. 134–146). Chicago: University of Chicago Press.

Manning, M. M., & Wainwright, L. D. (2010). The role of high-level play as a predictor social functioning in autism. *Journal of Autism and Developmental Disorders 40,* 523–533.

Manolitsi, M., & Botting, N. (2011). Language abilities in children with autism and language impairment: Using narrative as an additional source of clinical information. *Child Language Teaching and Therapy, 27,* 39–55.

Marcu, I., Oppenheim, D., Koren-Karie, N., Dolev, S., & Yirmiya, N. (2009). Attachment and symbolic play in preschoolers with autism spectrum disorders. *Journal of Autism and Developmental Disorders, 39,* 1321–1328.

Mason, R. M., Williams, D. L., Kana, R. K., Minshew, N., & Just, M. A. (2008). Theory of mind disruption and recruitment of the right hemisphere during narrative comprehension in autism. *Neuropsychologia, 46,* 269–280.

Matson, J. L., & Love, S. R. (1990). A comparison of parent-reported fear for autistic and nonhandicapped age-matched children and youth. *Australian and New Zealand Journal of Developmental Disabilities, 16,* 349–357.

Matson, J. L., & Nebel-Schwalm, M. S. (2007). Comorbid psychopathology with autism spectrum disorder in children: An overview. *Research in Developmental Disabilities, 28,* 341–352.

Mattila, M. L., Hurtig, T., Haapsamo, H., Jussila, K., Kuusikko-Gauffin, S., Kielinen,

M., et al. (2010). Comorbid psychiatric disorders associated with Asperger syndrome/high-functioning autism: A community and clinic-based study. *Journal of Autism and Developmental Disorders, 40,* 1080–1093.

Mayes, D. S., Calhoun, S. L., Mayes, R. D., & Molitoris, S. (2012). Autism and ADHD: Overlapping and discriminating symptoms. *Research in Autism Spectrum Disorder, 6,* 277–285.

Mayes, D. S., Calhoun, S. L., Murray, M. J., Ahuja, M., & Smith, A. S. (2011). Anxiety, depression, and irritability in children with autism relative to other neuropsychiatric disorders and typical development. *Research in Autism Spectrum Disorders, 5,* 474–485.

Mayes, S. D., & Calhoun, S. L. (2003a). Ability profiles in children with autism: Influence of age and IQ. *Autism, 6,* 65–80.

Mayes, S. D., & Calhoun, S. L. (2003b). Analysis of WISC-III, Stanford-Binet IV, and academic achievement test scores in children with autism. *Journal of Autism and Developmental Disorders, 33,* 329–341.

Mayes, S. D., & Calhoun, S. L. (2006). Frequency of reading, math, and writing disabilities in children with clinical disorders. *Learning and Individual Differences, 16,* 145–157.

Mazefsky, C. A. Anderson, R., Conner, C. M., & Minshew, N. (2011). Child Behavior Checklist scores for school-aged children with autism: Preliminary evidence of patterns suggesting the need for referral. *Journal of Psychopathology and Behavioral Assessment, 33,* 31–37.

Mazefsky, C. A., Conner, C. M., & Oswald, D. P. (2010). Association between depression and anxiety in high-functioning children with autism spectrum disorders and maternal mood symptoms. *Autism Research, 3,* 120–127.

Mazurek, M. O., & Kanne, N. (2010). Friendship and internalizing symptoms among children and adolescents with ASD. *Journal of Autism and Developmental Disorders, 40,* 1512–1520.

McCann, J., Peppe, S., Gibbon, F. E., O'Hare, A., & Rutherford, M. (2007). Prosody and its relationship to language in school-aged children with high-functioning autism. *International Journal of Language and Communication Disorders, 42,* 682–702.

McDonnell, J., Johnson, J. W., Polychronis, S., & Riesen, T. (2002). The effects of embedded instruction on students with moderate disabilities enrolled in general education classes. *Education and Training in Mental Retardation and Developmental Disabilities, 37,* 363–377.

McDuffie, A., Turner, L., Stone, W., Yoder, P., Wolery, M., & Ulman, T. (2007). Developmental correlates of different types of motor imitation in young children with autism spectrum disorders. *Journal of Autism and Developmental Disorders, 37,* 401–412.

McEvoy, R. E., Rogers, S. J., & Pennington, B. F. (1993). Executive function and social communication deficits in young autistic children. *Journal of Child Psychology and Psychiatry, 34,* 563–578.

McGee, G. G., Feldman, R., & Chernin, L. (1991). A comparison of emotional facial display by children with autism and typical preschoolers. *Journal of Early Intervention, 15,* 237–245.

McGovern, C. W., & Sigman, M. (2005). Continuity and change from early childhood to adolescence in autism. *Journal of Child Psychology and Psychiatry, 46,* 401–408.

McLennan, J. D., Lord, C., & Schopler, E. (1993). Sex differences in higher functioning people with autism. *Journal of Autism and Developmental Disorders, 23,* 217–227.

McPartland, J. C., Webb, S. J., Keehn, B., & Dawson, G. (2011). Patterns of visual attention to faces and objects in autism spectrum disorder. *Journal of Autism and Developmental Disorders, 41,* 148–157.

McPheeter, M. L., Davis, A., Navarre, J. R., & Scott, T. A. (2011). Family report of ASD concomitant with depression or anxiety among U.S. children. *Journal of Autism and Developmental Disorders, 41,* 646–653.

Meek, S. E., Robinson, L. T., & Jahromi, C. B. (2012). Parent–child predictors of social competence with peers in children with and without autism. *Research in Autism Spectrum Disorders, 6,* 815–823.[0]

Merikangas, K. R., He, J. P., Burstein, M., Swanson, S. A., Avenevoli, S., Cui, L., et al. (2010). Lifetime prevalence of mental disorders in U.S. adolescents: Results from the National Comorbidity Survey Replication—Adolescent Supplement (NCS-A). *Journal of the American Academy of Child and Adolescent Psychiatry, 49,* 980–989.

Mesibov, G., & Shea, V. (2011). Evidence-based practices and autism. *Autism, 15,* 114–133.

Mesibov, G., Shea, V., & Schopler, E. (2005). *The TEACCH approach to autism spectrum disorders.* New York: Plenum.

Meyer, J. A., Mundy, P. C., Van Hecke, A.V., & Durocher, J. S. (2006). Social attribution processes and comorbid psychiatric symptoms in children with Asperger syndrome. *Autism, 10,* 383–402.

Millward, C., Powell, S., Messer, D., & Jordan, R. (2000). Recall for self and other in autism: Children's memory for events experienced by themselves and their peers. *Journal of Autism and Developmental Disorders, 30,* 15–28.

Minshew, N. J., & Goldstein, G. (2001). The pattern of intact and impaired memory functions in autism. *Journal of Child Psychology and Psychiatry, 42,* 1095–1101.

Minshew, N. J., Turner, C. A., & Goldstein, G. (2005). The application of short forms of the Wechsler intelligence scales in adults and children with high functioning autism. *Journal of Autism and Developmental Disorders, 35,* 45–52.

Mitchell, S., Brian, J., Zwaigenbaum, L., Roberts, W., Szatmari, P., Smith, I., et al. (2006). Early language and communication development of infants later diagnosed with autism spectrum disorder. *Journal of Developmental and Behavioral Pediatrics, 27,* 69–78.

Moree, B. N., & Davis, T. E. (2010). Cognitive-behavioral therapy for anxiety in children diagnosed with autism spectrum disorders: Modification trends. *Research in Autism Spectrum Disorders, 4,* 346–354.

Morrison, L., Kamps, D., Garcia, J., & Parker, D. (2001). Peer mediation and monitoring strategies to improve initiations and social skills for students with autism. *Journal of Positive Behavior Interventions, 3,* 337–250.

Morsanyi, K., & Holyoak, K. J. (2010). Analogical reasoning ability in autistic and typically developing children. *Developmental Science, 13,* 578–587.

Moss, J., Magiati, I., Charman, T., & Howlin, P. (2008). Stability of the Autism Diagnostic Interview—Revised from pre-school to elementary school age in children with autism spectrum disorders. *Journal of Autism and Developmental Disorder, 38,* 1081–1091.

Mullen, E. M. (1995). *Mullen Scales of Early Learning* (AGS ed.). Circle Pines, MN: American Guidance Service.

Mundy, P. (1995). Joint attention and social-emotional approach behavior in children with autism. *Development and Psychopathology, 7,* 63–82.

Mundy, P., & Jarrold, W. (2010). Infant joint attention, neural networks and social cognition. *Neural Networks, 23,* 985–997.

Mundy, P., & Newell, L. C. (2007). Attention, joint attention, and social cognition. *Current Directions in Psychological Science, 16,* 269–274.

Mundy, P., & Sigman, M. (2006). Joint attention, social competence, and developmental psychopathology. In D. Cicchetti, & D. Cohen (Eds.), *Developmental psychopathology: Theory and methods* (2nd ed., Vol. 1, pp. 293–332). Hoboken, NJ: Wiley.

Mundy, P., Sigman, M., & Kasari, C. (1994). Joint attention, developmental level, and symptom presentation in autism. *Development and Psychopathology, 6,* 389–401.

Mundy, P., & Stella, J. (2001). Joint attention, social orientation, and communication in autism. In A. M. Wetherby & B. M. Prizant (Eds.), *Autism spectrum disorders: A transactional developmental perspective* (pp. 55–78). London: Brookes.

Mundy, P., Sullivan, L., & Mastergeorge, A. M. (2009). A parallel and distributed-processing model of joint attention, social cognition, and autism. *Autism Research, 2,* 2–21.

Murdock, L. C., & Hobbs, J. Q. (2011). Picture me playing: Increasing pretend play dialogue of children with autism spectrum disorders. *Journal of Autism and Developmental Disorders, 41,* 870–878.

Murray, M. J. (2010). Attention-deficit/hyperactivity disorder in the context of autism spectrum disorders. *Current Psychiatry Reports, 12,* 382–388.

Naber, F. B. A., Bakermans-Kranenburg, M. J., van IJzendoorn, M. H., Swinkels, S. H. N., Buitelaar, J. K., Dietz, C., et al. (2008). Play behavior and attachment in toddlers with autism. *Journal of Autism Developmental Disorders, 38,* 857–866.

Naber, F. B. A., Swinkels, S. H. N., Buitelaar, J. K., Bakermans-Kranenburg, M. J., van IJzendoorn, M. H., Dietz, C., et al. (2007). Attachment in toddlers with autism and other developmental disorders. *Journal of Autism and Developmental Disorders, 37,* 1123–1138.

Naber, F. B. A., Swinkels, S. H. N., Buitelaar, J. K., Dietz, C., van Daalen, E., Bakermans-Kranenburg, M. J., et al. (2007). Joint attention and attachment in toddlers with autism. *Journal of Abnormal Child Psychology, 35,* 899–911.

Nadig, A., Lee, I., Singh, L., Bosshart, K., & Ozonoff, S. (2010). How does the topic of conversation affect verbal exchange and eye gaze? A comparison between typical development and high-functioning autism. *Neuropsychologia, 48,* 2730–2739.

Nadig, A., Ozonoff, S., Young, G., Rozga, A., Sigman, M., & Rogers, S. (2007). A prospective study of response to name in infants at risk for autism. *Archives of Pediatric and Adolescent Medicine, 161,* 378–383.

Nah, Y., & Poon, K. (2011). The perception of social situations by children with autism spectrum disorders. *Autism, 15,* 185–203.

Nathan, M. J., Eilam, B., & Kim, S. (2007). To disagree, we must also agree: How intersubjectivity structures and perpetuates discourse in a mathematics classroom. *Journal of the Learning Sciences, 16,* 523–563.

Nation, K., Clarke, P., Wright, B., & Williams, C. (2006). Patterns of reading ability in children with autism spectrum disorder. *Journal of Autism and Developmental Disorders, 36,* 911–919.

Nation, K., & Penny, S. (2008). Sensitivity to eye gaze in autism: Is it normal? Is it automatic? Is it social? *Development and Psychopathology, 20,* 79–97.

National Research Council. (2001). *Educating children with autism.* Committee on Educational Interventions for Children with Autism, Division of Behavioral and Social Sciences and Education. Washington, DC: National Academy Press.

Neisser, U. (1988). Five kinds of self-knowledge. *Philosophical Psychology, 1,* 35–59.

Nelson, J. R., Benner, G. J., Lane, K., & Smith, B. W. (2004). Academic achievement of K–12 students with emotional and behavioral disorders. *Exceptional Children, 71,* 59–73.

Neuhaus, E., Beauchaine, T. B., & Bernier, R. (2010). Neurobiological correlates of social functioning in autism. *Clinical Psychology Review, 30,* 733–748.

New, J. J., Schultz, R. T., Wolf, J., Niehaus, J. L., Klin, A., German, T. C., et al. (2010). The scope of social attention deficits in autism: Prioritized orienting to people and animals in static natural scenes. *Neuropsychologia, 48,* 51–59.

References

299

Newcomb, A. F., & Bagwell, C. L. (1995). Children's friendship relations: A meta-analytic review. *Psychological Bulletin, 117,* 306–347.

Newman, T. M., Macomber, D., Naples, A. J., Babitz, T., Volkmar, F., & Grigorenko, E. L. (2007). Hyperlexia in children with autism spectrum disorders. *Journal of Autism and Developmental Disorders, 37,* 760–774.

Norbury, C. F. (2005). Barking up the wrong tree?: Lexical ambiguity resolution in children with language impairments and autistic spectrum disorders. *Journal of Experimental Child Psychology, 90,* 142–171.

Norbury, C. F., Griffiths, H., & Nation, K. (2010). Sound before meaning: Word learning in autistic disorders. *Neuropsychologia, 48,* 4012–4019.

Nuske, H. J., & Bavin, E. L. (2011). Narrative comprehension in 4–7-year-old children with autism: Testing the weak central coherence account. *International Journal of Language and Communication Disorders, 46,* 108–119.

O'Connor, I., & Klein, P. (2004). Explorations of strategies for facilitating the reading comprehension of high-functioning students with autism spectrum disorders. *Journal of Autism and Developmental Disorders, 34,* 115–127.

Odom, S. L., Collet-Klingenberg, L., Rogers, S., & Hatton, D. D. (2010). Evidence-based practices in interventions for children and youth with autism spectrum disorders. *Preventing School Failure, 54,* 275–282.

Oelwein, P. L. (1995). *Teaching reading to children with Down syndrome: A guide for parents and teachers.* Bethesda, MD: Woodbine House.

Oppenheim, D., Koren-Karie, N., Dolev, S., & Yirmiya, N. (2009). Maternal insightfulness and resolution of the diagnosis are associated with secure attachment in preschoolers with autism spectrum disorders. *Child Development, 80,* 519–527.

Orsmond, G., Krauss, M., & Seltzer, M. (2004). Peer relationships and social and recreational activities among adolescents and adults with autism. *Journal of Autism and Developmental Disabilities, 34,* 245–256.

Orsmond, G. I., & Kuo, H. (2011). The daily lives of adolescents with an autism spectrum disorder: Discretionary time use and activity partners. *Autism, 15,* 1–21.

Owen-DeSchryver, J., Carr, E., Cale, S., & Blakeley-Smith, A. (2008). Promoting social interactions between students with autism spectrum disorders and their peers in inclusive school settings. *Focus on Autism and Other Developmental Disabilities, 23,* 15–28.

Owens, G., Granader, Y., Humphrey, A., & Baron-Cohen, S (2008). LEGO® therapy and the social use of language program: An evaluation of two social skills interventions for children with high-functioning autism and Asperger syndrome. *Journal of Autism and Developmental Disorders, 38,* 1944–1957.

Ozonoff, S., Iosif, A. M., Baguio, F., Cook, I., Hill, M., Hutman, T., et al. (2010). A prospective study of the emergence of early behavioral signs of autism. *Journal of the American Academy of Child and Adolescent Psychiatry, 49,* 256–266.

Ozonoff, S., Macari, S., Young, G., Goldring, S., Thompson, M., & Rogers, S. (2008). Atypical object exploration at 12 months of age is associated with autism in a prosective sample. *Autism, 12,* 457–472.

Ozonoff, S., & Miller, J. N. (1995). Teaching theory of mind: A new approach to social skills training for individuals with autism. *Journal of Autism and Developmental Disorders, 25,* 415–433.

Ozonoff, S., Pennington, B. F., & Rogers, S. J. (1991). Executive function deficits in high-functioning autistic individuals: Relationship to theory of mind. *Journal of Child Psychology and Psychiatry, 32,* 1081–1105.

Ozonoff, S., South, M., & Provencal, S. (2005). Executive functions. In F. R. Volkmar, R. Paul, A. Klin, & D. Cohen (Eds.), *Handbook of autism and pervasive developmental disorders* (3rd ed., pp. 606–627). Hoboken, NJ: Wiley.

Ozonoff, S., & Strayer, D. L. (2001). Further evidence of intact working memory in autism. *Journal of Autism and Developmental Disorders, 31,* 257–263.

Palmen, A., Didden, R., & Arts, M. (2008). Improving question asking in high-functioning adolescents with autism spectrum disorders: Effectiveness of small-group training. *Autism, 12,* 83–98.

Pandolfi, V., Magyar, C. I., & Dill, C. A. (2009). Confirmatory factor analysis of the Child Behavior Checklist 1.5–5 in a sample of children with autism spectrum disorders. *Journal of Autism and Developmental Disorders, 39,* 986–995.

Pandolfi, V., Magyar, C. I., & Dill, C. A. (2012). An initial psychometric evaluation of the CBCL 6–18 in a sample of youth with autism spectrum disorders. *Research in Autism Spectrum Disorders, 33,* 134–145.

Parker, J., & Gottman, J. M. (1989). Social and emotional development in a relational context: Friendship interaction from early childhood to adolescence. In T. J. Berndt & G. W. Ladd (Eds.), *Peer relationships in child development* (pp. 95–131). New York: Wiley.

Paul, R. (2003). Promoting social communication in high-functioning individuals with autistic spectrum disorders. *Child and Adolescent Psychiatric Clinics, 12,* 87–106.

Paul, R., Orlovski, S. M., Marcinko, H. C., & Volkmar, F. (2009). Conversational behaviors in youth with high-functioning ASD and Asperger syndrome. *Journal of Autism and Developmental Disorders, 39,* 115–125.

Pellicano, E. (2007). Links between theory of mind and executive function in young children: Clues to developmental primacy. *Developmental Psychology, 43,* 974–990.

Pellicano, E., Maybery, M., Durkin, K., & Maley, A. (2006). Multiple cognitive capabilities/deficits in children with an autism spectrum disorder: "Weak" central coherence and its relationship to theory of mind and executive control. *Development and Psychopathology, 18,* 77–98.

Pennington, R. C. (2009). Exploring new waters: Writing instruction for students with autism spectrum disorders. *Beyond Behavior, 19,* 17–25.

Perkins, M. R., Dobbinson, S., Boucher, J., Bol, S., & Bloom, P. (2006). Lexical knowledge and lexical use in autism. *Journal of Autism and Developmental Disorders, 36,* 795–805.

Perner, J., & Wimmer, H. (1985). "John thinks that Mary thinks that . . ": Attribution of second-order beliefs by 5- to 10-year-old children. *Journal of Experimental Child Psychology, 39,* 437–471.

Persicke, A., Tarbox, A., Ranick, J., & St. Clair, M. (2012). Establishing metaphorical reasoning in children with autism. *Research in Autism Spectrum Disorders, 6,* 913–920.

Petersen, D. J., Bilenberg, N., Hoerder, K., & Gillberg, C. (2006). The population prevalence of child psychiatric disorders in Danish 8- to 9-year-old children. *European Child and Adolescent Psychiatry, 15,* 71–78.

Peterson, C. C., Garnett, M., Kelly, A., & Attwood, T. (2009). Everyday social and conversation applications of theory-of-mind understanding by children with autism-spectrum disorders or typical development. *European Child and Adolescent Psychiatry, 18,* 105–115.

Pexman, P. M., Rostad, K. R., McMorris, C. A., Climie, E. A., Stowkowy, J., & Glenwright, M. R. (2011). Processing of ironic language in children with high-functioning autism spectrum disorder. *Journal of Autism and Developmental Disorders, 41,* 1097–1112.

Phelan, H. L., Filliten, J. H., & Johnson, S. A. (2011). Brief report: Memory performance on the California Verbal Learning Test—Children's Version in autism spectrum disorder. *Journal of Autism and Developmental Disorders, 41,* 518–523.

Philip, R. C. M., Whalley, H. C., Stanfield, A. C., Sprengelmeyer, R., Santos, I. M., Young, A. W., et al. (2010). Deficits in facial, body movement and vocal emotional processing in autism spectrum disorder. *Psychological Medicine, 40,* 1919–1929.

Prizant, B. M., Wetherby, A. M., Rubin, E., Laurent, A. C., & Rydell, P. J. (2006). *The SCERTS model: Vol. II. Program planning and intervention.* Baltimore: Brookes.

Ramachandran, R., Mitchell, P., & Ropar, D. (2009). Do individuals with autism spectrum disorders infer traits from behavior? *Journal of Child Psychology and Psychiatry, 50,* 871–878.

Randi, J., Newman, T., & Grigorenko, E. L. (2010). Teaching children with autism to read for meaning: Challenges and possibilities. *Journal of Autism and Developmental Disorders, 40,* 890–902.

Raven, J. C., Court, J. H., & Raven, J. (1983). *Manual for Raven's Progressive Matrices and Vocabulary Scales: Advanced progressive matrices sets I and II.* London: H. K. Lewis.

Raven, J. C., Court, J. H., & Raven, J. (1990a). *Coloured Progressive Matrices.* Oxford, UK: Oxford University Press.

Raven, J. C., Court, J. H., & Raven, J. (1990b). *Standard Progressive Matrices.* Oxford, UK: Oxford University Press.

Reaven, J., Blakeley-Smith, A., Culhane-Shelburne, K., & Hepburn, S. (2012). Group cognitive behavior therapy for children with high-functioning autism spectrum disorders and anxiety: A randomized trial. *Journal of Child Psychology and Psychiatry, 53,* 410–419.

Reaven, J., Blakeley-Smith, A., Nichols, S., Dasari, M., Flanigan, E., & Hepburn, S. (2009). Cognitive behavioral group treatment for anxiety symptoms in children with high-functioning autism spectrum disorders: A pilot study. *Focus on Autism and Other Developmental Disabilities, 24,* 27–37.

Reaven, J., & Hepburn, S. (2003). Cognitive-behavioral treatment of obsessive–compulsive disorder in a child with Asperger syndrome. *Autism, 7,* 145–164.

Reed, T. (2002). Visual perspective taking as a measure of working memory in participants with autism. *Journal of Developmental and Physical Disabilities, 14,* 63–76.

Reichow, B. (2012). Overview of meta-analyses on early intensive behavioral intervention for young children with autism spectrum disorders. *Journal of Autism and Developmental Disorders, 42,* 512–520

Reichow, B., & Wolery, M. (2009). Comprehensive synthesis of early intensive behavioral interventions for young children with autism based on the UCLA Young Autism Project model. *Journal of Autism and Developmental Disorders, 39,* 23–41.

Reid, R., & Lienemann, T. O. (2006). Self-regulated strategy development for written expression with students with attention-deficit/hyperactivity disorder. *Exceptional Children, 73,* 53–68.

Reiersen, A. M., Constantino, J. N., Volk, H. E., & Todd, R. D. (2007). Autistic traits in a population-based ADHD twin sample. *Journal of Child Psychology and Psychiatry, 48,* 464–472.

Reiersen, A. M., & Todd. R. D. (2011). Attention-deficit/hyperactivity (ADHD). In D. G. Amaral, G. Dawson, & D. H. Geschwind (Eds.), *Autism spectrum disorders* (pp. 304–314). New York: Oxford University Press.

Reynhout, G., & Carter, M. (2006). Social stories for children with disabilities. *Journal of Autism and Developmental Disorders, 36,* 445–469.

Reynolds, C. R., & Kamphaus, R. W. (2004). *Behavior Assessment System for Children* (2nd ed.). Circle Pines, MN: American Guidance Service.

Riby, D., & Hancock, P. J. B. (2008). Viewing it differently: Social scene perception in Williams syndrome and autism. *Neuropsychologia, 46,* 2855–2860.

Riby, D., & Hancock, P. J. B. (2009). Do faces capture the attention of children with Williams syndrome or autism?: Evidence from tracking eye movements. *Journal of Autism and Developmental Disorders, 39,* 421–431.

Rieffe, C., Terwogt, M. M., & Kotronopoulou, K. (2007). Awareness of single and multiple emotions in high-functioning children with autism. *Journal of Autism and Developmental Disorders, 37,* 455–465.

Rieffe, C., Terwogt, M. M., & Stockmann, L. (2000). Understanding atypical emotions among children with autism. *Journal of Autism and Developmental Disorders, 30,* 195–203.

Roberts, V., & Joiner, R. (2007). Investigating the efficacy of concept mapping with pupils with autistic spectrum disorder. *British Journal of Special Education, 34,* 127–135.

Robinson, S., Goddard, L., Dritschel, B., Wisley, M., & Howlin, P. (2009). Executive functions in children with autism spectrum disorders. *Brain and Cognition, 71,* 362–368.

Rogers, S. (2000). Interventions that facilitate socialization in children with autism. *Journal of Autism and Developmental Disorders, 30,* 399–409.

Rogers, S. R., & Bennetto, L. (2001). Intersubjectivity in autism: The role of imitation and executive function. In A. M. Wetherby & B. M. Prizant (Eds.), *Autism spectrum disorders: A transactional developmental perspective* (Vol. 9, pp. 79–107). Baltimore: Brookes.

Rogers, S. R., Ozonoff, S., & Maslin-Cole, C. (1991). A comparative study of attachment behavior in young children with autism or other psychiatric development. *Journal of the American Academy of Child and Adolescent Psychiatry, 30,* 483–488.

Rogers, S. R., Ozonoff, S., & Maslin-Cole, C. (1993). Developmental aspects of attachment behavior in young children with pervasive developmental disorder. *Journal of the American Academy of Child and Adolescent Psychiatry, 32,* 1274–1282.

Rogers, S. R., & Pennington, B. F. (1991). A theoretical approach to the deficits in infantile autism. *Development and Psychopathology, 3,* 137–162.

Roid, G. H., & Miller, L. J. (1997). *Leiter International Performance Scale—Revised.* Wood Dale, IL: Stoelting.

Ronald, A., Simonoff, E., Kuntsi, J., Asherson, P., & Plomin, R. (2008). Evidence for overlapping genetic influences on autistic and ADHD behaviors in a community twin sample. *Journal of Child Psychology and Psychiatry, 49,* 535–542.

Ronen, T. (1998). Linking development and emotional elements into child and family cognitive-behavioral therapy. In P. Graham (Ed.), *Cognitive-behavior therapy for children and families* (pp. 1–17). New York: Cambridge University Press.

Rotheram-Fuller, E., Kasari, C., Chamberlain, B., & Locke, J. (2010). Social involvement of children with autism spectrum disorders in elementary school classrooms, *Journal of Child Psychology and Psychiatry, 51,* 1227–1234.

Rubin, E., & Laurent, A. C. (2004). Implementing a curriculum-based assessment to prioritize learning objectives in Asperger syndrome and high-functioning autism. *Topics in Language Disorders, 24,* 298–315.

Rubin, E., & Lennon, L. (2004). Challenges in social communication in Asperger syndrome and high-functioning autism. *Topics in Language Disorders, 24,* 271–285.

Rubin, K. H., Bukowski, W. M., & Laursen, B. (Eds.). (2009). *Handbook of peer interaction, relationships and groups.* New York: Guilford Press

Rump, K. M., Giovannelli, J. L., Minshew, N. J., & Strauss, M. S. (2009). The development of emotion recognition in individuals with autism. *Child Development, 80,* 1434–1447.

Rundblad, G., & Annaz, D. (2010). The atypical development of metaphor and metonymy comprehension in children. *Autism, 14,* 29–36.

Russell, E., & Sofronoff, K. (2005). Anxiety and social worries in children with Asperger syndrome. *Australasian and New Zealand Journal of Psychiatry, 39,* 633–638.

Rutgers, A. H., Bakermans-Kranenburg, M. J., van IJzendoorn, M. H., & van Bercke-laer-Onnes, I. A. (2004). Autism and attachment: A meta-analytic review. *Journal of Child Psychology and Psychiatry, 45*, 1123–1134.

Rutherford, M. D., & Rogers, S. J. (2003). The cognitive underpinnings of pretend play in autism. *Journal of Autism and Developmental Disorders, 33*, 289–302.

Rutherford, M. D., Young, G. S., Hepburn, S., & Rogers, S. J. (2007). A longitudinal study of pretend play in autism. *Journal of Autism and Developmental Disorders, 37*, 1024–1039.

Rutter, M., Le Couteur, A., & Lord, C. (2003). *The Autism Diagnostic Interview—Revised (ADI-R) manual.* Los Angeles: Western Psychological Services.

Ryan, C., & Charragáin, C. N. (2010). Teaching emotion recognition skills to children with autism. *Journal of Autism and Developmental Disorders, 40*, 1505–1511.

Saarni, C. (1999). *The development of emotional competence.* New York: Guilford Press.

Saldana, D., & Frith, U. (2007). Do readers with autism make bridging inferences from world knowledge? *Journal of Experimental Child Psychology, 96*, 310–319.

Samson, A. C., Huber, O., & Ruch, W. (2011). Teasing, ridiculing and the relation to the fear of being laughed at in individuals with Asperger's syndrome. *Journal of Autism and Developmental Disorders, 41*, 475–483.

Scahill, L., McDougle, C. J., Williams, S. K., Dimitropoulos, A., Aman, M. G., McCracken, J. T., et al. (2006). Children's Yale–Brown Obsessive–Compulsive Scale modified for pervasive developmental disorders. *Journal of the American Academy of Child and Adolescent Psychiatry, 45*, 1114–1123.

Scahill, L., Riddle, M., McSwiggin-Hardin, M., Ort, S., King, R., Goodman, W. K., et al. (1997). Children's Yale–Brown Obsessive–Compulsive Scale: Reliability and validity. *Journal of the American Academy of Child and Adolescent Psychiatry, 36*, 844–852.

Scarpa, A., & Reyes, N. M. (2011). Improving emotion regulation with CBT in young children with high-functioning autism spectrum disorders: A pilot study. *Behavioral and Cognitive Psychotherapy, 39*, 495–500.

Scheeren, A. M., Koot, H. M., & Begeer, S. (2012). Social interaction style of children and adolescents with high-functioning autism spectrum disorder. *Journal of Autism and Developmental Disorders, 42*, 2046–2055.

Schietecatte, I., Roeyers, H., & Warreyn, P. (2012). Exploring the nature of joint attention impairments in young children with autism spectrum disorder: Associated social and cognitive skills. *Journal of Autism and Developmental Disorders, 42*, 1–12.

Schopler, E., & Reichler, R. J. (1971). Developmental therapy by parents with their own autistic child. In M. Rutter (Ed.), *Infantile autism: Concepts, characteristics, and treatment* (pp. 206–227). London: Churchill Livingstone.

Schroeder, J. H., Desrocher, M., Bebko, J. M., & Cappadocia, M. C. (2010). The neurobiology of autism: Theoretical applications. *Research in Autism Spectrum Disorders 4*, 555–564.

Schroeder, J. H., Weiss, J., & Bebko, J. (2011). CBCL profiles of children and adolescents with Asperger syndrome: A review and pilot study. *Journal on Developmental Disabilities, 17*, 26–37.

Schuler, A. (2003). Beyond echoplaylia: Promoting language in children with autism. *Autism, 7*, 455–469.

Schuler, A. L., & Wolfberg, P. J. (2000). Promoting peer play and socialization: The art of scaffolding. In A. Wetherby & B. M. Prizant (Eds.), *Transactional foundations of language intervention* (pp. 251–277). Baltimore: Brookes.

Schwartz, C. B., Henderson, H. A., Inge, A. P., Zahka, N. E., Coman, D. C., Kojkowski, N. M., et al. (2009). Temperament as a predictor of symptomatology and adaptive functioning in adolescents with high-functioning autism. *Journal of Autism and Developmental Disorders, 39,* 842–855.

Secan, K. E., Egel, A. L., & Tilley, C. S. (1989). Acquisition, generalization and maintenance of question-answering in autistic children. *Journal of Applied Behavior Analysis, 22,* 181–196.

Seltzer, M. M., Krauss, M. W., Shattuck, P. T., Orsmond, G., Swe, A., & Lord, C. (2003). The symptoms of autism spectrum disorders in adolescence and adulthood. *Journal of Autism and Developmental Disorders, 33,* 565–581.

Semrud-Clikeman, M., Walkowiak, J., Wilkinson, A., & Butcher, B. (2010). Executive functioning in children with Asperger syndrome, ADHD-combined type, ADHD-predominately inattentive type, and controls. *Journal of Autism and Developmental Disorders, 40,* 1017–1027.

Semrud-Clikeman, M., Walkowiak, J., Wilkinson, A., & Portman Minne, E. (2010). Direct and indirect measures of social perception, behavior, and emotional functioning in children with Asperger's disorder, nonverbal learning disability, or ADHD. *Journal of Abnormal Child Psychology, 38,* 509–519.

Seskin, L., Feliciano, E., Tippy, G., Yedloutschnig, R., Sossin, M., & Yasik, A. (2010). Attachment and autism: Parental attachment representations and relational behaviors in the parent–child dyad. *Journal of Abnormal Child Psychology, 38,* 949–960.

Shaffer, D., Fisher, P., Lucas, C., Dulcan, M., & Schwab-Stone, M. (2000). NIMH Diagnostic Interview Schedule for Children Version IV (NIMH DISC-IV): Description, differences from previous versions, and reliability of some common diagnoses. *Journal of the American Academy of Child and Adolescent Psychiatry, 39,* 28–38.

Shallice, T. (1982). Specific impairments of planning. *Philosophical Transactions of the Royal Society B: Biological Sciences, 298,* 199–209.

Shapiro, T., Sherman, M., Calamari, G., & Koch, D. (1987). Attachment in autism and other developmental disorders. *Journal of American Academy of Child and Adolescent Psychiatry, 26,* 480–484.

Shattuck, P. T., Seltzer, M. M., Greenberg, J. S., Orsmond, G., Bolt, D., Kring, S., et al. (2007). Change in autism symptoms and maladaptive behaviors in adolescents and adults with an autism spectrum disorder. *Journal of Autism and Developmental Disorders, 37,* 1735–1747.

Shih, P., Shen, M., Ottl, B., Keehn, B., Gaffrey, M. S., & Muller, R. A. (2010). Atypical network connectivity for imitation in autism spectrum disorder. *Neuropsychologia, 48,* 2931–2939.

Shores, R. L. (1987). Overview of research on social interaction: A historical and personal perspective. *Behavioral Disorders, 12,* 233–241.

Shure, M. B. (1981). Social competence as a problem-solving skill. In J. D. Wine & M. D. Smye (Eds.), *Social competence* (pp. 158–185). New York: Guilford Press.

Sigman, M., Kasari, C., Kwon, J. H., & Yirmiya, N. (1992). Responses to the negative emotions of others by autistic, mentally retarded, and normal children. *Child Development, 63,* 796–807.

Sigman, M., & McGovern, C. W. (2005). Improvement in cognitive and language skills from preschool to adolescence in autism. *Journal of Autism and Developmental Disorders, 35,* 15–23.

Sigman, M., & Mundy, P. (1989). Social attachment in autistic children. *Journal of the American Academy of Child and Adolescent Psychiatry, 28,* 74–81.

Sigman, M., & Ruskin, E. (1999). Continuity and change in the social competence of children with autism, Down syndrome, and developmental delays. *Monographs of the Society for Research in Child Development, 64*(1), 1–139.

Sigman, M., & Ungerer, J. (1984). Attachment behaviors in autistic children. *Journal of Autism and Developmental Disorders, 14,* 231–243.

Sikora, D. M., Haley, P., Edwards, J., & Butler, R. W. (2002). Tower of London test performance in children with poor arithmetic skills. *Developmental Neuropsychology, 21,* 243–254.

Simonoff, E., Pickles, A., Charman, T., Chandler, S., Loucas, T., & Baird, G. (2008). Psychiatric disorders in children with autism spectrum disorders: Prevalence, comorbidity, and associated factors in a population-derived sample. *Journal of the American Academy of Child and Adolescent Psychiatry, 47,* 921–929.

Smith, B. J., Gardiner, J. M., & Bowler, D. M. (2007). Deficits in free recall persist in Asperger's syndrome despite training in the use of list-appropriate learning strategies. *Journal of Autism and Developmental Disorders, 37,* 445–454.

Smith, L., Montagne, B., Perrett, D. I., Gill, M., & Gallagher, L. (2010). Detecting subtle facial emotion recognition deficits in high-functioning autism using dynamic stimuli of varying intensities. *Neuropsychologia, 48,* 2777–2781.

Smith-Myles, B., Hilgenfeld, T. D., Barnhill, G., Griswold, D., Hagiwara, T., & Simpson, R. (2002). Analysis of reading skills in individuals with Asperger syndrome. *Focus on Autism and Other Developmental Disabilities, 17,* 44–47.

Snowling, M., & Frith, U. (1986). Comprehension in "hyperlexic" readers. *Journal of Experimental Child Psychology, 42,* 392–415.

Sofronoff, K., Attwood, T., & Hinton, S. (2005). A randomized controlled trail of a CBT intervention for anxiety in children with Asperger syndrome. *Journal of Child Psychology and Psychiatry, 45,* 1–9.

Sofronoff, K., Attwood, T., Hinton, S., & Levin, I. (2007). A randomized controlled trial of a cognitive behavioral intervention for anger management in children diagnosed with Asperger syndrome. *Journal of Autism and Developmental Disorders, 37,* 1203–1214.

Solish, A., Perry, A., & Minnes, P. (2010). Participation of children with and without disabilities in social, recreational and leisure activities. *Journal of Applied Research in Intellectual Disabilities, 23,* 226–236.

Solomon, M., Bauminger, N., & Rogers, S. (2011). Abstract reasoning and friendship in high-functioning preadolescents with autism spectrum disorders. *Journal of Autism and Developmental Disorders, 41,* 32–43.

Solomon, M., Goodlin-Jones, B. L., & Anders, T. F. (2004). A social adjustment enhancement intervention for high-functioning autism, Asperger's syndrome, and pervasive developmental disorder NOS. *Journal of Autism and Developmental Disorders, 34,* 649–668.

Solomon, M., Miller, M., Taylor, S. L., Hinshaw, S. P., & Carter, C. S. (2012). Autism symptoms and internalizing psychopathology in girls and boys with autism spectrum disorders. *Journal of Autism and Developmental Disorders, 49,* 48–59.

Solomon, O. (2004). Narrative introductions: Discourse competence of children with autistic spectrum disorders. *Discourse Studies, 6,* 253–276.

Sontag, J. C. (1996). Toward a comprehensive theoretical framework for disability research: Bronfenbrenner revisited. *Journal of Special Education, 30,* 319–344.

South, M., Ozonoff, S., & McMahon, W. M. (2007). The relationship between executive functioning, central coherence, and repetitive behaviors in the high-functioning autism spectrum. *Autism, 11,* 441–455.

Southwick, J. S., Bigler, E. D., Froehlich, A., DuBray, M. B., Alexander, A. L., Lange, S., et al. (2011). Memory functioning in children and adolescents with autism. *Neuropsychology, 25,* 701–710.

Sparrow, S., Balla, D. A., & Cicchetti, D. V. (1984). *Vineland Adaptive Behavior Scales.* Circle Pines, MN: American Guidance Service.

Spector, J. E. (2011). Sight word instruction for students with autism: An evaluation of the evidence base. *Journal of Autism and Developmental Disorders, 41,* 1411–1422.

Speer, L. L., Cook, A. E., McMahon, W. M., & Clark, E. (2007). Face processing in children with autism: Effects of stimulus contents and type. *Autism, 11,* 265–277.

Spence, S. H. (2003). Social skills training with children and young people: Theory, evidence and practice. *Child and Adolescent Mental Health, 8,* 84–96.

Spence, S. H., & Donovan, C. (1998). Interpersonal problems. In P. Graham (Ed.), *Cognitive-behavior therapy for children and families* (pp. 217–245). New York: Cambridge University Press.

Spencer, T. D., & Slocum, T. A. (2010). The effect of a narrative intervention on story retelling and personal story generation skills of preschoolers with risk factors and narrative language delays. *Journal of Early Intervention, 32,* 178–199.

Spiker, M. A., Lin, C. E., Van Dyke, M., & Wood, J. J. (2012). Restricted interests and anxiety in children with autism. *Autism, 16,* 306–320.

Spivack, G., & Shure, M. B. (1974). *Social adjustment of young children: A cognitive approach to solving real-life problems.* San Francisco: Jossey-Bass.

Sprafkin, J., Volpe, R. J., Gadow, K. D., Nolan, E. E., & Keely, K. (2002). A DSM-IV-referenced screening instrument for preschool children: The Early Childhood Inventory—4. *Journal of the American Academy of Child and Adolescent Psychiatry, 41,* 604–612.

St. Clair-Thompson, H., & Gathercole, S. E. (2006). Executive functions and achievements in school: Shifting, updating, inhibition, and working memory. *Quarterly Journal of Experimental Psychology, 59,* 745–759.

Starr, E., Szatmari, P., Bryson, S., & Zweigenbaum, L. (2003). Stability and change among high-functioning children with pervasive developmental disorders: A 2-year outcome study. *Journal of Autism and Developmental Disorders, 33,* 15–22.

Steele, S., Minshew, N., Luna, B., & Sweeney, J. (2007). Spatial working memory deficits in autism. *Journal of Autism and Developmental Disorders, 37,* 605–612.

Stefanatos, G. A., & Baron, I. S. (2011). The ontogenesis of language impairment in autism: A neuropsychological perspective. *Neuropsychology Review, 21,* 252–270.

Sterling, L., Dawson, G., Estes, A., & Greenson, J. (2008). Characteristics associated with presence of depressive symptoms in adults with autism spectrum disorder. *Journal of Autism and Developmental Disorders, 38,* 1011–1018.

Stewart, M., Barnard, L., Pearson, J., Hasan, R., & O'Brien, G. (2006). Presentation of depression in autism and Asperger syndrome: A review. *Autism, 10,* 103–116.

Stichter, J. P., Herzog, M. J., Visovsky, K., Schmidt, C., Randolph, J., Schultz, T., et al. (2010). Social competence intervention for youth with Asperger syndrome and high-functioning autism: An initial investigation. *Journal of Autism and Developmental Disorders, 40,* 1067–1079.

Stone, W. L., & Caro-Martinez, L. M. (1990). Naturalistic observations of spontaneous communication in autistic children. *Journal of Autism and Developmental Disorders, 20,* 437–453.

Stringfield, S. G., Luscre, D., & Gast, D. L. (2011). Effects of a story map on accelerated reader postreading test scores in students with high-functioning autism. *Focus on Autism and Other Developmental Disabilities, 26,* 218–229.

Sturm, H., Fernell, E., & Gillberg, C. (2004). Autism spectrum disorders in children with normal intellectual levels: Associated impairments and subgroups. *Developmental Medicine and Child Neurology, 46,* 444–447.

Su, H. F. (2002). Project MIND: Math is not difficult. *Journal of Mathematics Education Leadership, 5,* 26–29.

Su, H. F., Lai, L., & Rivera, J. (2010). Using an exploratory approach to help children with autism learn mathematics. *Creative Education, 1,* 149–153.

Subiaul, F., Lurie, H., Romansky, K., Klein, T., Holmes, D., & Terrace, H. (2007). Cognitive imitation in typically developing 3- and 4-year olds and individuals with autism. *Cognitive Development, 22,* 230–243.

Sukhodolsky, D. G., Scahill, L., Gadow, K. D., Arnold, L. E., Aman, M. G., McDougle, C. J., et al. (2008). Parent-rated anxiety symptoms in children with pervasive developmental disorders: Frequency and association with core autism symptoms and cognitive functioning. *Journal of Abnormal Child Psychology, 36,* 117–128.

Sung, M., Ooi, Y, Goh, T. J., Pathy, P., Fung, D., Ang, R. P., et al. (2011). Effects of cognitive-behavioral therapy on anxiety in children with autism spectrum disorders: A randomized controlled trial. *Child Psychiatry and Human Development, 42,* 634–649.

Swanson, H. L. (1999). Reading comprehension and working memory in learning-disabled readers: Is the phonological loop more important than the executive system? *Journal of Experimental Child Psychology, 72,* 1–31.

Swettenham, J., Baron-Cohen, S., Charman, T., Cox, A., Baird, G., Drew, A., et al. (1998). The frequency and distribution of spontaneous attention shifts between social and nonsocial stimuli in autistic, typically developing and nonautistic developmentally delayed infants. *Journal of Child Psychology and Psychiatry, 39,* 747–753.

Szatmari, P., Bryson, S. E., Boyle, M. H., Streiner, D. L., & Duku, E. (2003). Predictors of outcome among high-functioning children with autism and Asperger syndrome. *Journal of Child Psychology and Psychiatry, 44,* 520–528.

Szatmari, P., & McConnell, B. (2011). Anxiety and mood disorders in individuals with autism spectrum disorders. In D. G. Amaral, G. Dawson, & D. H. Geschwind (Eds.), *Autism spectrum disorders* (pp. 330–338). New York: Oxford University Press.

Sze, K. M., & Wood, J. J. (2007). Cognitive behavioral treatment of comorbid anxiety disorders and social difficulties in children with high-functioning autism: A case report. *Journal of Contemporary Psychotherapy, 37,* 133–143.

Tager-Flusberg, H. (2001a). A reexamination of the theory of mind hypothesis of autism. In J. Burack, T. Charman, N. Yirmiya, & P. Zelazo (Eds.), *Development and autism: Perspectives from theory and research* (pp. 173–193). Hillsdale, NJ: Erlbaum.

Tager-Flusberg, H. (2001b). Understanding the language and communicative impairments in autism. *International Review of Research in Mental Retardation, 23,* 185–205.

Tager-Flusberg, H. (2008). Cognitive neuroscience of autism. *Journal of the International Neuropsychological Society, 14,* 917–921.

Tager-Flusberg, H. (2010). The origins of social impairments in autism spectrum disorder: Studies of infants at risk. *Neural Networks, 23,* 1072–1076.

Tager-Flusberg, H., Paul, R., & Lord, C. (2005). Language and communication in autism. In F. Volkmar, R. Paul, A. Kline, & D. J. Cohen (Eds.), *Handbook of autism and pervasive developmental disorders* (3rd ed., pp. 335–364). New York: Wiley.

Tager-Flusberg, H., & Sullivan, K. (1995). Attributing mental states to story characters: A comparison of narratives produced by autistic and mentally retarded individuals. *Applied Psycholinguistics, 16,* 241–256.

Tannock, R. (2013). Rethinking ADHD and LD in DSM-5: Proposed changes in diagnostic criteria. *Journal of Learning Disabilities, 46,* 5–25.

Taylor, B. P., & Hollander, E. (2011). Comorbid obsessive-compulsive disorders. In D. G. Amaral, G. Dawson, & D. H. Geschwind (Eds.), *Autism spectrum disorders* (pp. 270–284). New York: Oxford University Press.

Taylor, J. L., & Seltzer, M. M. (2010). Changes in the autism behavioral phenotype during the transition to adulthood. *Journal of Autism and Developmental Disorders, 40,* 1431–1446.

Taylor, J. L., & Seltzer, M. M. (2011a). Changes in the mother–child relationship during the transition to adulthood for youth with autism spectrum disorders. *Journal of Autism and Developmental Disorders, 41,* 1397–1410.

Taylor, J. L., & Seltzer, M. M. (2011b). Employment and post-secondary educational activities for young adults with autism spectrum disorders during the transition to adulthood. *Journal of Autism and Developmental Disorders, 41,* 566–574.

Terpstra, J. E., Higgins, K., & Pierce, T. (2002). Can I play?: Classroom-based interventions for teaching play skills to children with autism. *Focus on Autism and Other Developmental Disabilities, 17,* 119–126.

Tharpe, A. M., Bess, F. H., Sladen, D. P., Schissel, H., Couch, S., & Schery, T. (2006). Auditory characteristics of children with autism. *Ear and Hearing, 27,* 430–441.

Thiemann, K. S., & Goldstein, S. (2004). Effects of peer training and written text cueing on social communication of school-age children with PDD. *Journal of Speech, Language, and Hearing Research, 47,* 126–144.

Toichi, M., & Kamio, Y. (2002). Long-term memory and levels of processing in autism. *Neuropsychologia, 40,* 964–969.

Toichi, M., & Kamio, Y. (2003). Long-term memory in high-functioning autism: Controversy on episodic memory in autism reconsidered. *Journal of Autism and Developmental Disorders, 33,* 151–161.

Toth, K., Munson, J., Meltzoff, N., & Dawson, G. (2006). Early predictors of communication development in young children with autism spectrum disorder: Joint attention, imitation, and toy play. *Journal of Autism and Developmental Disorders, 36,* 993–1005.

Tracy, J. L., Robins, R. W., Schriber, R. A., & Solomon, M. (2011). Is emotion recognition impaired in individuals with autism spectrum disorders? *Journal of Autism and Developmental Disorders, 41,* 102–109.

Travis, L. L., & Sigman, M. (1998). Social deficits and interpersonal relationships in autism. *Mental Retardation and Developmental Disabilities Research Reviews, 4,* 65–72.

Trevarthen, C. (1979). Communication and co-operation in early infancy: A description of primary intersubjectivity. In M. Bullowa (Ed.), *Before speech: The beginning of interpersonal communication* (pp. 321–343). Cambridge, UK: Cambridge University Press.

Trevarthen, C., & Aitken, K. J. (2001). Infant intersubjectivity: Research, theory, and clinical implications. *Journal of Child Psychology and Psychiatry, 42,* 3–48.

Troia, G. A., & Graham, S. (2003). Effective writing instruction across the grades: What every educational consultant should know. *Journal of Educational and Psychological Consultation, 14,* 75–89.

Turner, M. A. (1999). Generating novel ideas: Fluency performance in high-functioning and learning-disabled individuals with autism. *Journal of Child Psychology and Psychiatry, 40,* 189–201.

Uono, S., Sato, W. S., & Toichi, M. (2009). Dynamic fearful gaze does not enhance attention orienting in individuals with Asperger's disorder. *Brain and Cognition, 71,* 229–233.

van der Geest, J. N., Kemner, C., Camfferman, G., Verbaten, M. N., & van Engeland, H. (2002). Looking at images with human figures: Comparison between autistic and normal children. *Journal of Autism and Developmental Disorders, 32,* 69–75.

van der Geest, J. N., Kemner, C., Verbaten, M. N., & van Engeland, H. (2002). Gaze behavior of children with pervasive developmental disorder toward human faces: A fixation time study. *Journal of Child Psychology and Psychiatry, 43,* 669–678.

van IJzendoorn, M. H., Rutgers, A. H., Bakermans-Kranenburg, M. J., Swinkels, S. H. N., van Daalen, E., Dietz, C., et al. (2007). Parental sensitivity and attachment in children with autism spectrum disorder: Comparison with children with mental retardation, with language delays, and with typical development. *Child Development, 78,* 597–608.

van Roekel, E., Scholte, E., & Didden, R. H. (2010). Bullying among adolescents with autism spectrum disorders: Prevalence and perception. *Journal of Autism and Developmental Disorders, 40,* 63–73.

Verté, S., Geurts, H. M., Roeyers, H., Oosterlaan, J., & Sergeant, J. A. (2006). Executive functioning in children with an autism spectrum disorder: Can we differentiate within the spectrum? *Journal of Autism and Developmental Disorders, 36,* 351–372.

Vital, P. M., Ronald, A., Wallace, G. L., & Happé, F. (2009). Relationship between special abilities and autistic-like traits in a large population-based sample of 8-year-olds. *Journal of Child Psychology and Psychiatry, 50,* 1093–1101.

Vitaro, F., Boivin, M., & Bukowski, W. M. (2009). The role of friendship in child and adolescent psychosocial development. In K. H. Rubin, W. M. Bukowski, & B. Laursen (Eds.), *Handbook of peer interactions, relationships, and groups* (pp. 568–588). New York: Guilford Press.

Vivanti, G., Nadig, A., Ozonoff, S., & Rogers, S. J. (2008). What do children with autism attend to during imitation tasks? *Journal of Experimental Child Psychology, 101,* 186–205.

Volker, M. A., Lopata, E. C., Smerbeck, A. M., Knoll, V. M., Thomeer, M. L., & Toomey, J. A. (2010). BASC-2 PRS profiles for students with high-functioning autism spectrum disorders. *Journal of Autism and Developmental Disorders, 40,* 188–199.

Volkmar, F. R., State, M., & Klin, A. (2009). Autism and autism spectrum disorders: Diagnostic issues for the coming decade. *Journal of Child Psychology and Psychiatry, 50,* 108–115.

Volkmar, F. R., Szatmari, P., & Sparrow, S. S. (1993). Sex differences in pervasive developmental disorders. *Journal of Autism and Developmental Disorders, 23,* 579–591.

Volling, B. L., McElwain, N. L., & Miller, A. (2002). Emotion regulation in context: The jealousy complex between young siblings and its relations with child and family characteristics. *Child Development, 73,* 581–600.

Vygotsky, L. S. (1962). *Thought and language.* Cambridge, MA: MIT Press. (Original work published 1934 in Russian)

Wahlberg, T., & Magliano, J. P. (2004). The ability of high function individuals with autism to comprehend written discourse. *Discourse Processes, 38,* 119–144.

Wainscot, J. J., Naylor, P., Sutcliffe, P., Tantam, D., & Williams, J. V. (2008). Relationships with peers and use of the school environment of mainstream secondary school pupils with Asperger syndrome (high-functioning autism): A case-control study. *International Journal of Psychology and Psychological Therapy, 8,* 25–38.

Wechsler, D. (1974). *Wechsler Intelligence Scale for Children—Revised.* New York: Psychological Corporation.

Wechsler, D. (1981). *Wechsler Adult Intelligence Scale—Revised.* New York: Psychological Corporation.

Wechsler, D. (1989). *Wechsler Preschool and Primary Scale for Intelligence—Revised.* San Antonio, TX: Psychological Corporation.

Wechsler, D. (1991). *Wechsler Intelligence Scale for Children* (3rd ed.). San Antonio, TX: Psychological Corporation.

Wechsler, D. (1992). *Wechsler Intelligence Scale For Children* (3rd U.K. ed.). London: Psychological Corporation.

Wechsler, D. (1997). *Wechsler Adult Intelligence Scale* (3rd ed.). San Antonio, TX: Psychological Corporation.

Wechsler, D. (1999). *Wechsler Abbreviated Scale of Intelligence.* San Antonio, TX: Psychological Corporation.

Wellman, H. M. (1993). Early understanding of mind: The normal case. In S. Baron-Cohen, H. Tager-Flusberg, & D. J. Cohen (Eds.), *Understanding of other minds: Perspectives from autism* (pp. 10–39). Oxford, UK: Oxford University Press.

Wetherell, D., Botting, N., & Conti-Ramsden, G. (2007). Narrative skills in adolescents with a history of SLI in relation to non-verbal IQ scores. *Child Language Teaching and Therapy, 23,* 95–113.

Whalon, K. J., Al Otaiba, S., & Delano, M. E. (2009). Evidence-based reading instruction for individuals with autism spectrum disorders. *Focus on Autism and Other Developmental Disabilities, 24,* 3–16.

Whalon, K. J., & Hanline, M. F. (2008). Effects of a reciprocal questioning intervention on the question generation and responding of children with autism spectrum disorder. *Education and Training in Developmental Disabilities, 43,* 367–387.

Whitby, P. J. S., & Mancil, G. R. (2009). Academic achievement profiles of children with high-functioning autism and Asperger syndrome: A review of the literature. *Education and Training in Developmental Disabilities, 44,* 551–560.

Whitby, P. J. S., Travers, J. C., & Harnik, J. (2009). Academic achievement and strategy instruction to support the learning of children with high-functioning autism. *Beyond Behavior, 19,* 3–9.

White, S. J., & Saldan, D. (2011). Performance of children with autism on the Embedded Figures Test: A closer look at a popular task. *Journal of Autism and Developmental Disorders, 41,* 1565–1572.

White, S. W., Albano, A. M., Johnson, C. R., Kasari, C., Ollendick, T., Klin, A., et al. (2010). Development of a cognitive-behavioral intervention program to treat anxiety and social deficits in teens with high-functioning autism. *Clinical Child and Family Psychology Review, 13,* 77–90.

White, S. W., Ollendick., T., & Bray, B. (2011). College students on the autism spectrum: Prevalence and associated problems. *Autism, 15,* 683–701.

White, S. W., Oswald, D., Ollendick, T., & Scahill, L. (2009). Anxiety in children and adolescents with autism spectrum disorders. *Clinical Psychology Review, 29,* 216–229.

White, S. W., & Roberson-Nay, R. (2009). Anxiety, social deficits, and loneliness in youth with autism spectrum disorders. *Journal of Autism and Developmental Disorders, 39,* 1006–1013.

Whitehouse, A. J. O., Maybery, M. T., & Durkin, K. (2007). Evidence against poor semantic encoding in individuals with autism. *Autism, 11,* 241–254.

Willemsen-Swinkels, S. H. N., Bakermans-Kranenburg, M. J., Buitelaar, J. K, van IJzendoorn, M. H., & van Engeland, H. (2000). Insecure and disorganized attachment in children with pervasive developmental disorder: Relationship with social interaction and heart rate. *Journal of Child Psychology and Psychiatry, 41,* 759–767.

Williams, D., & Happé, F. (2010). Recognising "social" and "non-social" emotions in self and others: A study of autism. *Autism, 14,* 285–304.

Williams, D. L., Goldstein, G., Carpenter, P. A., & Minshew, N. (2005). Verbal and spatial working memory in autism. *Journal of Autism and Developmental Disorders, 35,* 747–756.

Williams, D. L., Goldstein, G., & Minshew, N. (2006a). Neuropsychological functioning in children with autism: Further evidence for disordered complex information processing. *Child Neuropsychology, 12,* 279–298.

Williams, D. L., Goldstein, G., & Minshew, N. (2006b). The profile of memory function in children with autism. *Neuropsychology, 20,* 21–29.

Williams, J., Whitten,, A., & Singh, T. (2004). A systematic review of action imitation in autistic spectrum disorder. *Journal of Autism and Developmental Disorders, 34,* 285–296.

Williams, M. A., Moss, S. A., Bradshaw, J. L., & Rinehart, N. J. (2002). Random number generation in autism. *Journal of Autism and Developmental Disorders, 32*, 43–47.

Willoughby, K. A., Desrocher, M., Levine, B., & Rovet, J. F. (2012). Episodic and semantic autobiographical memory and everyday memory during late childhood and early adolescence. *Frontiers in Psychology, 3*, 1–15.

Wilson, C. E., Brock, J., & Palermo, R. (2010). Attention to social stimuli and facial identity recognition skills in autism spectrum disorder. *Journal of Intellectual Disability Research, 54*, 1104–1115.

Wimmer, H., & Perner, J. (1983). Beliefs about beliefs: Representation and constraining function of wrong beliefs in children's understanding of deception. *Cognition, 13*, 103–128.

Wing, L. (1981). Asperger's syndrome: A clinical account. *Psychological Medicine, 11*, 115–130.

Wing, L., & Gould, J. (1979). Severe impairments of social interaction and associated abnormalities in children: Epidemiology and classification. *Journal of Autism and Developmental Disorders, 9*, 11–29.

Wing, L., Gould, J., & Gillberg, C. (2011). Autism spectrum disorders in the DSM-5: Better or worse than the DSM-IV? *Research in Developmental Disabilities, 32*, 768–773.

Witkin, H. A., Ottman, R. K., Raskin, E., & Karp, S. A. (1971). *A manual for the Embedded Figures Test.* Palo Alto, CA: Consulting Psychologists Press.

Wolfberg, P. J. (1999). *Play and imagination in children with autism.* New York: Teachers College Press.

Wood, J. J. (2012, May). *Enhanced cognitive behavioral treatment for anxiety in youth with ASD.* Paper presented at the International Conference for Autism (IMFAR), Toronto, Ontario, Canada.

Wood, J. J., Drahota, A., Sze, K., Har, K., Chiu, A., & Langer, D. A. (2009). Cognitive behavioral therapy for anxiety in children with autism spectrum disorders: A randomized, controlled trial. *Journal of Child Psychology and Psychiatry, 50*, 224–234.

Wood, J. J., Drahota, A., Sze, K. M., Van Dyke, M., Decker, K., Fujii, C., et al. (2009). Effects of cognitive behavioral therapy on parent-reported autism symptoms in school-age children with high-functioning autism. *Journal of Autism and Developmental Disorders, 39*, 1608–1612.

Wood, J. J., & Gadow, K. D. (2010). Exploring the nature and function of anxiety in youth with autism spectrum disorders. *Clinical Psychology: Science and Practice, 17*, 281–292.

World Health Organization. (1992). *The ICD-10 classification of mental and behavioral disorders: Clinical descriptions and diagnostic guidelines.* Geneva, Switzerland: Author.

World Health Organization. (2001). *The world health report 2001—Mental health: New understanding, new hope.* Geneva, Switzerland: Author.

Yirmiya, N., & Charman, T. (2010). The prodrome of autism: Early behavioral and biological signs, regression, peri- and post-natal development and genetics. *Journal of Child Psychology and Psychiatry, 51*, 432–458.

Yirmiya, N., Sigman, M. D., Kasari, C., & Mundy, P. (1992). Empathy and cognition in high-functioning children with autism. *Child Development, 63*, 150–160.

Yirmiya, N., Solomonica-Levi, D., Shulman, C., & Pilowsky, T. (1996). Theory of mind abilities in individuals with autism, Down syndrome, and mental retardation of unknown etiology: The role of age and intelligence. *Journal of Child Psychology and Psychiatry, 37*, 1003–1014.

Yoshida, Y., & Uchiyama, T. (2004). The clinical necessity for assessing attention deficit/hyperactivity disorder (AD/HD) symptoms in children with high-functioning pervasive developmental disorder (PDD). *European Child and Adolescent Psychiatry, 13,* 307–314.

Young, G., Merin, N., Rogers, S., & Ozonoff, S. (2009). Gaze behavior and affect at 6 months: Predicting clinical outcomes and language development in typically developing infants and infants at risk for autism. *Developmental Science, 12,* 798–814.

Zandt, F., Prior, M., & Kyrios, M. (2009). Similarities and differences between children and adolescents with autism spectrum disorder and those with obsessive–compulsive disorder: Executive functioning and repetitive behaviour. *Autism, 13,* 43–57.

Zingerevich, C., & LaVesser, P. D. (2009). The contribution of executive functions to participation in school activities of children with high-functioning autism spectrum disorders. *Research in Autism Spectrum Disorders, 3,* 429–437.

Zwaigenbaum, L., Bryson, S., Rogers, T., Roberts, W., Brian, J., & Szatmari, P. (2005). Behavioral manifestations of autism in the first year of life. *International Journal of Developmental Neuroscience, 23,* 143–152.

Index

f indicates a figure; *t* indicates a table.

Academic abilities/achievement, 121–130; *see also* Cognitive-academic capabilities; specific academic areas
  joint attention and, 12
  in mathematics, 129–130
  in reading, 123–128
  in writing, 128–129
Adaptive skills, assessment of, 100–103
Adolescence to adulthood transition, 103–108
Affect, weak central coherence and, 25–26
Affective disorders, HFASD and, 3–4
Affective education
  CBE interventions for, 245*t*
  definition/aim and examples of, 236*t*–237*t*
Affective Matching Measure, aim and description of, 255*t*
Affective theory, 8–9
Age, friendship qualities and, 82
Age of onset, in DSM-5, 7
Aloneness; *see also* Loneliness
  Kanner's observations about, 59, 86
Analogical reasoning, weak central coherence and, 27
Anaphoric cueing, 202, 205
  relevant intervention and definition for, 211*t*
Anxiety disorders
  comorbidity with HFASD
    differential diagnosis in, 139–141
    prevalence of, 141–144
  definition of, 139
Asperger, Hans, 4
Asperger syndrome, 4
  ADHD and, 133–135
  adult dependence and, 106–107
  anxiety disorders and, 142, 178–179
  DSM-IV-TR and, 5–6
  DSM-5 and, 6–8
  early social-deficit markers and, 92–93
  educational social outcomes and, 105–107
  emotion recognition and, 46

false-belief tests and, 15
gelotophobia and, 155
mood disorders and, 137–138
peer bullying and, 63
psychopathology measures and, 145, 149
reading comprehension and, 126
social information processing and, 37–38
study findings for, 101–102
Assessment measures
  for attachment, 252*t*
  for comorbidity, 144–150
    Behavior Assessment System for Children–2nd ed., 147–148
    Child Behavior Checklist, 144–145
    Child Symptom Inventory–IV, 148–149
    Diagnostic Interview Schedule for Children–IV, 148
    general measures, 144–149
    Schedule for Affective Disorders and Schizophrenia for School-Age Children (6–18), 145–147
  for specific psychopathologies, 149–150
  for emotional expressiveness/responsiveness, 253*t*–254*t*
  for executive function, 258*t*–259*t*
  for friendship, 260*t*–262*t*
  for social cognition: problem solving, 263*t*–264*t*
  for social cognition: ToM, 265*t*–266*t*
  for social competence/adjustment, 267*t*–271*t*
  for social interaction, 272*t*–274*t*
Attachment
  in ASD, 72–76
  assessment measures for, 252*t*
  caregiver characteristics and, 75–76
  caregiver–stranger differentiation and, 72–74
  security of, 9, 55
    friendship and, 82–83
    individual differences in, 74–75
    ToM and, 223
  in TYP, 60, 73–74, 223

313

Attention-deficit/hyperactivity disorder
(ADHD), 132–135
   comorbidity with HFASD
      differential diagnosis of, 133
      prevalence of, 133–135
   defined, 132
Autism Behavior Checklist, 101–102
Autism Comorbidity Interview–Present and
   Lifetime Version (ACI-PL), 146–147
Autism Diagnosis Interview (ADI)
   for measuring repetitive/stereotyped
      behaviors, 22
   for measuring social deficits in preschoolers,
      101
Autism Diagnostic Interview–Revised (ADI-R), 6
   aim and description, 267t
Autism Diagnostic Observation Schedule
   (ADOS), 6
   aim and description, 267t
Autism spectrum disorders (ASD)
   attachment in, 72–76 (see also Attachment)
   comorbid conditions and, 7 (see also
      Comorbid conditions)
   desire for peer relations and, 59
   DSM-IV approach to, 6–7
   DSM-IV-TR criteria for, 59–60
   DSM-5 criteria for, 28, 59–60
   IQ definition of, 8
   Kanner's perception of, 8–9, 59
   sensory behaviors and, 7
   ToM hypothesis and, 15–16
Autobiographical memory, 116–118
   episodic, 117
   everyday, 117–118
   impairments in, 194

B

Behavior Assessment System for Children
   (BASC-2 PRS)
   aim and description, 268t
   for assessing comorbidity, 147–148
Behavior Rating Inventory of Executive
   Function (BRIEF), aim and description
   of, 258t
Behavioral interventions
   for cognitive/academic functioning, 189–190
   for social-interactive behaviors, definition/
      aim and examples of, 237t–239t
Behavioral rehearsal, definition/aim and
   examples of, 238t
Behaviors, restricted and repetitive; see
   Restricted and repetitive behaviors
Beliefs, first- versus high-order, 13–14
Bodily cues, in emotion recognition, 50
Bullying, by peers, 62–63, 182, 218, 222

C

Cambridge Mindreading Face–Voice Battery–
   Children Version (CAM-C), aim and
   description of, 255t
Caregiver
   characteristics of, 75–76

child's attachment security and, 72–74, 76
child's jealousy and, 17, 55
TYP attachment and, 60
Caregiver–child interaction, joint attention and,
   10–11
Caregiver–stranger differentiation, attachment
   quality and, 72–74
Central coherence theory, 23, 40; see also Weak
   central coherence
Child and Adolescent Social Perception
   Measure (CASP), aim and description of,
   256t
Child Behavior Checklist (CBCL)
   aim and description, 269t
   for assessing comorbidity, 144–145
Child Symptom Inventory–IV, for assessing
   comorbidity, 148
Children's Depression Inventory (CDI), 149
   aim and description of, 253t
Children's Yale–Brown Obsessive Compulsive
   Scale, 149–150
Cloze tasks, 202–203
   relevant intervention and definition for, 211t
Cognitive characteristics, 111–121
   language and narrative ability, 120–121
   memory, 113–119 (see also Memory)
Cognitive compensation, 43
   example of, 158
Cognitive compensation hypothesis, 3, 5,
   57–58, 84–85
Cognitive functioning; see also Cognitive-
   academic capabilities
   concrete versus abstract, 111
   imitation skills and, 119
   language and narrative abilities and,
      120–121
   peer relations and, 84
   social participation and, 61
   tools for assessing, 111
Cognitive reconstruction techniques
   definition/aim and examples, 234t
   for enhancing social-cognition capabilities,
      definition/aim and examples, 234t–237t
Cognitive theories, 18–27
   of executive functioning, 18–23 (see also
      Executive functioning)
   of weak central coherence, 23–27
Cognitive-academic capabilities
   current understanding of, 225–226
   executive functioning and, 18–19, 21
   theory of mind and, 14–15
Cognitive-academic interventions, 187–211
   behavioral interventions, 189–190
   frequently used strategies for, 188
   future directions for, 226–228
   general strategies, 190–191
   glossary of professional terms for, 211t–214t
   for mathematics skills, 209–210
   for memory skills, 191–194
   for question asking and answering, 194–197
   for reading, 197–206
      for comprehension, 199–206 (see also
         Reading comprehension strategies)
      using visual learning, 197–199

selecting strategies for, 210
structured teaching, 188–191
writing strategies, 206–209
Cognitive-behavioral treatment (CBT)
background of, 157
definition/aim and examples of, 234t–239t
impact on comorbid anxiety, 179–181
impacts on social functioning, 181
modifications of, for HFASD, 180–181
social skills training and, 156
studies of, 159–163
techniques and settings for, 241f
Cognitive-behavioral-ecological interventions
(CBE), 156, 158, 163–178
adult facilitators of, 170–171
criteria for selecting peer aides in, 246t
curriculum topics for, 244t–245t
design of, 164–175
dual treatment modes of, 165–166
dyadic, 165–166
ecological basis for, 169–173
efficacy studies of, 175–178
emphases of, 168–169
generalization and maintenance of, 173–175
group, 166
impacts on anxiety, 179–181
impacts on social functioning, 181
model for, 247f
overview of, 163–164
parents and, 173
peers and, 171–173
procedures for, 166–167
social implications for, 178–181
Cognitive-oriented training, theory of mind
and, 159–160
Collaborative problem solving (CPS); see also
Problem solving
social-cognitive skills and, 98–99
in study of friendship in preschoolers, 97–99
Collateral skills, relevant intervention and
definition for, 211t
Color-coded organizers, relevant intervention
and definition for, 211t
Communication capabilities, as social deficit
predictor, 101–102
Communication impairment; see also
Sociocommunicative domain
in HFA, 5
Comorbid conditions, 7, 131–151; see also
specific conditions
ADHD, 132–135
anxiety disorders, 139–144
assessment measures for, 144–150 (see also
Assessment measures, for comorbidity;
specific assessment measures)
defined, 131
differential diagnosis and, 132
mood disorders, 135–138
Composition abilities, 128–129; see also
Writing
Computer games, for social interventions, 163
Computer-mediated story construction,
207–208

Concept clarification techniques, definition/aim
and examples, 234t
Concept formation, 111–112
Concept mapping, 205
for reading comprehension, 200
relevant intervention and definition for, 211t
Concrete–representational–abstract strategy,
relevant intervention and definition for,
211t
Conners 3rd Edition, 149
Construction game scenario, 77
Contextual cueing, 205
relevant intervention and definition for, 211t
Conversation, social versus functional-
informational, 65
Conversation skills, group, CBE interventions
for, 245t
Cooperative play, 65–67
Cooperative skills, CBE interventions for, 245t
Cueing
anaphoric, relevant intervention and
definition for, 211t
contextual, 205
relevant intervention and definition for,
211t
external, relevant intervention and definition
for, 212t
pictorial, relevant intervention and definition
for, 213t
verbal, relevant intervention and definition
for, 214t
Cueing strategies
for cognitive-academic functioning, 191
for facilitating memory performance, 193
for reading comprehension, 202–203

D

Decoding skills, 124–125
relevant intervention and definition for,
212t
Delis Kaplan Executive Function System
(D-KEFS), aim and description of, 258t
Delta Messages program, 198–199
Depression
diagnostic criteria and differential diagnosis,
136–137
prevalence in HFASD, 137–138
Development of self, 16–17
Developmental changes in social function,
88–109
CBE approach and, 168–169
early markers of, 90–93
in HFASD, 89–90
school transitions and, 100–103
school, "real"-world transitions and,
103–108
in toddler and preschool years, 93–100
in TYP, 88–89
Diagnostic Analysis of Non-Verbal Accuracy–2,
aim and description of, 256t
Diagnostic and Statistical Manual of Mental
Disorders (DSM-IV-TR), ASD in, 5–6,
59–60

Diagnostic and Statistical Manual of Mental Disorders (DSM-5), ASD in, 6–8, 28, 59–60
Diagnostic criteria, 4–8
  cognitive theories and, 18–27
  DSM-IV-TR, 5–6
  DSM-5, 6–8
  social-cognitive theories and, 13–17
  social-communicative theories and, 8–13
Diagnostic Interview Schedule for Children–IV (DISC-IV), for assessing comorbidity, 148
Drawing game scenario, 77–78
Dyadic Relationships Q-Set (DRQ), aim and description of, 260*t*
Dyadic treatment mode, 165–166

E

Early Childhood Friendship Survey, aim and description of, 260*t*
Echolalia, 5, 95, 101
Educational outcomes, prospects for, 105–106
Embarrassment, recognition of, 49
Embedded instruction
  for cognitive-academic functioning, 191
  as question answering strategy, 196–197
  relevant intervention and definition for, 212*t*
Emergent literacy, relevant intervention and definition for, 212*t*
Emotion Inventory, aim and description of, 257*t*
Emotion recognition
  of basic emotions, 45–48
  of complex emotions, 48–50
Emotional competencies, 40–57
  current understanding of, 219–221
  emotional expressiveness and responsiveness, 52–57
  versus emotional understanding in TYP, 40–42
  higher emotion-understanding capabilities, 50–51
  summary of, 50–51
  understanding of emotions in others, 45–50
  understanding of emotions in self, 42–45
Emotional expressiveness/responsiveness, 52–57
  assessment measures for, 253*t*–254*t*
  empathy and, 56–57
  jealousy and, 54–56
  loneliness and, 56
  social rules about, 50–51
  social-cognitive deficits and, 53–54
Emotional understanding/recognition
  aim and description of, 255*t*–257*t*
  CBE interventions for, 244*t*
  in HFASD, 42–52
  higher, 50–62
  of others, 45–50
  physiological measures of, 54
  of self, 42–45
  summary of, 52
  in TYP, 40–42, 45–51

Emotions
  complex, 41
  hidden, 41–42, 50–51
  mixed, 41
  social, 17
  spontaneous, 53
Empathy Quotient and Systemizing Quotient, aim and description of, 253*t*
Empathy/emotional responsiveness, 56–57
Employment, difficulties with, 105–107
Environmental factors
  in friendships, 83
  in peer relations, 85, 86
Episodic memory, 117
Executive functioning
  assessment measures for, 258*t*–259*t*
  collaborative problem solving and, 99
  correlates of, 20–22
  disorders associated with, 22
  HFASD and, 19–20
  processes of, 18
  summary of, 22–23
  typical development of, 18–19
External cueing, relevant intervention and definition for, 212*t*
Eye contact
  atypical, as social-deficit marker, 5, 92
  friendship dyads and, 78
  joint attention and, 11
  peer interactions and, 68
  prosocial behaviors and, 64

F

Facial cues, processing of, 45–46, 50
Facial expression, 5
  in differential diagnosis, 133, 136–137
  in HFASD/Asperger's, 101, 105
  versus TYP, 53–54
  in PDD-NOS, 92
  social cognition and, 32
  understanding, 45–48, 50
Factual knowledge, relevant intervention and definition for, 212*t*
False-belief research, 14
Family factors, friendship qualities and, 83
Faux Pas Stories, aim and description, 265*t*
Feedback and reinforcement techniques, definition/aim and examples of, 238*t*
Figurative language, 203–206
Flowchart, relevant intervention and definition for, 212*t*
Friendship, 76–84
  assessment measures for, 260*t*–262*t*
  contributors to, 81–83
  current understanding of, 221–224
  nature and quality in, 77–79
  partners in, 79–81
  predictors of, 81
  toddler/preschooler, 96–100
  understanding importance of, 52, 165
Friendship Nominations and Peer Acceptance, aim and description of, 261*t*

Friendship Observation Scale (FOS), aim and description of, 261*t*
Friendship Qualities Scale (FQS), aim and description of, 262*t*

G

Gelotophobia, 155
Gender, differences based on, 230–231
Genetic–environmental factors, 229
Global attribution style, in Asperger's syndrome, 38
Graphic maps, relevant intervention and definition for, 212*t*
Graphic organizers, 205
    relevant intervention and definition for, 212*t*
Group conversation skills, CBE interventions for, 245*t*
Group interventions, change agents in, 240*t*
Group stress, coping with, CBE interventions for, 245*t*
Group treatment, 166

H

Handwriting ability, 128–129
High-functioning autism (HFA), 4
    characteristics of, 5
    DSM-5 and, 6
    false-belief tests and, 15
High-functioning autism spectrum disorders (HFASD)
    characteristics of, 3–4
    definitions and theoretical explanations, 3–28 (*see also* Diagnostic criteria)
Homework, for social-interactive behaviors, definition/aim and examples of, 239*t*
Homographs, 205
Hyperlexia, 127–128

I

Identification theory, 10
Imitation skills, 119
Index of Empathy for Children and Adolescents (IECA), aim and description of, 254*t*
Infant
    with ASD, 90–91, 93
    attachment of, 72 (*see also* Attachment)
    social-emotional deficit in, markers of, 90–91
    typical development (TYP) in, 9–12
Inferential knowledge, relevant intervention and definition for, 212*t*
Information processing, memory links with, 118–119
Intelligence scores, executive functioning and, 20
Interactions; *see* Peer interactions; Social interactions
Interpersonal situations, experiencing *versus* understanding, 17
Intersubjectivity theory, 9
Intrinsic reinforcers, relevant intervention and definition for, 212*t*

Inventory of Parent and Peer Attachment, aim and description of, 252*t*
IQ; *see also* Cognitive functioning
    academic achievement and, 122
    adaptive capability and, 102–103
    adult psychosocial adjustment and, 107–108
    and anxiety in HFASD, 143
    and depression in ASD, 135
    empathy and, 57
    friendship qualities and, 81–82, 84
    jealousy and, 55
    mathematical ability and, 129
    as social deficit predictor, 101–102
    social participation and, 61
    tools for assessing, 111
IQ testing, findings of, 111–113
Irony, understanding, 51

J

Jealousy, 17, 54–56
John and Mary Ice-Cream Van Story, aim and description, 265*t*
Joint attention
    academic implications of, 12
    attachment security and, 74–75
    play performance and, 94
    responding *versus* initiating, 11–12
    social competence and, 85, 89–92, 108
Joint attention theory, 10–12
Junior Detective, 163
Junior Hayling Test, aim and description of, 258*t*

K

Kanner, Leo, 4, 8–9, 59, 86
Kerns Security Scale (KSS), aim and description of, 252*t*

L

Language
    figurative, 203–206
    role of, 231–232
Language abilities, 120–121
    as social deficit predictor, 101
Language impairment, weak central coherence and, 26–27
Language scores, as social-deficit markers, 92
Learning, joint attention and, 12
Listening, social, 165
Literacy; *see* Reading; Writing
Loneliness
    emotional expressiveness/responsiveness and, 56
    lack of friendships and, 84
Loneliness Rating Scale, aim and description of, 254*t*
Low-functioning autism (LFA)
    anxiety disorders and, 142–143
    developmental changes in social functioning and, 102–104, 106, 108–109

Low-functioning autism (LFA) (*continued*)
  DSM-5 and, 6
    hyperlexia and, 128
    social conversation and, 66
    social involvement and, 61
  emotional responsiveness and, 57
  executive function and, 21
  friendship and, 81
  IQ definition of, 8
  memory and, 115
  memory skill strategies and, 192
  mood disorders and, 137
  multiple-exemplar training and, 190
  reading strategies and, 198
  and recognition of facial expression, 45
  social attention deficit and, 33
  social conversation and, 66
  social involvement and, 61
  and understanding of social situations, 17

M

Mathematical abilities, 129–130
"Mathematics Interventions for Students with
    High-Functioning Autism/Asperger's
    Syndrome" (Donaldson and Zager), 209
Mathematics strategies, 209–210
Mediation
  adult–child, role description of, 240*t*
  dyadic peer, role description of, 240*t*
Memory, 113–119
  autobiographical, 116–117
  episodic, 117
  everyday, 117–118
  links with information processing, 118–119
  spatial working, 114
  summary of, 118
  temporal, 114–115
  verbal working, 115–116
  working, 113–114
Memory skills, strategies targeting, 191–194
Mental imagery
  for facilitating memory performance,
    192–193
  relevant intervention and definition for, 212*t*
Metaphors, 204–205, 206
Metarepresentation, 13–14
Metonymies, 203–204, 206
Mnemonics, relevant intervention and definition
    for, 213*t*
Modeling techniques, definition/aim and
    examples of, 237*t*
Mood disorders
  comorbidity with HFASD, 135–138
  definition of, 135–136
Mother–adolescent relationships, 104
Multimodal interventions, 160–163
Multiple-exemplar training/instruction (MET/
    MEI)
  for cognitive/academic functioning, 189–
    190
  figurative language and, 204–206
Multisensory approach, relevant intervention
    and definition for, 213*t*

N

Narrative abilities, 120–121
Narrative processing, weak central coherence
    and, 25
Natural environment, relevant intervention and
    definition for, 213*t*
Neurobiological issues, 217, 230
Neurological findings, 229–230
Neuropsychological characteristics, 229
Nonsocial objects, visual attention to, 32–33

O

Obsessive–compulsive disorder, *versus* HFASD,
    140–141

P

Parents; *see also* Caregiver
  role in CBE interventions, 173
  role in CBT interventions, 180
PDD-NOS, 4
  ADHD and, 133–134
  anxiety disorders and, 143
  versus autism, 92
  DSM-IV-TR and, 6
  DSM-5 and, 6–8
  psychopathology measures and, 145
Peer aides, selection criteria for, 246*t*
Peer Interaction Observation Schedule (PIOS),
    aim and description of, 272*t*
Peer interactions; *see also* Peer relations; Social
    interactions
  of toddlers and preschoolers, 96–100
Peer mediation, dyadic, role description of,
    240*t*
Peer relations, 59–87
  and attachment in HFASD, 72–76
  bullying in, 62–63, 182, 218, 222
  current understanding of, 221–224
  defined, 60
  ecological perspective on, 85
  and friendship in HFASD, 76–84
  integrative thoughts about, 84–86
  partner's role in, 67–69
  predictors of, 85
  similarities between HFASD and TYP
    groups, 86
  social interaction in HFASD and, 60–72 (*see
    also* Social interaction in HFASD)
  social interventions in, 86
  struggle with, 217–218
  in TYP, 59
  with TYP partners, 68–69
Peers, role in CBE interventions, 171–
    173
Pervasive developmental disorders not
    otherwise specified (PDD-NOS), 4; *see*
    PDD-NOS
Phobias, *versus* HFASD, 141
Phonological awareness, 125
Pictorial cues, relevant intervention and
    definition for, 213*t*

Pictures of Facial Affect System, aim and description of, 257*t*
Pivotal response training (PRT)
  for cognitive/academic functioning, 189
  relevant intervention and definition for, 213*t*
Pivotal skills, relevant intervention and definition for, 213*t*
Play
  nonsocial, 67
  social, 65–67, 93–95
  symbolic, 74–75
Playground
  aloneness on, 67
  social demands on, 67–68
Playground Observation of Peer Engagement (POPE), aim and description of, 272*t*
Pragmatic Rating Scale (PRS) Coding, aim and description of, 273*t*
Preschoolers
  friendship and peer interaction in, 96–100
  social-emotional deficit in, markers of, 90–91
Problem solving
  assessment measures of, 263*t*–264*t*
  social, 39
  social-interpersonal, CBE interventions for, 244*t*
Problem-Solving Measure (PSM), aim and description, 263*t*
Problem-solving techniques, definition/aim and examples of, 235*t*–236*t*
Program for the Evaluation and Enrichment of Relational Skills (PEERS), 182–183
Project MIND (Math Is Not Difficult), 209
Prompt, relevant intervention and definition for, 213*t*
Psychopathology
  comorbidity with HFASD (*see* Comorbid conditions)
  measures for assessing, 149–150

Q

Quality of Play Questionnaire (QPQ), aim and description of, 274*t*
Question answering, strategies targeting, 195–197
Question asking, strategies targeting, 194–195
Question-related skills, summary of, 197

R

Reading, 123–128
  comprehension skills in, 126–127
  decoding skills in, 124–125
  hyperlexia and, 127–128
  phonological awareness skills in, 125
  sight-word skills in, 124
Reading comprehension, weak central coherence and, 26
Reading comprehension strategies, 199–206
  cueing, 202–203
  for figurative language, 203–205
  using visual support, 200–202

Reading Mind in the Eyes Test–Child Revised Version, aim and description, 266*t*
Reading strategies, 197–206; *see also* Reading comprehension strategies
Reading the Mind in Films–Child Version, 48–49
  aim and description of, 257*t*
Real and Deceptive Emotion Task, aim and description, 266*t*
Recall task, relevant intervention and definition for, 213*t*
Rehearsal
  for facilitating memory performance, 192
  relevant intervention and definition for, 213*t*
Relaxation and exposure techniques, definition/aim and examples of, 239*t*
Repeated storybook-reading technique, relevant intervention and definition for, 213*t*
Repetitive behaviors, 4–7
  as early social deficit marker, 91, 93
  executive function and, 19–22
  frequency of play activity and, 94
  ToM and, 16
  transitions and, 101–104
Repetitive behaviors/interests
  in DSM-5, 6–7
  executive functioning and, 19, 21–22
Restricted and repetitive behaviors; *see* Repetitive behaviors
Retrieval stage, relevant intervention and definition for, 213*t*
Rhyming strategy, relevant intervention and definition for, 214*t*
Ridicule, fear of, 155

S

Sarcasm, understanding, 51
Savant skills, 26, 122
Scaffolding strategies
  applications of, 227
  for cognitive-academic functioning, 190
  for emotional and social exchanges, 221
  reading instruction and, 198–199, 201
  relevant intervention and definition for, 214*t*
  responsive communication and, 95
  in social interventions, 166
  writing instruction and, 206
Schedule for Affective Disorders and Schizophrenia for School-Age Children (6–18), for assessing comorbidity, 145–147
School success; *see also* Academic abilities/achievement
  executive functioning and, 21
School transitions
  ADI and VAB results and, 102–103
  social challenges of, 89
  trajectories and predictors of, 100–103
Schoolyard; *see* Playground
Self-instruction techniques, definition/aim and examples of, 235*t*
Self-Perception Profile for Children (SPPC), aim and description, 269*t*

Self-regulated strategy development (SRSD), for writing instruction, 206–207
Self-regulating strategy, relevant intervention and definition for, 214t
Self-talk techniques, definition/aim and examples of, 235t
Semantic cueing, for facilitating memory performance, 193
Sensory behaviors
in DSM-5, 7
social impairment and, 85
Sight-word instruction, 197–198
Sight-word skills, 124
Social appropriateness, judging, 38–39
Social attention, 32–36
to dynamic *versus* static stimuli, 35
research summary, 36
to social *versus* nonsocial stimuli, 33–35
Social behavior; *see also* Peer relations
with adults *versus* peers, 60
Social challenges, during TYP, 88–89
Social cognition, 32–36
assessment measures of, 263t–266t
collaborative problem solving and, 98–99
defining, 32
multimodal interventions and, 161–163
social attention and, 32–36
social information processing and, 37–40
Social Communication Emotion Regulation Training System model (SCERTS), 182–183
Social Communication Questionnaire (SCQ), aim and description, 269t
Social communicative theories, 8–13
affective theory, 8–9
identification, 9
intersubjective theory, 9
joint attention, 9–12
summary of, 13
Social Competence Inventory (SCI), aim and description, 270t
Social competence/adjustment, assessment measures of, 267t–271t
Social constructions, integrating with experience, 166–167
Social contact, initiation and responses in, 63–65
Social conversation, 65–67
curriculum unit for, 248f–249f
versus functional–informational, 65
Social deficits, 5
multidimensional nature of, 218
predictors of, 85
trajectories and predictors of, 100–103
Social emotions, experiencing *versus* understanding, 17
Social environment, role of, 69–70
Social functioning
CBT-based interventions and, 181
developmental changes in (*see* Developmental changes in social functioning)
neurobiological correlates of, 229–230

Social functioning interventions, future directions for, 217–225
for emotional competence, 219–221
for peer relations, 221–224
for social-cognitive capabilities, 218–219
Social information processing (SIP), 37–40
in Asperger syndrome, 37–38
Social initiations, teaching, 165–166
Social interaction, 60–72; *see also* Social relationships
assessment measures of, 272t–274t
current understanding of, 221–224
individual differences in, 70–71
initiations and responses in, 63–65
multimodal interventions and, 161–163
nature and profile of, 63–67
negative–nonadaptive, 64
participation in, 61–63
partner's role in, 67–69
positive–adaptive, 63–64
research themes for, 60–61
social conversation and social play in, 65–67
social environment/social situation in, 69–70
social involvement and, 61–63
Social Interaction Observation Scale, aim and description of, 273t
Social interventions, 155–186
CBE-based, 163–178
adult facilitators of, 170–171
design of, 164–175
dual treatment modes of, 165–166
dyadic, 165–166
ecological basis for, 169–173
efficacy studies of, 175–178
emphases of, 168–169
generalization and maintenance of, 173–175
group, 166
impacts on anxiety, 179–181
impacts on social functioning, 181
overview of, 163–164
parents and, 173
peers and, 171–173
procedures for, 166–167
social implications for, 178–181
CBT-based studies of, 159–163
on cognitive-oriented training, 159–160
on multimodal training, 160–161
on social cognition/interaction, 161–163
challenges and components of, 155–156
change agents in, 240t
conceptual basis of, 156–158
curriculum content for, 184
future directions in, 183–186, 224–225
for improving social relationships, 182–183
interaction quality and, 184
in peer relations, 86
settings and personnel for, 185–186
techniques used in, needed research on, 184–185
Social involvement, 61–63
Social isolation, prevalence of, 155
Social listening, 165
Social phobia, *versus* HFASD, 141

Social play, 65–67, 93–95
Social problem-solving, 39
Social relationships; *see also* Attachment;
        Friendship
    interventions for improving, 182–183
    jealousy and, 54–55
Social Responsiveness Scale (SRS), aim and
        description, 270*t*
Social situations
    intuitive reading of, deficiencies in, 66
    nonstructured, 70
Social skills
    friendship for enhancing, 78
    learning, integration with experiencing,
        166–167
Social Skills Rating Scale (SSRS), aim and
        description, 270*t*
Social skills training (SST); *see also* Cognitive-
        behavioral treatment (CBT)
    developments in, 156–158
    theory of mind and, 160–161
Social story techniques, definition/aim and
        examples of, 237*t*
Social Support Scale for Children (SSSC), aim
        and description of, 262*t*
Social understanding
    CBE interventions for, 244*t*
    deficits in, 52
Social-cognitive capabilities
    current understanding of, 218–219
    peer relations and, 85–86
    techniques for enhancing, 234*t*–237*t*
Social-cognitive deficits, emotional
        expressiveness and, 53–54
Social-cognitive theories, 13–17
    contributions of, 28
    development of self, 16–17
    summary of, 17
    theory of mind, 13–16
Social communication disorder, 7
Social-communicative behaviors, in infants,
        90–91
Social-communicative theories, contributions
        of, 28
Social-deficit markers
    in children at varying levels of cognitive
        functioning, 91–92
    in infants and toddlers, 90–91
    summary of, 93
Social-emotional capabilities, friendship
        qualities and, 82–83
Social-emotional deficit, early markers of, from
        infancy through preschool years, 90–93
Social-emotional understanding, CBE
        interventions for, 245*t*
Social-interpersonal problem solving, CBE
        interventions for, 244*t*
Sociocommunicative domain
    in DSM-5, 6–7
    executive functioning and, 19–20
Source monitoring, 21
Spatial working memory, 114
Story maps, 205
    for reading comprehension, 200

relevant intervention and definition for, 214*t*
Storybook-reading technique, repeated, relevant
        intervention and definition for, 213*t*
Strange Situation, 73
Strange story measure, aim and description,
        266*t*
Symbolic play, 74–75

T

Teacher, training for CBE interventions,
        170–171
Teacher Perception Measure, aim and
        description, 271*t*
Temporal memory, 114–115
Test of Problem Solving–3 (TOPS-3), aim and
        description, 263*t*
Thematic interventions, 201, 205
    relevant intervention and definition for,
        214*t*
Theory of mind, 13–16, 19, 20, 28
    assessment measures of, 265*t*–266*t*
    bullying victims and, 63
    CBE interventions and, 167, 172, 174, 176
    cognitive functioning and, 110
    cognitive-academic capabilities and, 14–15
    cognitive-oriented training and, 159–160
    collaborative problem solving and, 98–99
    emotional understanding and, 42, 48–49
    empathy and, 56
    executive function and, 20
    false-belief research and, 14
    friendships and, 72, 82–83
    future research needs for, 219–224
    language abilities and, 121
    limitations of, 15–16
    neurological influences on, 229
    reading skills and, 123, 126
    social cognition and, 161–162
    social functioning and, 63, 72, 82–83, 100,
        108
    social play and, 93–94
    social skills training and, 160–161
    toddlers/preschoolers and, 100
    in TYP, 89
    weak central coherence and, 24–25, 27
    writing skills and, 121
Toddlers
    friendship and peer interaction in, 96–100
    social-emotional deficit markers in, 91
Tower of Hanoi, aim and description of, 259*t*
Transitions
    adolescence to adulthood, 103–108
    CBE ecological perspective and, 169–170
    school, 100–103
Treatment and Education of Autistic and
        Related Communication-Handicapped
        Children (TEACCH), 188
Typical development (TYP), 9–10
    attachment classification in, 73–74
    emotional understanding in, 40–42, 45–50
    of executive functioning, 18–19
    peers and, 59
    social challenges during, 88–89